Nutrition in Aging

Nutrition in Aging

ELEANOR D. SCHLENKER, Ph.D., R.D.

Associate Professor, and Chairman,
Department of Human Nutrition and Foods,
College of Agriculture,
University of Vermont,
Burlington, Vermont

With **30** illustrations

TIMES MIRROR/MOSBY College Publishing

St. Louis • Toronto • Santa Clara   1984

Editor: Nancy K. Roberson
Assistant editor: Catherine H. Converse
Editing supervisor: Lin Dempsey
Manuscript editor: Sheila Walker
Design: Diane M. Beasley
Production: Judith Bamert, Linda R. Stalnaker

Library of Congress Cataloging in Publication Data

Schlenker, Eleanor D.
   Nutrition in aging.

   Includes bibliographical references and index.
      1.   Aging—Nutritional aspects.   2.   Aged—Nutrition.
3.   Nutritional disorders—Age factors.   I.   Title.   [DNLM:
1.   Nutrition—In old age.   2.   Aging.   WT 100 S341n]
QP86.S35   1984   613.2′0880565   83-27038
ISBN 0-8016-4379-1

GW/VH/VH   9   8   7   6   5   4   3   03/C/286

Preface

Have you considered the career opportunities in nutrition, dietetics, or health education working with older people? As the older population continues to expand, professionals in health care facilities and community programs will be expected to develop nutrition standards and resources to meet the food needs of this age group and to provide constructive advice to help clients solve their food-related problems.

At present research exploring nutrient requirements and metabolism in older people has been limited. Nutrient needs in older people are complicated by the presence of chronic disease and physical problems that often require dietary modification. Food selection is made difficult by social, economic, and physiologic factors that interfere with food shopping or meal preparation.

Nutrition in Aging has been developed to prepare the prospective nutrition or other health professional with a basic knowledge necessary to make informed decisions regarding the particular nutrition and food needs of older people. I have deliberately employed a positive approach: although older people may have a different set of problems than younger people, these problems are not insurmountable. Emphasis is placed on seeking alternatives and evaluating each client as an individual.

When selecting subject matter for inclusion in this text, the following were important considerations.

Comprehensive Coverage of Topics

In working with older people, it is necessary to have a basic understanding of the demographic, biologic, and physiologic factors related to the aging process, as well as their effect on fundamental nutrition processes. The opening chapters therefore focus on socioeconomic and health characteristics of the older person and the relationship of lifelong nutrition practices to both morbidity and mortality. Age-related physiologic and biochemical changes that affect nutrient digestion, absorption, metabolism, and excretion are discussed in detail.

The middle chapters focus on the requirements of older people for the macronutrients, vitamins, and minerals, including factors that influence these requirements and practical aspects of food selection. Nutrient-related disorders and the nutritional influence of drugs are discussed in relation to nutrient intake and requirements.

The later chapters discuss application of theories and principles in nutrition practice. Methods for evaluation of nutritional status and nutrition education are presented for implementation in community and institutional settings. Factors influencing food behavior in older people that must be kept in mind when one is considering food selection for either individuals or groups are described, along with their nutritional implications.

Balance of Scientific and Applied Information

Working with older clients demands clear comprehension of both nutrition theory and practical aspects of the individual's particular situation. The health professional needs to understand why a problem exists, how it can be solved, and the alternatives available. To provide a conceptual framework of both past and current thinking, classic studies in the field as well as representative findings from contemporary literature are included. Where appropriate, experimental data have been presented to allow students to understand the basis on which conclusions have been developed. It is pointed out that solutions to the food-related problems of older people may require compromise between ideal and realistic options.

Existence of Controversy

At present there are many unanswered questions relating to nutrient requirements, absorption, and metabolism and aspects such as vitamin supplementation and mental function in the aged. Currently, many different opinions exist regarding these questions. I have attempted to present alternative points of view and describe the experimental supporting evidence allowing the student to reach his or her own conclusions. For many of these issues there is no clear-cut solution at this time.

Resources for Future Use

To make this text useful as a reference when the student has gone on to a professional situation, I have provided extensive bibliographies, including both current and classical references in the field, that could serve to answer questions or provide more information as needed. The tools for evaluation of dietary status can be adapted to a variety of community situations. The government and professional organizations included are sources of further information regarding needs of and services for older people.

Pedagogical Aids

Various components have been included to facilitate use of this text by both faculty and students.

Chapter Introduction: This section provides an overview of the topics to be covered and the questions that must be considered in evaluation of the material presented.

Chapter Summary: The student's attention is directed to the main concepts developed within the chapter to reinforce these ideas and serve as an outline for continued study.

Review Questions: These questions can aid in study or discussion, allowing students to focus on what information should have been retained from the chapter. Applying the theories and principles to practical situations is emphasized. Students are given the opportunity to deal with current controversies and cite reasons for their decisions.

Glossary: Common terms relating to both aging and nutrition literature are defined in the context of this text.

I am indebted to many people for their help and support in preparation of this manuscript. Both the content and organization of this text were improved immeasurably by the many helpful comments and suggestions of the reviewers listed below who dedicated much time and effort to this task.

Ruth E. Eshleman, Ph.D.
University of Rhode Island

P. Vincent Hegarty, Ph.D.
University of Houston

Barbara B. North, M.S.
North Dakota State University

JoAnn Prophet, R.D., M.S.
University of California, Davis

Helen Smiciklas Wright, Ph.D.
Pennsylvania State University

Agnes Powell, Professor Emerita, University of Vermont, developed part of the material relating to drug-nutrient interactions; Joseph Carlin, M.S., R.D., Nutritionist, Region 1, Administration on Aging, Boston, Mass., provided many helpful materials and review comments for Chapter 12; and Dr. William Tisdale, Professor of Medicine, University of Vermont contributed many helpful notes regarding accuracy and content throughout. The resourcefulness and encouragement of Catherine Converse, my developmental editor, at Times Mirror/Mosby and the creativity of Sue Storey, my illustrator, added to this manuscript.

The many individuals at the University of Vermont who contributed to this effort include the librarians in the Documents Section, Bailey-Howe Library and Dana Medical Library; present and former students who made helpful suggestions and devoted innumerable hours to painstaking tasks; secretaries who gave conscientious effort and infinite patience to the preparation of this manuscript; the faculty of the Department of Human Nutrition and Foods who provided continued encouragement and cheerfully dealt with my overcommitments during the last year; and the administration of the College of Agriculture, who agreed to and supported this project.

Eleanor D. Schlenker

Contents

Chapter 1

Demographic and Biologic Aspects of Aging

Advances in the treatment of infectious disease and improvements in health practices, quality of diet, and sanitation have led to significant increases in life expectancy in this century. There are now more older persons in the world than at any time in history. One of every nine persons in the United States is age 65 or over.[89] Unfortunately, we are only beginning to examine the particular nutrient needs, nutrition problems, and socioeconomic and health factors influencing the food choices of older persons. Other considerations in food selection are the biologic and physiologic changes occurring as part of the aging process. Such alterations can lead to chronic disorders requiring dietary management. Effective nutrition intervention requires evaluation and understanding of the many complex variables affecting both the nutritional status of the aged and their nutritional care.

POPULATION TRENDS

Definition of Age

In legal matters age is defined on the basis of chronologic age or the number of years a person has lived. Reaching a particular age determines eligibility for benefits or services, although standards are not consistent. One can participate in the congregate meal program and other services mandated under the Older Americans Act at age 60 and receive Medicare and full Social Security benefits at age 65.[10,90]

Hickey[27] pointed out the limitations of current census statistics, which group all persons over age 64. Although the degree of change occurring over a 20-year interval is easily recognized at younger ages, changes occurring over the 20-year period between ages 65 and 85 are also significant. For example, health-related problems are less important in those recently retired; major functional limitations become more prevalent beyond age 75.[27] Only 1% of those age 65 to 74, as compared to 25% of those above age 85, reside in nursing homes.[84] As the number of older persons continues to increase, the collection and representation of population data by 5- or 10-year intervals would allow examination of age-related differences and appropriate planning for needed services.

Increase in Numbers

Persons over age 65 are the most rapidly expanding segment of the population, comprising 11% of the total, or 25.5 million persons.[63,65,89] In contrast, at the turn of the century only 4% of the population, or 3 million persons, were age 65 or over (Fig. 1-1). This age group has increased eightfold since 1900, whereas the general population has increased about threefold.[89] Furthermore, this increase in number will continue. Over the next 40 years (by the year 2020) the number of persons age 65 and over will about double.[63,70] At present the net increase in the older population is 1600 per day,[89] as about 5200 persons reach age 65 and about 3600 persons above age 65 die. As this continues the most rapid growth will be among the oldest.[71]

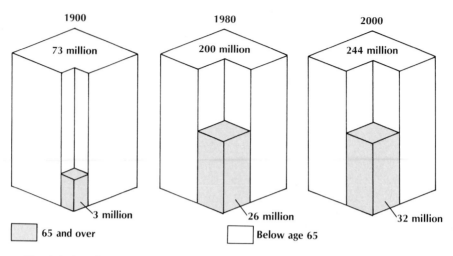

Fig. 1-1. Age distribution of the U.S. population. (Data from references 70 and 89.)

Those age 75 to 84 will increase by 50%; the group age 85 and above will double.

Several factors have contributed to the change in both the absolute number and the proportion of older persons in the general population.[63] The high birth rate at the beginning of this century is, in part, responsible. The present decline in birth rates resulting in fewer persons in younger age groups has brought about an increase in the proportion of older persons in our society.[63] Improvements in health care leading to increased life expectancy and decreased death rates have been a secondary influence on the growth of the older population.

Composition of the Older Population

The majority of older people are women, whereas younger age groups contain about the same number of men and women.[71] There are nearly two women per man among those age 75 and over. This divergence in sex ratio reflects the increasing life expectancy of women since 1900; men have benefited less from decreasing death rates. Similarly, over 90% of older persons are white.[73] This relates to not only the greater number of whites in the general population but also the differential mortality rates between whites and nonwhites.[65,71]

Implications of Present Trends

The increase in number and proportion of older persons has implications for both the family and the society as a whole. A concept used in planning for future services is the dependency ratio—the number of persons age 65 and over divided by the number of persons of working age (18 to 64 years). This ratio is now about 1:5 (1 person age 65 and over for every 5 persons age 18 to 64). By the year 2020 the ratio will have risen to 1:4.[64] Increasing ratios are resulting in changes in the funding structure and policies of the federal Social Security system and will influence private pension plans as well.[90]

As the birth rate declines, aged parents will have fewer children and grandchildren to provide economic and emotional support, or assistance with shopping and transportation. Shanas and Hauser,[55] evaluating the impact of zero population growth, concluded that the types of support now provided by family members will have to be assumed by

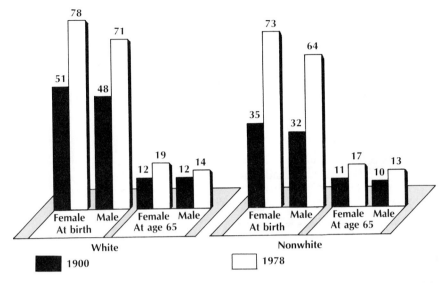

Fig. 1-2. Increases in life expectancy according to age, sex, and race. (Data from United States Department of Health and Human Services: Life tables: Vital statistics of the U.S., 1978, vol. II, section 5, DHHS Publication No. (PHS) 81-1104, Hyattsville, Md., 1980, U.S. Government Printing Office.

government or private sources as the numbers of older persons without families begin to rise.

Another consideration is health care, since older persons are the largest users of health services such as physicians' visits, hospital care, and prescription drugs.[7,78] Although persons above age 65 represent only 11% of the population, they incur 30% of health care expenditures.[78] In the future they will require an ever-growing share of both public and private health insurance resources. Preventive health services including a nutritionally adequate diet could reduce both hospitalization or institutionalization.[77]

TRENDS IN MORTALITY AND MORBIDITY

Decreasing mortality rates and increasing life expectancy define the life span quantitatively.[63] Incidence of chronic disease and utilization of health resources provide an indication of the general quality of life. Both aspects need to be considered when evaluating the older population.

Changes in Life Expectancy

Basis of Change in Life Expectancy. Life expectancy defines in years the average remaining lifetime for a person of a given age.[63,75] The increase in the proportion of older persons in the general population is often attributed to the fact that people are living longer. In fact more people are living to advanced ages as compared to the number who managed to survive the hazards of infancy, childhood, and young adulthood in earlier times. However, an individual who reached the age of 60 in colonial times could expect to live about 16 more years.[69] This life expectancy was about the same as for a 60-year-old in 1978.[79]

The dramatic increase in life expectancy since

1900 has occurred primarily in infancy and childhood (Fig. 1-2). Surprisingly, there has been little change in life expectancy at older ages. Despite the improvements in medical care since 1900, life expectancy at age 65 has increased by only 2 years in men, although by 7 years in women. The increasing number of older persons therefore does not reflect an increase in *maximum* life span but the extended life span of those individuals who in the past died prematurely.[63]

Differences in Life Expectancy Among Population Groups. Gains in the average life span have not been uniform among all groups (Fig. 1-2). Women have made increasing strides in life expectancy as compared to men. Although expected years of life at birth differed by only 3 years in 1900, women can now expect to live 7 to 9 years longer, depending on their particular race or ethnic group.[79] This increase in life expectancy among adult women could reflect to some extent the decrease in deaths related to childbearing; however, in past years men were often employed in hazardous situations and occupation-related accidents were frequent.[63]

The differential between men and women could be genetic, environmental, or a combination of both. In an effort to resolve this question, Madigan[38] examined the mortality records and life spans of 10,000 men and 32,000 women living in Catholic teaching orders over a 50-year period. In those groups women lived longer. Since living situations (and presumably environmental stress) were considered to be similar, the sex differential in mortality was believed to reflect biologic differences; social stress was thought to play only a minor role. Madigan concluded that women were equally susceptible to infectious disease but had a biologic resistance to degenerative diseases leading to earlier deaths in men. Although this study has several limitations (i.e., possible use of tobacco or alcohol by men and not women; adjustment to life in a religious order may be more difficult for men),[93] it represents a major effort to evaluate life expectancy in humans in a controlled environment.

Behavior and environment influence mortality patterns in men and in future years may alter life expectancy in women.[92] Increased use of cigarettes among women of all ages is resulting in higher death rates from lung cancer (rate tripled between 1950 and 1977).[88] In 1972 it was estimated that about two thirds of the mortality differential between men and women at middle age and beyond was explained by difference in smoking habits.[46] A current influence on the mortality differential is heart disease; the mortality rate for men is twice that for women.[74] It has been confirmed that female hormones do exert a protective role against coronary heart disease in women during the child-bearing years.[92] Differing vulnerability of men and women to specific degenerative diseases will most likely continue to widen the gap in life expectancy.

Race, education, and income influence life expectancy.[29,43] As described in Fig. 1-2, nonwhites at all ages have decreased life expectancies. Within all races education and income are inversely related to mortality. The lower mean income levels of nonwhites can result in diets of poorer quality, decreased medical care, and inferior living conditions. Nonwhites are also more likely to reside in poorer neighborhoods characterized by high rates of crime and victimization. Furthermore, nonwhites have higher death rates from particular chronic diseases including diabetes mellitus and cerebrovascular disease.[74] Limited medical care for management of diabetes or hypertension could contribute to the increased probability of death.

Leading Causes of Death

The most common causes of death in 1900 and 1979 are compared in Table 1-1. Not only were total death rates higher in 1900 but also the primary causes of death differed.[75,86] The death rate per 100,000 persons was nearly twice as high in 1900 (1719 versus 870) and people were more likely to die at younger ages. Infant mortality was nearly six times higher in 1900 than in 1979. The dramatic

Table 1-1. Leading causes of death in 1900 and 1979

Cause of Death	Death Rate (per 100,000 population)	
	1900	1979
Diseases of the heart	137	333
Cancer	64	183
Cerebrovascular disease	107	77
Accidents	72	48
Influenza and pneumonia	202	20
Infant deaths	63	11
Diabetes mellitus	11	15
Arteriosclerosis	*	13
Liver disease and cirrhosis	12	14
Pulmonary disease	49	23

*Unknown.

Data from references 75 and 86.

decrease in deaths from infectious diseases (i.e., influenza and pneumonia) has resulted from the development of antibiotic drugs. Fewer deaths from accidents can be attributed to improvement in both working and living conditions, although automobile accidents are a leading cause of death among young men. In contrast, the number of cancer deaths has increased nearly threefold. Sophisticated methods now diagnose malignancy that may have gone undetected in 1900.[63] In addition, persons living longer and exposed to potential carcinogens over a lifetime are more likely to develop cancer. The significant increase in smoking since 1900 further contributes to the high death rate; lung cancer accounts for 25% of all cancer deaths.[81]

The dramatic rise in deaths from chronic disease is a consequence of degenerative changes associated with the aging process. Individuals who in 1900 died of infectious disease at an early age now survive to develop chronic disease. Heart disease, cancer, or cerebrovascular disease causes three of every four deaths in persons age 65 or above.[65]

Eliminating each of these causes would have a different effect on life expectancy at older ages. Eliminating cancer would have little effect, increasing the average life span by only 1.4 years. Eliminating cardiovascular diseases would add over 11 years to life expectancy in the over 65 group.

Although the possibility of completely eradicating deaths from cardiovascular disorders is unlikely, death rates can be reduced by following a prudent diet, regular physical exercise, avoidance of smoking and excessive use of alcohol, and regular medical check-ups.[76] Such appropriate behavior is believed to have contributed to the 17% decrease in mortality from heart disease observed over the past decade.[78]

Future Trends

Despite the fact that preventive health habits decrease the incidence of degenerative disease, life expectancy may not increase if present trends are continued. Waldron[92] proposes that as women continue to enter the labor force and adopt an aggressive life-style, considered to be detrimental to health, vulnerability to coronary death will increase. If present smoking habits continue, lung cancer will surpass breast cancer as the leading cancer in women by the mid-1980s.[77]

Cigarette smoking is considered to be the greatest single preventable cause of illness and premature death in the United States.[77] It has been suggested that coronary deaths would decrease by 30% if all Americans stopped smoking; smokers have a 70% greater risk of death from all causes than nonsmokers.[77] Although the percentage of adults who smoke has declined over the past 15 years (with the exception of women age 65 and over), those who continue to smoke are more likely to be heavy smokers.[81] One third of male smokers and about one fourth of female smokers use over two packs per day.

Of greater impact on mortality trends in the next 30 years will be the current smoking habits of teenagers, if continued. More than one fifth of girls and boys age 12 to 17 are regular smokers.[81] A behavior pattern including a diet high in sucrose, fat, and sodium; use of cigarettes; excessive use of alcohol; and limited exercise promotes the early development of health problems and may result in significant changes in mortality. The adoption of positive health habits early in life is essential to reduce chronic disease in the expanding older population of future decades.

SOCIOECONOMIC CHARACTERISTICS OF THE OLDER POPULATION

Living Arrangements

The general public associates old age with poor health, illness, and disability,[19] which often leads to the assumption that the majority of older persons live in institutions. In fact 95% of all aged live within the community with either a spouse or other family members or alone.[71] Seventy-five percent of older men are married. In contrast, over half of older women are widows.[71] This difference in marital status is reflected in the living arrangements of older persons (Fig. 1-3). About one third of older women live alone and about one fourth live with someone other than their spouse.

About 5% of persons age 65 and above are institutionalized (See Fig. 1-3). The majority (about 1 million persons) of the institutionalized live in nursing homes,[72] although about one sixth are in hospitals or community homes designed for the mentally handicapped or psychiatric patient. Over half of those in nursing homes are at least 80 years of age.

Older persons are more likely to live in rural or suburban locations than in densely populated areas. Although over 60% reside in metropolitan areas, less than one third live in central cities, with the others in surrounding communities.[89]

Living arrangements can contribute to the food problems of older people. An individual who lives alone and is bored or depressed may not bother to prepare a meal. An aged widow who never learned to drive and lives in a rural area is dependent on friends or relatives for transportation to a food store. Although older people in the inner city have

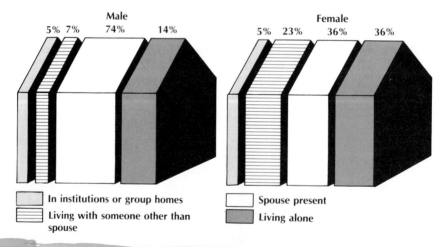

Fig. 1-3. Living arrangements of people age 65 and above. (Data from United States Bureau of the Census: Demographic aspects of aging and the older population in the U.S., Current Population Reports, Special Studies Series P-23, No. 59, Revised, Washington, D.C., 1978, U.S. Government Printing Office.)

greater access to services, they are less visible and therefore easily overlooked.[1]

Level of Income

Based on the assumption that living expenses and personal wants decrease, it is commonly believed[10,45] that older persons require less money to live on than younger persons. In fact, basic needs of food, housing, and transportation change very little, and health care is an ever-increasing expense. Unfortunately, financial problems are a source of anxiety for many older individuals. In a national survey of 2800 persons above age 65, 40% indicated that not having enough money to live on was a serious problem.[19] When retired people were asked how they would spend an additional $100 per month, about half referred to basic items such as food, clothes, health care, or paying old bills.[90] Spending additional money on food was the most frequent response.

Social Security is the principal income of the majority of older Americans. Since 1975 Social Security benefits have increased annually according to the increase in the Consumer Price Index (CPI) for the previous year. Despite this rise in mean income, a disproportionate number of older persons and families have incomes below the poverty line (amount of money required to provide basic necessities). Thirteen percent of the general population, as compared to 16% of older persons, are poor.[89] Women and minority groups are more likely to fall below the poverty line (Fig. 1-4). Over 40% of all black women and about one third of all black men are in this category. Current estimates of poverty among the aged may indeed be conservative,[89] as institutionalized poor and older persons with reduced incomes who live with relatives are excluded.

Individuals who have been retired for a number of years tend to have less adequate financial re-

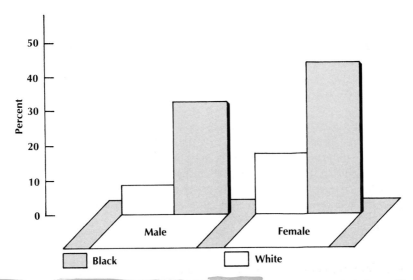

Fig. 1-4. Percent of aged falling below the poverty line. (Data from United States House of Representatives Select Committee on Aging: Every ninth American (1982 Edition), Comm. Pub. No. 97-332, Washington, D.C., 1982, U.S. Government Printing Office.)

sources than those recently retired.[8] The latter had higher average earnings and therefore receive higher Social Security and pension benefits than those retired for several years. When Social Security benefits are lower, the cost-of-living adjustments also represent a smaller amount of money. As a result individuals retired for 7 years and above age 70 were found to have lost buying power (4%), despite the fact that the over-65 group as a whole gained in buying power (10%).[8] Usually couples have a more adequate income than single individuals. Older clients should be encouraged to participate in programs such as Food Stamps or Title III-C congregate meals from which they might benefit (see Chapter 12).

GOVERNMENT AGENCIES SERVING THE OLDER POPULATION

At the federal level aging activities focus on both research and delivery of services. The National Institute on Aging (NIA), established in 1974, conducts research directed toward improving the quality of life for older persons.[11] Biomedical and behavioral research concerned with the physiologic, psychologic, social, and health aspects of aging seeks information for the development of both preventive and therapeutic approaches to the needs and problems of elders. Although some of this research is carried on by NIA, other funds are awarded to universities and scientific foundations for carrying out approved research plans.

Delivery of services to older persons using funds appropriated under the Older Americans Act and other legislation is the responsibility of the Administration on Aging within the Department of Health and Human Services. Funds are usually delegated to the state agency on aging, which administers programs at the state and local level. Programs may include nutrition services, transportation services, development of senior centers, senior housing, or help with seeking employment. At all levels an important role of these agencies is advocacy—efforts to influence both legislative bodies and other government agencies to respond to the needs of the aged. Listings of both public and private agencies and organizations serving older persons can be found in Appendix A.

BIOLOGIC ASPECTS OF AGING

Characteristics of the Aging Process

Although the progression of biologic and physiologic events occurring over the life span has been observed for centuries, only recently has the study of aging emerged as a science.[12] Gerontology is the study of normal aging, whereas geriatrics deals with the physical health and medical problems of older people.

In broad terms the study of aging encompasses all structural and functional changes occurring throughout the life span from embryonic development through maturation to senescence.[50] In our context aging refers to the time-dependent biologic and physiologic changes beginning about age 30 that are degenerative in nature and lead to increased vulnerability.[69] The pattern and sequence of changes associated with normal aging are the same in all members of a species, although the rate of progression will differ from one individual to another.

Comfort[12] postulates that if individuals remained as able throughout life to handle physiologic stress and resist disease as they are at age 10, half of the population would have a life expectancy of 700 years. As a result of degenerative changes in body structure and function, and the progressive nature of these events, the likelihood of death doubles every 8 years after maturation is complete.[94] The death rate among persons age 30 is 20 per 1000 population; by age 80 the death rate has accelerated to 130 per 1000.[58]

Factors Affecting the Aging Process

Intrinsic Factors. Oliver Wendell Holmes in his treatise on how to live 3 score and 10 years facetiously recommended that individuals advertise for parents from families whose members survive to age 80 or 90.[44] The genetic material combined at the moment of fertilization is a primary determinant of rate of aging and ultimate life span.[48] One obvious genetic characteristic influencing longevity is sex; in most species, including humans, females live longer than males.[12] People living to age 70 or beyond are more likely to have had parents who also survived to that age, than are the general population.[44]

Although it is generally recognized that biologic make-up exerts a major influence on the life span, the mechanism of genetic control is not understood. Two areas proposed for further study are (1) the regulation of protein synthesis and (2) the effectiveness of the immune system. As pointed out by Weksler[95] the individual producing high density versus low density lipoproteins has a reduced probability of cardiovascular attack. Age-associated alterations in body defense mechanisms increase vulnerability to infectious and toxic agents and autoimmune activity with increased tissue destruction and degenerative disease.

Current evidence suggests that impaired immune function does increase the risk of death in older individuals. Older people are considered more susceptible to infections than younger people, and pneumonia is still a major cause of death among the aged despite treatment with antibiotics.[28] An on-going population study of 3500 persons in Western Australia revealed an increase in serum auto-antibodies up to age 70 and then a decline.[37] This finding could be interpreted as reflecting increased mortality among those with higher autoantibody activity. Preserving normal immune response may prove to be a means of preventing deterioration and enhancing human life span.

Extrinsic Factors. Environmental factors are known to modify the genetic program in both animal models and humans. In animals exposed to irradiation, aging is accelerated as a result of genetic mutation and the subsequent replication of imperfect proteins. Chronic exposure to sunlight or an ultraviolet lamp increases the rate of normal changes in skin collagen[4] that result in characteristic skin wrinkling. Excessive exposure is associated with an increased incidence of skin cancer.[80]

Level of nutrition appears to have the greatest potential for positive alteration of the genetic program. Not only can dietary manipulation extend the life span[5] but also it acts at an early stage, prolonging the period of youth and vitality. The influence of nutrition on life span will be discussed in Chapter 2.

Aging at the Cellular Level

Although it is generally agreed that age-related structural and functional impairments relate to alterations at the cellular level, these relationships are poorly understood. The classic work in cellular aging was performed by Hayflick,[22,24-25] who developed a model in vitro system using fibroblasts from connective tissue cultured on a nutrient medium. These experiments revealed that all normal cells are limited to a finite number of divisions. The number of divisions reflects the life span of that species. Cells taken from a mouse with a life expectancy of 3.5 years will divide about 21 times; cells from a human with a life expectancy of 70 years will divide about 50 times. Human fibroblasts preserved at sub-zero temperatures for as long as 12 years resumed division when thawed and cultured; however, the total number of divisions still equalled about 50, confirming that this characteristic is inherent in the cell.

Recent work has determined that the number of cell divisions is also related to donor age.[24,54] Cultures derived from donors age 65 and over produced fewer cells than those from young donors age 20 to 35. While 60% of cells obtained from young donors divided at least eight times over a 2-week period, this was true for only 2% of cells from older donors.[54] Further studies will explore the relationship between cell proliferative capacity and the physiologic health of the donor.

Although these studies provide a conceptual framework for understanding the aging process and changes at the cellular level, limited proliferative capacity is not generally considered the basis of age-related changes in organs and tissues.[24,60,66] Highly differentiated cells in muscle or neural tissue lose mitotic ability early in life. Liver and kidney cells retain the ability to divide, but they do not under normal circumstances. Organs composed of nonproliferating cells lose tissue as a result of cell death and functional changes in remaining cells. Although cell loss may result in the observed changes in both organ function and control systems, the reverse might also be true: alterations in control molecules could lead to changes at the cellular level. Strehler[66] concludes that both mechanisms are likely to be involved in the aging process.

Present knowledge regarding structural and biochemical changes in the aging cell is limited. The nucleus appears to change in shape and increase in DNA content. Small vacuoles filled with fluid appear in the cytoplasm.[31] Although some reports suggest a change in enzyme levels, one cannot generalize as to the direction of change or the particular enzyme involved.[52] The most obvious change is the accumulation of golden brown fluorescent granules in the cytoplasm of nonproliferating cells.[31] This pigment, called lipofuscin (from the name of the stain used in microscopic examination), ceroid, or aging pigment,[66] has been identified in various tissues including brain, heart, and skeletal muscle; accumulation over adulthood is directly proportional to age. Chemically, lipofuscin is composed of lipid and protein.

The origin of lipofuscin and its physiologic significance is a matter of controversy. Strehler,[66] after extensive review, concluded that lipofuscin is the oxidation product of unsaturated lipids from various membranes within the cell. Whether this is a result of normal aging or the product of a lifetime of environmental insults has not been resolved. Another question still unanswered is the possible effect of lipofuscin accumulation on cell function or mortality.

Theories of Aging

Approaches to Aging. In the past, theories describing the aging process focused on functional aspects such as the decline in homeostatic control of organ systems or alterations in immune response.[31] The cross-linking theory proposed that chemical reactions producing hydrogen bonds and disulfide bridges resulted in insoluble aggregates that interfered with normal cell processes and the passage of nutrients or waste products. Studies of proliferating cells have emphasized the genetic mechanism in the aging process. As the site of control is the transcription and translation of the genetic material, current theories focus on those events.[23]

Two different opinions exist concerning the fundamental control of the aging process. Some believe that aging represents a programmed series of events that is an extension of growth and maturation.[23] The codon-restriction theory is based on this hypothesis. An opposing point of view suggests that aging is the result of random insults, with consequent mutations in the genetic material and synthesis of abnormal proteins.[23] The error and redundant message theories represent this point of view.

Error Theory. The error theory proposes that over a lifetime the genetic messages reproduced as RNA and DNA are increasingly subject to error as a result of "wear and tear" or environmental influences such as exposure to radiation.[23,25] The molecules produced from faulty DNA do not perform as expected, leaving the cell impaired in ability to carry on essential functions. Studies of single cell organisms suggest that when errors accumulate to a certain point, death ensues. Although cells contain enzymes for repair of DNA, this process becomes less efficient as the cell ages. However, species with longer life spans tend to have increased capacity for DNA repair.[21]

Hayflick[25] illustrated this concept by comparing the human organism to a household appliance. Both machines could operate indefinitely if replacement parts were available. When complete repair is no longer possible, the appliance or organism ceases to function.

Redundant Message Theory. Particular DNA sequences are selectively repeated within the cell nucleus. It has been estimated that less than 1% of available genetic information is used by a cell in its lifetime.[25] When the gene used for replicating a particular sequence becomes damaged, another gene possessing the correct sequence is used, preventing the synthesis of nonfunctional proteins. According to the redundant message theory, when all genes containing the correct message are exhausted, age changes become apparent.

Programmed Aging and Code Restriction. The code restriction hypothesis suggests that cellular changes reflect a continuation of the genetic program.[23,25] Special "aging genes" may repress particular DNA sequences, preventing their duplication. The point of control may be the production of transfer RNA synthetases. A cell uses those code sequences for which transfer RNA is available. Repression of specific synthetases and transfer RNA halts the synthesis of protein from that code. When the existing supply of the required protein is exhausted, structural and functional changes become apparent. An alternative mechanism of repression may be enhanced binding of certain proteins on the DNA strand, increasing the energy required to separate the two strands. Consequently, transcription does not proceed, and that sequence of the genetic code is lost.

In summary, there is no single theory that fully explains aging phenomena. Each of the theories described is compatible with the biochemical and physiologic changes observed in both aging cells and intact animals. It is possible that all three processes are acting simultaneously, as none is mutually exclusive. Hayflick[23] observes that genetic direction is a more likely explanation than environmental causes since the variation in average life span between species is greater than the range of individual life spans within species. Furthermore,

animals maintained in protected environments (i.e., pathogen-free, pollution-free) and fed optimum diets still undergo biologic aging.

PHYSIOLOGIC ASPECTS OF AGING

Physical Health

Functional Assessment. Although changes in physical appearance (graying of the hair or use of a walking cane) provide clues as to chronologic age, functional age is less easily defined.[94] At present criteria have not been developed for realistic assessment of older versus younger individuals. In younger persons assessment may focus on the absence of disease. Hickey[27] maintains that for one who has undergone the wear and tear of 60 or 70 years of living, use of such a model is inappropriate. Andres[3] suggested a model comparing individuals of similar age. Older persons would be rated as to their functional performance according to standards derived from their peer group. Chronologic age is the least reliable measure of functional capability.

Presence of Chronic Disease. Although chronic problems are uncommon in younger persons, they increase in frequency through middle age. Seventy-two percent of those between ages 45 and 64 and 86% of those age 65 and over have at least one chronic physical problem.[41] Watkin[94] quotes a survey of congregate meal participants that indicated 60% had one to six chronic disorders. The most common physical problems among older persons are arthritis (38%), impaired hearing (29%), impaired vision (20%), hypertension (20%), and heart conditions (20%).[41]

Impaired mobility as a result of arthritis or poor vision can hinder the older person in both shopping and meal preparation. Failing eyesight may preclude driving or walking to a food store. As noted above, at least 20% of older people have conditions that require sodium restriction, weight control, or drug therapy (i.e., diuretics, analgesics) in their management, indicating a need for dietary counseling.

Most older people consider themselves to be in good health despite the presence of chronic disease. In a National Health Survey of 40,000 households representative of the general population, nearly 70% of those age 65 and above considered their health to be excellent or good.[76] Less than 10% reported their health as poor. Positive attitudes toward health, however, do not preclude some degree of functional disability. Nearly half of those above age 65 living in the community have some limitation in physical activity, and for many the limitation is major.[82]

Any degree of activity limitation has serious implications regarding the older individual's ability to remain independent. People unable to carry on major activity cannot perform household tasks, go food shopping, or prepare meals.[82] For those who are limited in ability to carry on major activity, such tasks may still be difficult.

On the average older people have 39 restricted-activity days and 14 bed-rest days each year, about twice that reported by younger people.[87] For the older individual living alone, nutrient intake can be severely reduced on days when usual activities must be curtailed, if neighbors or family members are not available to provide meals. Dehydration as well as limited food intake can be a problem. Couples have an advantage in that one can provide food for the other on disability days.

Access to Medical Care. Utilization of health services relates to sex and income as well as age. Because older women live longer, they continue to develop more physical problems requiring medical attention. Low income individuals may not seek medical attention even though it is indicated if they lack insurance and cannot afford to pay for the service.[85,87] According to current estimates, individuals age 65 or above visit a physician about six times a year, as compared to about five for younger age groups.[87] As a result of severe chronic disease requiring specialized treatment or surgery, an older person is more likely to be hospitalized at least once during the year than is a younger adult, and will stay longer if admitted.

Integration of Physiologic Systems

Changes in Physiologic Function. A characteristic of physiologic aging is decreased ability to respond to changes in either the internal or external environment.[61] Rate of recovery or return to homeostasis following displacement is slowed in the older individual. Impaired adaptation can result from altered sensitivity of control receptors or changes in organs or tissues.

Fig. 1-5 describes the age-related decline in physiologic systems occurring between ages 30 and 80. These data were obtained from a longitudinal study of adult males being carried on at the Gerontology Research Center of the National Institute on Aging located in Baltimore. Although these values represent cross-sectional comparisons of one age group with another, the long-range goal is to examine age-related changes occurring within individuals over adult life.[61] In Fig. 1-5 the functional capacity of adults at age 30 is considered to equal 100%; decline in function is rated accordingly.

Physiologic responses differ in their rate of change according to the degree of systems coordination required. The fasting blood glucose level shows little change under resting conditions. Nerve conduction velocity, a function involving one organ system, decreases by about 15%. Resting cardiac output requiring both neural and muscular input declines by 30%. When the desired response involves many organ systems, as for example maximum work rate, age-related decline is substantial (70%).

In general, changes are most evident when comparing simple versus complex behavior.[61] As a system becomes more complex, requiring greater integration of functional parts, impairment becomes more apparent. For example, an older person may walk with comparative ease on a level surface whereas climbing stairs, requiring more complicated muscular motions and compensation for greater oxygen expenditure, will demand heavy effort. Food preparation procedures requiring both visual and motor coordination, such as peeling veg-

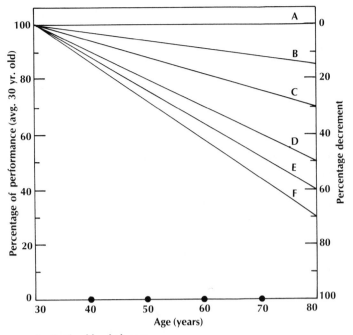

A. Fasting blood glucose
B. Nerve conduction velocity and some cellular enzyme activities
C. Cardiac index (resting)
D. Vital capacity and renal blood flow
E. Maximum breathing capacity
F. Maximum work rate and maximum O₂ uptake

Fig. 1-5. Age-related decrements in physiological function. (From Shock, N.W.: Energy metabolism, caloric intake, and physical activity of the aging. In Carlson, L.A., ed.: Nutrition in old age, Symposia Swedish Nutrition Foundation X, Stockholm, Sweden, 1972, Almqvist & Wiksell.)

etables, may become difficult. Neuromuscular control is believed to contribute significantly to the loss of muscle coordination, as performance on a bicycle begins to decline by age 40 when individual muscle strength is still unchanged.[61]

Despite known decrements in physiologic parameters, most older persons function quite well on a day-to-day basis under normal or resting conditions. For most organ systems, the general ratio of maximum functional capacity to average physiologic demand ranges from 7 to 11; thus some

degree of loss can occur with no noticeable change in function.[67] However, when extreme demands are placed on the system, or when functional losses are excessive, problems become evident. As described in later chapters, physiologic considerations enter into dietary recommendations for older persons.

Variability Among Individuals. Although normal aging leads to changes *in the same direction* in all persons, the rate of change is unique to each individual. In fact the variability between individuals of the same age may actually exceed that observed between persons of different ages.[42] This reflects both genetic constitution and lifelong experiences influencing physical well-being. Dietary habits, level of medical care, exposure to disease or pollution, use of alcohol, smoking, obesity, degree of exercise, and psychologic stress all exert an effect. Since no two persons experience the same combination of variables, by age 60 all individuals are remarkably different. On this basis older persons differ more from one another than do younger persons.

In an evaluation of maximum breathing capacity in men age 20 to 90, one individual age 30 had a functional capacity equal to that of males between ages 80 and 90; in contrast, a 90-year-old performed at the level of those age 40.[42] Such differences underscore the need to assess each client as an individual and not on the basis of chronologic age.

AGING AND NEUROENDOCRINE FUNCTION

Brain and Neural Tissue

Structural Aspects. The structural units comprising the central nervous system are the neurons and the glia (structural and functional supporting cells). Neurons lose the capacity to divide following differentiation; glial cells, on the other hand, continue to divide throughout life. The change in proportion of neurons to glia has been associated with changes in motor function and coordination. Pathologic alterations in neural RNA, observed in parkinsonism, are first apparent in the glia.[91]

The age-related loss of neurons was first demonstrated in the classic work of Brody,[9] who counted the cells in the cerebral cortex (obtained at autopsy) of 20 persons from newborn to 95 years of age. All were considered free of neurologic disease. Although degree of cell loss varied between cortical sections, differences in cell numbers between younger and older persons were 30% to 50%.

Although there is general agreement concerning loss of neurons in advanced age, questions regarding age-related changes in brain weight are still not resolved. Cross-sectional data obtained at autopsy suggest a 10% to 12% decrease in brain weight by age 90; however, this could be a secular effect.[68] Because brain weight is related to body size, which has increased with successive generations, smaller brain weights may represent smaller individuals rather than changes within individuals. According to Terry,[68] such data present a misleading impression of cerebral atrophy. Moreover, neither brain weight nor cell number appears to be a factor in Alzheimer-type senile dementia (see Chapter 9).

Biochemical Aspects. Biochemical as well as structural changes may contribute to loss of integrative function by the aging nervous system. Makman and coworkers[39] observed a 30% to 40% decrease in dopamine receptor sites in the hypothalamus, cortex, and striatum of older animals; however, these findings have not been confirmed with humans. These brain regions, however, are known to influence motor control, neuroendocrine response, cognitive function, and memory.

Decreased synthesis of neurotransmitters may contribute to functional changes in the aging brain.[36] Conduction of neural impulses requires the release of a chemical transmitter (i.e., dopamine, serotonin, acetylcholine) believed to be synthesized in the neuron. Sufficient numbers of transmitter molecules must be present to activate the adjoining cell. Two common transmitters, dopamine and norepinephrine, are derived from tyrosine; serotonin is derived from tryptophan. Recent evidence suggests that enzymes required for these conversions—tyrosine hydroxylase and aromatic amino acid decarboxylase—are reduced in neurons of older people.[36]

Findings of decreased levels of transmitters further support the suggestion that synthesis is diminished. At the same time enzymes involved in catecholamine catabolism increase. Robinson[47] observed enhanced levels of both monoamine oxidase and catecholamine degradation products in older humans. Decreasing synthesis and accelerated catabolism, acting simultaneously, can bring about significantly reduced transmitter levels.[36]

Changes in number or structure of neural cells, loss of membrane receptor sites, and still unknown factors may all be involved in altered neurotransmission and brain function. The most striking reductions in neural transmitters, however, occur in the hypothalamus and cerebral cortex, which control functions exhibiting age-related alterations. Moreover, a dopamine analogue (levodopa) is used to control parkinsonism. Thus neurotransmitter availability and possible replacement should continue to be explored with age-related changes in neural function.

Behavioral Aspects. Chronic disease is associated with functional changes in the aging brain.[96] Older persons with cardiovascular disease had lower scores on tests of both psychomotor function and cognitive skills than healthy persons of similar age.[26] The cardiovascular group was especially disadvantaged in tests allowing limited time for completion. Goldfarb,[15] evaluating intellectual and functional ability in older patients, found that individuals with reduced brain blood flow and oxygen utilization were more likely to be incontinent, score poorly on mental status tests (i.e., "How old are you?" "Where are we now?") and have reduced life expectancy as compared to normal controls of similar age. Further work with humans should evaluate the behavioral implications of biochemical and structural changes in the aging brain.

Endocrine System

Information is limited regarding age-related changes in hormone levels or the mechanisms involved. A review by Gregerman and Bierman[17] indicates that blood levels of some hormones (aldosterone) decrease, whereas others (thyroxin) do not appear to change (Table 1-2). Decreased secretion can result from either impaired synthesis or faulty release of the hormone. Alternatively, reduced hormone utilization or slowed excretion would limit hormone release through homeostatic mechanisms. For example, loss of lean body mass is considered the basis for the age-related change in secretion and metabolic conversion of thyroid hormone. (This will be discussed further in Chapter 3.) Alterations in synthesis of plasma proteins serving as transport molecules could influence not only blood hormone concentrations but also rate of conversion to active forms.[17]

Current research on endocrine function in aging is being directed toward the hypothalamic-pituitary axis regulating hormone secretion. Preliminary work with animal models suggests that neural sen-

Table 1-2. Age-related changes in endocrine secretion

	Plasma Level	Response to Stimulation	Sensitivity of Target Organ
Thyrotropin (TSH)	Unchanged	Decreased	Unchanged
Thyroxin (T_4)	Unchanged	Unchanged	Increased
Triiodothyronine (T_3)	Decreased	*	*
Parathyroid hormone	Decreased	*	Increased
Aldosterone	Decreased	*	*
Insulin	Unchanged	Decreased	Unchanged

*No information presently available.

Modified from Gregerman, R.I., and Bierman, E.L.: Aging and hormones. In Williams, R.H., ed.: Textbook of endocrinology, ed. 5, Philadelphia, 1974, W.B. Saunders Co.

sors within the aged hypothalamus are less sensitive to messages received and release of tropic hormones is delayed, although this may not be true for all hormone systems.[30] The pituitary of older animals appears able to respond to tropic hormones as released from the hypothalamus.

Impaired response of target tissues to hormone secretion could relate to a decrease in hormone receptors on the cell membrane. Roth[51] observed age-related losses in receptor concentrations in various animal tissues. In some cases decreases in hormone response closely parallel decreases in receptor sites, although findings are not consistent among hormones. Whether these observations in animals are also true in humans has not been determined.

Loss of Adaptive Mechanisms

Adaptive response frequently requires induction of an enzyme to bring about a return to homeostasis. An increase in blood glucose level, for example, results in secretion of insulin and a subsequent increase in hepatic glucokinase required for the first step in metabolism of glucose. Enzyme induction, however, is altered with age.[2] This modification in enzyme induction is characterized by an increase in time between the initial stimulus and appearance of the enzyme. Animal studies evaluating glucokinase response to a glucose load revealed a threefold increase in lag time among older (24 months of age) as compared to younger (2 months of age) animals. Young fasted animals, on refeeding, reached normal glucokinase levels within 8 hours; older animals required at least 24 hours.

The problem in enzyme adaptation relates to the control mechanism, not a failure in protein synthesis.[53] In the case of glucokinase, beta cells of the pancreas are less sensitive to blood glucose and insulin release is delayed. Although relatively few hormone-enzyme systems have been studied in depth, age-related alterations in enzyme induction have been related to defects in glucagon, insulin, adrenal glucocorticoid, and thyroxin regulation.[53]

Impaired hormonal regulation has nutritional implications for glucose and energy metabolism and protein utilization. Impaired glucose tolerance is a frequent observation among older individuals (see Chapter 8). The role of insulin in protein utilization and storage may be particularly important among those with borderline intakes or excessive losses of protein. Such alterations could contribute to the impaired ability of some older persons to adapt to changes in nutrient intake.

AGING IN ORGAN SYSTEMS

Cardiovascular System

Heart Structure and Function. Age-related changes in the heart and circulatory system involve both structure and function. At one time it was believed that the heart muscle atrophied in later years as a result of reduced physical activity.[20] Hypertrophy of the heart muscle was thought to result from cardiovascular disease and increased work load. Recent examinations of nonhypertensive men and women representing both sedentary and active occupations have shown an age-related hypertrophy of the left ventricle occurring between 25 and 80 years of age.[32] This is consistent with autopsy data suggesting that heart mass increases 1 to 1.5 gm per year between the ages of 30 and 90.[32]

According to Lakatta,[32] age-related cardiac hypertrophy is poorly understood. One theory suggests that the gradual increase in both systolic and diastolic blood pressure occurring over adulthood stimulates hypertrophy. Severe hypertension does lead to exaggerated hypertrophy; age-related changes are, however, less obvious. Increased peripheral resistance to blood flow caused by atherosclerotic deposition, coupled with loss of arterial elasticity, also adds to the work load of the heart. It is possible that various factors are involved in the changes observed.

Despite a small increase in size, the effectiveness of the heart as a pump is significantly reduced as the strength of contraction is diminished.[20] As the volume of blood pumped with each stroke decreases,[56] resting cardiac output is significantly lowered (from 6.5 to 3.8 liters/minute between ages 25 and 85). This results in longer circulation time (19 to 29 seconds) for blood to pass through the peripheral vascular system and return to the heart. With decreased cardiac output, blood flow through the coronary arteries supplying nutrients to the heart muscle itself drops by one third.[20] The aging heart also appears less able to use oxygen, which no doubt contributes to the decrease in muscular strength.[20] Therefore strain on the heart increases as nutrients become less available.

Response to Stress. The aged heart poorly tolerates stress arising from either physiologic or emotional causes. Harris[20] points out that many older persons who function well under ordinary conditions develop simple tachycardia with emotional stress, fever, or exercise. This indicates the importance of medical evaluation of older people prior to initiation of a strenuous exercise program, as well as a gradual approach to length and intensity of exercise among those previously sedentary.

The reduced ability of the heart to respond to stress has been related to reduced sensitivity to adrenergic stimulation.[33] Heart rates following strenuous exercise are 20% lower in men age 75 than in those age 20.[32] Chemoreceptor systems may also be impaired, as heart rate increased to a greater extent in younger versus older men breathing gas with a low oxygen content.[32]

Decreased cardiac output and increased circulatory time mean that nutrients are less efficiently delivered to the cells. Tissue oxygen concentration is considered to be the primary regulator of cardiac function.[18] The apparent decrease in sensitivity of the chemoreceptors to reduced oxygen pressure could result in an oxygen deficit contributing to cell dysfunction or death, although this has not been explored.

Of further importance is the effect of reduced cardiac output on other organ systems.[57] Cerebral blood flow decreases by 20% and renal blood flow by about 60%. A diminished supply of blood and oxygen to the brain has been implicated in loss of mental function in older persons.[96] Removal of waste products is less efficient with a reduced glomerular filtration rate. Altered cardiovascular function therefore has far-reaching consequences for the functional capability of the aged individual.

Hypertension. Age-related changes in cardiovascular function contribute to the increase in blood pressure observed through adulthood. Systolic blood pressure tends to increase gradually in both sexes up to age 70; resting diastolic pressure rises to a lesser extent.[34] A blood pressure of 120/75 at age 25 is likely to rise to 160/90 by age 65.[49]

In a national health survey of over 22,000 persons mean systolic blood pressure rose from 121 mm Hg in those age 25 to 34 to 151 mm Hg in those age 65 to 74.[83] After age 44 systolic pressure increased by about 0.9 mm Hg per year. Between ages 25 and 44 systolic pressure was higher in men; between ages 45 and 64 both sexes were equal; at age 65 and over systolic pressures of women exceeded those of men by 6 mm Hg. Diastolic pressures increased from 78 mm Hg to 86 mm Hg over the age range studied. For men, diastolic levels were highest between ages 45 and 54; for women diastolic pressure increased until age 64.

Hypertension is a significant medical and nutritional problem among older persons. Thirty-four percent of persons age 65 to 74 have definite hypertension (systolic pressure ≥160 mm Hg or diastolic pressure ≥95 mm Hg).[83] When those with borderline hypertension are included (systolic pressure between 140 and 159 mm Hg and diastolic pressure between 90 and 94 mm Hg), approximately two thirds of all older persons can be considered hypertensive. High blood pressure increases the risk of both cerebrovascular accidents, or strokes, and coronary artery disease in persons of all ages. Treatment of hypertension involves sodium restriction, weight control, and diuretics, all of which can present dietary problems (see Chapter 9).

Renal System

Kidney function deteriorates with age as a result of both loss of nephrons and decrease in blood flow. Goldman[16] suggests the total number of nephrons declines by 30% to 40%; kidney weight declines by about the same amount. Decreased blood perfusion as a result of a change in cardiac output is most apparent in the cortex, whereas the medulla shows less change.[13]

The decline in functional nephrons brings about an equivalent decline in functional measurements. The estimated reduction in glomerular filtration rate (GFR) ranges from 30% to 40%[13] to as high as 46%.[16] This may reflect both differences in study populations (independent-living versus institutionalized or hospitalized aged) and the variability among individuals.[13]

Observed changes in tubular functions parallel the changes in kidney mass. Reabsorption of glucose and secretion of para-aminohippuric acid decline in about the same ratio as GFR.[35] Therefore decreased renal function most likely results from the decline in numbers of nephrons, with most remaining nephrons functioning normally. Even damaged nephrons appear to contribute to urine formation. Observed changes at the cellular level in aged rats include decreased functioning mitochondria and sodium-potassium ATPase activity.[35]

The aged kidney is less able to adjust either urine flow rate or urine osmolality. The ability to form concentrated urine after 12 hours of restricted fluid intake was significantly less in older versus younger or middle age persons.[13] The differences in solute excretion did not relate to differences in salt or protein intake, nor did decline in GFR appear to be the major cause of the observed differences in ability to concentrate urine. Defects in the countercurrent system or solute transport out of the lumen have been postulated as contributing factors.

Other work evaluating fluid regulation suggests that osmoreceptors in the hypothalamic-neurohypophyseal region increase in sensitivity to serum osmolality in later adulthood.[13] Vasopressin secretion was nearly doubled in older versus younger individuals given hypertonic saline. As pointed out by Epstein,[13] changes in kidney function and vasopressin regulation have serious implications for water balance in the older person. When fluid intake is restricted hypernatremia leading to delirium and eventual death is a danger. At the other extreme enhanced secretion of vasopressin coupled with drugs that further augment vasopressin activity raises the possibility of water intoxication.

Age-related changes in kidney function have many nutritional implications for conservation of nutrients and excretion of waste. Required nutrients actively reabsorbed in the kidney tubule include glucose, amino acids, ascorbic acid, and plasma proteins.[60] Excessive protein intake producing nitrogenous waste and hydrogen ions burdens a less efficient kidney. Blood urea nitrogen (BUN) increases with age and normal healthy older persons can have levels above 20 mg/100 ml.[14] In dehydration, BUN levels may rise to 200 mg/100 ml or more. Megadoses of vitamins, prescribed for the older individual on the assumption that what is not needed can be readily excreted, may accumulate at high levels while awaiting excretion. Drug dosages may also need to be adjusted in light of altered excretion rates.

Pulmonary System

Structural changes in the lung result in loss of alveolar surface area and decrease in elasticity.[40] Alveolar membranes weaken and stretch, air sacs become larger, and surface area for gas exchange declines by as much as 30% between ages 20 and 80. Cross-linking of elastin may be responsible for the loss of elasticity at all lung volumes. Because the chest wall is less easily expanded, the work of breathing is increased.

Although total lung capacity does not change, the proportion of alveolar space ventilated with each breath decreases and residual volume increases. Even when corrected for sex, height, and weight, vital capacity decreases with age; residual volume at age 60 is about 20% greater than at age 20.[40] Increasing resistance to air flow in the passages contributes to reduced ventilation. Gas exchange is also less efficient because of thickening and subsequent decreasing permeability of the alveolar membranes, reduced capillary blood flow, and limited surface area. As a result, oxygen partial pressure in arterial blood decreases; oxyhemoglobin saturation is only about 90% in advanced age, as compared to 96% at younger ages.[56]

The biochemical and mechanical changes in pulmonary function are magnified during exercise. In a young man (age 20) the blood may take up 4 liters of oxygen per minute; in an older man (age 75) this drops to 1.5 liters per minute, thus curtailing the physical endurance of the older individual.[57] Reduced blood flow to the lungs no doubt contributes to this difference in oxygen uptake.

Internal Environment

Body cells require a fluid environment maintained within narrow limits of pH, oxygen content, and electrolyte composition. Extensive work[61] has demonstrated that blood plasma constituents exhibit little variation at *resting levels* between older and younger persons. Fasting blood glucose levels are unchanged in healthy aged. Blood pH was slightly lower in men between ages 40 and 89 as compared to those age 20 to 29 (7.37 versus 7.40), although differences were significant only in the oldest age group (80 to 89 years).[62] Serum bicarbonate and arterial and red cell carbon dioxide did not change with age.

The return to resting levels following an acid or base load, however, is slowed in advanced age as a result of altered lung and kidney response. As the older individual is less able to maintain high rates of respiration, even under stress, carbon dioxide is less easily removed. Following administration of 10 gm ammonium chloride,[59] young adults (age 20 to 25) returned to equilibrium levels within 8 to 10 hours; older men (age 75 to 85) required 24 to 48 hours. Measurements of GFR confirmed

that reduced renal blood flow rather than impaired mechanisms for ammonia secretion was responsible for the increased time required.

An important point, however, is that older persons are able to return to normal resting levels, although additional time is required. Excessive use of self-prescribed drugs (i.e., antacids) or supplements adding to the normal acid-base load could stress homeostatic mechanisms in the older adult.

Measurement of Biologic Age

Measurements used to assess biologic age have included motor reaction time, graying of hair, and acuity of sensory organs. Because of the differing rates of aging among organ systems, however, efforts to formulate an equation to calculate a statistic have generally been unsuccessful. The most successful attempt has been a profile of physical measurements including pulmonary function, body composition, work capacity (involving muscle, lung and cardiovascular response), psychomotor function, and visual perception. Each was evaluated on a 12-point scale in nearly 1100 healthy adult men.[6] When examined by a physician not associated with the study, those men considered to appear older than their chronologic age were also older in biologic age on the basis of their physiologic profile.

Follow-up over a 19-year period confirmed that survivors had been rated younger in biologic age, regardless of chronologic age. Those who died over the 19-year interval had reduced lung capacity, higher blood pressure, decreased plasma protein, and impaired psychomotor function when evaluated earlier. Contrary to what might have been expected, the deceased had been rated higher in work capacity and had exhibited less change in sensory function or body composition.

Borkan and Norris[6] suggest that certain functions are more vulnerable to age-associated deterioration. Further evaluation will consider differences in biologic age as related to nutrition, life-style, and aspects of preventive health. Identification of those physiologic and biochemical parameters that most closely parallel molecular aging processes could make possible the adoption of appropriate preventive measures.

SUMMARY

Persons age 65 and over are the fastest growing segment of the population. As a result of improved sanitation, health care, and antibiotic drugs, those who previously died prematurely now survive to advanced ages. Gains in life expectancy have occurred at younger ages; life expectancy at age 65 has not changed in the last century. Females and whites have benefited most from these trends.

Ninety-five percent of older persons live within the community. The majority of women are widowed and many live alone; most men are married and live with their spouse. Despite cost-of-living increases in Social Security, 16% of older Americans fall below the poverty line. Females, blacks, and those above age 70 are most likely to be poor.

Older persons are the largest users of health care with more physician visits per year, more hospital admissions, and more days of restricted activity or bed rest. Chronic disease results in some limitation of activity for nearly half of those over age 65.

Biologic aging processes resulting in loss of cells and impaired function in some remaining cells lead to physiologic changes in organ systems. The ability to respond to changes in the environment is reduced; the time required for enzyme induction increases and hormonal control is altered.

Organ systems differ in degree of age-related change; the more complex the response, the greater the decline. The heart decreases in both strength and rate of contraction; the consequent reduction in cardiac output reduces the blood supply to the lung, kidney, and coronary arteries. The lungs decrease in compliance and elasticity with a loss of alveolar surface for gas exchange and an increase in residual volume.

Age-related changes in kidney function include decreased glomerular filtration rate, reduced ability to excrete solute, and less efficient reabsorption of water and nutrients. Under resting conditions concentrations of blood constituents including glucose, bicarbonate, and hydrogen ions do not change, although return to equilibrium following displacement is slowed. These physiologic alterations become clinically significant under various conditions including emotional stress, physical exercise, dehydration, or inappropriate drug dosage.

REVIEW QUESTIONS

1. What factors have contributed to the increase in both the number and proportion of older people in the general population? Will life expectancy continue to rise indefinitely? Explain.
2. Describe socioeconomic factors that may influence food intake in older people.
3. How is increasing age related to physical health? Is it appropriate to compare younger and older people on the basis of physical health or functional capability?
4. Older individuals are less able to respond to changes in either the external or internal environment. What biochemical, cellular, and/or physiologic changes contribute to loss of adaptive mechanisms?
5. What are major age-related alterations in the (a) cardiovascular, (b) renal, (c) pulmonary, and (d) endocrine systems? Discuss the nutritional implications of these changes.

REFERENCES

1. Abrams, M.: The SRO elderly from the perspective of a hotel owner. In The invisible elderly, Washington, D.C., 1976, National Council on the Aging.
2. Adelman, R.C.: An age-dependent modification of enzyme regulation, J. Biol. Chem. **245:**1032, 1970.
3. Andres, R.: Aging and carbohydrate metabolism. In Carlson, L.A., ed.: Nutrition in old age, Symposia Swedish Nutrition Foundation X, Stockholm, 1972, Almqvist & Wiksell.
4. Andrew, W.: The anatomy of aging in man and animals, New York, 1971, Grune and Stratton.
5. Barrows, C.H.: Ecology of aging and the aging process, biological parameters, Gerontologist **8:**84, 1968.
6. Borkan, G.A., and Norris, A.H.: Assessment of biological age using a profile of physical parameters, J. Gerontol. **35:**177, 1980.
7. Brehm, H.P.: Organization and financing of health care for the aged: Future implications. In Haynes, S.G., and Feinleib, M., eds.: Epidemiology of aging, DHHS Publication

No. (NIH) 80-969, Washington, D.C., 1980, U.S. Government Printing Office.

8. Bridges, B., and Packard, M.D.: Price and income changes for the elderly, Social Security Bull. **44**(1):3, 1981.

9. Brody, H.: Organization of the cerebral cortex. III. A study of aging in the human cerebral cortex, J. Comp. Neurol. **102**:511, 1955.

10. Butler, R.N.: Why survive? Being old in America, New York, 1975, Harper and Row, Publishers.

11. Butler, R.N.: Mission of the National Institute on Aging, J. Am. Geriatr. Soc. **25**(3):97, 1977.

12. Comfort, A.: The biology of senescence, ed. 3, New York, 1979, Elsevier North Holland, Inc.

13. Epstein, M.: Effects of aging on the kidney, Fed. Proc. **38**:168, 1979.

14. Feinstein, E.I., and Friedman, E.A.: Renal disease in the elderly. In Rossman, I., ed.: Clinical geriatrics, ed. 2, Philadelphia, 1979, J.B. Lippincott Co.

15. Goldfarb, A.V.: Memory and aging. In Goldman, R., and Rockstein, M., eds.: The physiology and pathology of human aging, New York, 1975, Academic Press, Inc.

16. Goldman, R.: Decline in organ function with aging. In Rossman, I., ed.: Clinical geriatrics, ed. 2, Philadelphia, 1979, J.B. Lippincott Co.

17. Gregerman, R.I., and Bierman, E.L.: Aging and hormones. In Williams, R.H., ed.: Textbook of endocrinology, ed. 5, Philadelphia, 1974, W.B. Saunders Co.

18. Guyton, A.C.: Textbook of medical physiology, ed. 3, New York, 1966, W.B. Saunders Co.

19. Harris, L., and Associates, Inc.: The myth and reality of aging in America, Washington, D.C., 1975, National Council on the Aging.

20. Harris, R.: Cardiac changes with age. In Goldman, R., and Rockstein, M., eds.: The physiology and pathology of human aging, New York, 1975, Academic Press Inc.

21. Hart, R.W., and Setlow, R.B.: Correlation between deoxyribonucleic acid excision-repair and life-span in a number of mammalian species, Proc. Natl. Acad. Sci. USA **71**:2169, 1974.

22. Hayflick, L.: The longevity of cultured human cells, J. Am. Geriatr. Soc. **22**:1, 1974.

23. Hayflick, L.: Current theories of biological aging, Fed. Proc. **34**:9, 1975.

24. Hayflick, L.: Cell aging. In Cherkin, A., and others, eds.: Physiology and cell biology of aging (Aging, vol. 8), New York, 1979, Raven Press.

25. Hayflick, L.: The cell biology of human aging, Sci. Am. **242**(1):58, 1980.

26. Hertzog, C., Schaie, K.W., and Gribbin, K.: Cardiovascular disease and changes in intellectual functioning from middle to old age, J. Gerontol. **33**:872, 1978.

27. Hickey, T.: Health and aging, Monterey, Calif., 1980, Brooks/Cole Publishing Co.

28. Hijmans, W., and Hollander, C.F.: The pathogenic role of age-related immune dysfunctions. In Makinodan, T., and Yunis, E., eds.: Immunology and aging, New York, 1977, Plenum Medical Book Co.

29. Kitagawa, E.M., and Houser, P.M.: Differential mortality in the U.S.: A study of socioeconomic epidemiology, Cambridge, Mass., 1973, Harvard University Press.

30. Klug, T.L., and Adelman, R.C.: Altered hypothalamic-pituitary regulation of thyrotropin in male rats during aging, Endocrinology **104**:1136, 1979.

31. Kohn, R.R.: Principles of mammalian aging, Englewood Cliffs, N.J., 1971, Prentice-Hall.

32. Lakatta, E.G.: Alterations in the cardiovascular system that occur in advanced age, Fed. Proc. **38**:163, 1979.

33. Lakatta, E.G.: Age-related alterations in the cardiovascular response to adrenergic mediated stress, Fed. Proc. **39**:3173, 1980.

34. Lasser, R.P., and Master, A.M.: Observation of frequency distribution curves of blood pressure in persons aged 20 to 106 years, Geriatrics **14**:345, 1959.

35. Lindeman, R.D.: Age changes in renal function. In Goldman, R., and Rockstein, M., eds.: The physiology and pathology of human aging, New York, 1975, Academic Press, Inc.

36. Lytle, L.D., and Altar, A.: Diet, central nervous system, and aging, Fed. Proc. **38**:2017, 1979.

37. Mackay, I.R., Whittingham, S.F., and Mathews, J.D.: The immunoepidemiology of aging. In Makinodan, T., and Yunis, E., eds.: Immunology and aging, New York, 1977, Plenum Medical Book Co.

38. Madigan, F.C.: Are sex mortality differentials biologically caused? Milbank Mem. Fund Q. **35**:203, 1957.

39. Makman, M.H., and others: Aging and monoamine receptors in brain, Fed. Proc. **38**:1922, 1979.

40. Mauderly, J.L.: Effect of age on pulmonary structure and function of immature and adult animals and man, Fed. Proc. **38**:173, 1979.

41. National Council on the Aging: Fact book on aging: A profile of America's older population, Washington, D.C., 1978, National Council on the Aging.

42. Norris, A.H., and Shock, N.W.: Aging and variability, Ann. N.Y. Acad. Sci. **134**:591, 1966.

43. Palmore, E.: Predictors of longevity. In Haynes, S.G., and Feinleib, M., eds.: Epidemiology of aging, DHHS Publication No. (NIH) 80-969, Washington, D.C., 1980, U.S. Government Printing Office.

44. Pearl, R.: Studies on human longevity. 4. The inheritance of longevity: Preliminary report. Hum. Biol. **3**:245, 1931.

45. Reingold, J., Wolk, R., and Schwartz, S.: A gerontological sheltered workshop: The aged person's attitude about money, J. Am. Geriatr. Soc. **19**:315, 1971.

46. Retherford, R.D.: Tobacco smoking and sex mortality differential, Demography **9**(2):203, 1972.

47. Robinson, D.S.: Changes in monoamine oxidase and monoamines with human development and aging, Fed. Proc. **34**:103, 1975.

48. Rockstein, M.: The genetic basis for longevity. In Rockstein, M., ed.: Theoretical aspects of aging, New York, 1974, Academic Press, Inc.

49. Rockstein, M.: The biology of aging in humans: An overview. In Goldman, R., and Rockstein, M., eds.: The physiology and pathology of human aging, New York, 1975, Academic Press, Inc.

50. Rockstein, M., Chesky, J., and Sussman, M.: Comparative biology and evolution of aging, In Finch, C.E., and Hayflick, L., eds.: Handbook of the biology of aging, New York, 1977, Van Nostrand Reinhold Co.

51. Roth, G.S.: Hormone receptor changes during adulthood and senescence: Significance for aging research, Fed. Proc. **38**:1910, 1979.

52. Sanadi, D.R.: Metabolic changes and their significance in aging. In Finch, C.E., and Hayflick, L., eds.: Handbook of the biology of aging, New York, 1977, Van Nostrand Reinhold Co.

53. Sartin, J., and others: The role of hormones in changing adaptive mechanisms during aging, Fed. Proc. **39**:3163, 1980.

54. Schneider, E.L.: Cell replication and aging: In vitro and in vivo studies, Fed. Proc. **38**:1857, 1979.

55. Shanas, E. and Hauser, P.M.: Zero population growth and the family life of older people, J. Social Issues **30**(4):79, 1974.

56. Shock, N.W.: Physiological aspects of aging in man, Annu. Rev. Physiol. **23**:97, 1961.

57. Shock, N.W.: The physiology of aging, Sci. Am. **206**:100, 1962.

58. Shock, N.W.: Biologic concepts of aging, Psych. Res. Rep. **23**:1, 1968.

59. Shock, N.W.: Homeostatic disturbances and adaptations in aging, Bull. Schweiz. Akad. Med. Wiss. **24**:284, 1968.

60. Shock, N.W.: Physiologic aspects of aging, J. Am. Diet. Assoc. **56**:491, 1970.

61. Shock, N.W.: Systems integration. In Finch, C.E., and Hayflick, L., eds.: Handbook of the biology of aging, New York, 1977, Van Nostrand Reinhold Co.

62. Shock, N.W., and Yiengst, M.J.: Age changes in the acid-base equilibrium of the blood of males, J. Gerontol. **5**:1, 1950.

63. Siegel, J.S.: Prospective trends in the size and structure of the elderly population; impact of mortality trends and some implications, Current Population Reports, Special Studies Series P-23, No. 78, Washington, D.C., 1979, U.S. Bureau of Census.

64. Siegel, J.S.: The future of the American family, Current Population Reports, Special Studies, Series P-23, No. 78, Washington, D.C., 1979, U.S. Bureau of the Census.

65. Siegel, J.S.: Recent and prospective demographic trends for the elderly population and some implications for health care. In Haynes, S.G., and Feinleib, M., eds.: Epidemiology of aging, DHHS Publication No. (NIH) 80-969, Washington, D.C., 1980, U.S. Government Printing Office.

66. Strehler, B.L.: Time, cells, and aging, ed. 2, New York, 1977, Academic Press, Inc.

67. Strehler, B.L., and Mildvan, A.S.: General theory of mortality and aging, Science **132**:14, 1960.

68. Terry, R.D.: Senile dementia, Fed. Proc. **37**:2837, 1978.

69. United States Bureau of the Census: Historical statistics of the United States: Colonial times to 1970, Part I, Washington, D.C., 1975, U.S. Government Printing Office.

70. United States Bureau of the Census: Projections of the population of the United States: 1977 to 2050, Current Population Reports, Series P-25, No. 704, Washington, D.C., 1977, U.S. Government Printing Office.

71. United States Bureau of the Census: Demographic aspects of aging and the older population in the U.S., Current Population Reports, Special Studies Series P-23, No. 59, Revised, Washington, D.C., 1978, U.S. Government Printing Office.

72. United States Bureau of the Census, Social and economic characteristics of the older population: 1978, Current Population Reports, Special Studies Series P-23, No. 85, Washington, D.C., 1979, U.S. Government Printing Office.

73. United States Bureau of the Census: Population profile of the United States: 1981, Current Population Reports, Series P-20, No. 374, Washington, D.C., 1982, U.S. Government Printing Office.

74. United States Department of Health, Education, and Welfare: Mortality trends: Age, color, and sex, United States: 1950-69, DHEW Publication No. (HRA) 74-1852, Rockville, Md., 1973, U.S. Government Printing Office.

75. United States Department of Health, Education and Welfare: Facts of life and death, DHEW Publication No. (PHS) 79-1222, Washington, D.C., 1978, U.S. Government Printing Office.

76. United States Department of Health, Education and Welfare: Health: United States, 1978, DHEW Publication No. (PHS) 78-1252, Hyattsville, Md., 1978, U.S. Government Printing Office.

77. United States Department of Health, Education, and Welfare: Healthy people: The Surgeon General's report on health promotion and disease prevention, 1979, DHEW Publication No. (PHS) 79-55071, Washington, D.C., 1980, U.S. Government Printing Office.

78. United States Department of Health and Human Services: Health: United States, 1980, DHHS Publication No. (PHS) 81-1232, Hyattsville, Md., U.S. Government Printing Office.

79. United States Department of Health and Human Services: Life tables: Vital statistics of the U.S., 1978, vol. II, Section 5, DHHS Publication No. (PHS) 81-1104, Hyattsville, Md., 1980, U.S. Government Printing Office.

80. United States Department of Health and Human Services: Age Page. Skin: Getting the wrinkles out of aging, Washington, D.C., 1981, National Institute on Aging.

81. United States Department of Health and Human Services: Health: United States, 1981, DHHS Publication No. (PHS) 82-1232, Hyattsville, Md., 1981, U.S. Government Printing Office.

82. United States Department of Health and Human Services: Health characteristics of persons with chronic activity limitation: United States, 1979, DHHS Publication No. (PHS) 82-1565, Hyattsville, Md., 1981, U.S. Government Printing Office.

83. United States Department of Health and Human Services: Hypertension in adults 25-74 years of age, United States, 1971-1975, DHHS Publication No. (PHS) 81-1671, Washington, D.C., 1981, U.S. Government Printing Office.

84. United States Department of Health and Human Services: Long term care: Background and future directions, DHHS Publication No. (HCFA) 81-20047, Washington, D.C., 1981, U.S. Government Printing Office.

85. United States Department of Health and Human Services: Use of health services by women 65 years of age and over: United States, DHHS Publication No. (PHS) 81-1720, Hyattsville, Md., 1981, U.S. Government Printing Office.

86. United States Department of Health and Human Services: Advance report of final mortality statistics, 1979, Monthly Vital Stat. Rep. **31**(6):suppl., Sept. 30, 1982.

87. United States Department of Health and Human Services: Current estimates from the National Health Interview Survey: United States, 1981, DHHS Publication No. (PHS) 83-1569, Hyattsville, Md., 1982, U.S. Government Printing Office.

88. United States Department of Health and Human Services: Mortality from diseases associated with smoking: United States, 1960-1977, DHHS Publication No. (PHS) 82-1854, Hyattsville, Md., 1982, U.S. Government Printing Office.

89. United States House of Representatives Select Committee on Aging: Every ninth American (1982 Edition), Comm. Pub. No. 97-332, Washington, D.C., 1982, U.S. Government Printing Office.

90. United States Senate Special Committee on Aging: Summary of recommendations and surveys on social security and pension policies, Washington, D.C., 1980, U.S. Government Printing Office.

91. Vernadakis, A.: Neuronal-glial interactions during development and aging, Fed. Proc. **34**:89, 1975.

92. Waldron, I.: Sex differences in longevity. In Haynes, S.G., and Feinleib, M., eds: Epidemiology of aging, DHHS Publication No. (NIH) 80-969, Washington, D.C., 1980, U.S. Government Printing Office.

93. Waldron, I.: Discussion. In Haynes, S.G., and Feinleib, M., eds.: Epidemiology of aging, DHHS Publication No. (NIH) 80-969, p. 314, Washington, D.C., 1980, U.S. Government Printing Office.

94. Watkin, D.M.: The physiology of aging, Am. J. Clin. Nutr. **36**(suppl.):750, 1982.

95. Weksler, M.E.: Genetic and immunologic determinants of aging. In Haynes, S.G., and Feinleib, M., eds.: Epidemiology of aging, DHHS Publication No. (NIH) 80-969, Washington, D.C., 1980, U.S. Government Printing Office.

96. Wilkie, F.L.: Blood pressure and cognitive functioning. In Haynes, S.G., and Feinleib, M., eds.: Epidemiology of aging, DHHS Publication No. (NIH) 80-969, Washington, D.C., 1980, U.S. Government Printing Office.

Chapter 2

Nutrition and the Life Span

Since antiquity people have been searching for potions to preserve youth and prolong life. Early explorers came to the New World seeking the "fountain of youth." Today hormone and vitamin preparations promising to retard aging or restore physical health receive widespread attention. Long-lived individuals are sought after for their secrets regarding food, drink, and daily habits. Unfortunately, there has been little attempt to follow individuals over a period of years to obtain information relating to state of health and years of life. Most of what is known regarding the influence of nutrition upon the aging process has come from animal studies exploring the effects of both quantitative and qualitative dietary manipulations.

HISTORICAL PERSPECTIVE

Historical writings contain many directives for maintenance of good health and prolongation of life. Cornaro,[18] whose book *The Art of Living Long* was published in the 1500s, became an ardent advocate of temperate diet after becoming ill with fever, pains in the stomach, and perpetual thirst. Previously given to excessive food and drink, he from that time on ate sparingly of bread, meat, milk, egg yolk, and soup and at age 95 wrote his final treatise on the wisdom of a moderate diet. Cornaro recognized that one needs less food as the body grows older. He limited himself to 12 ounces of food per day and exhorted younger people to avoid overindulgence.

Francis Bacon (1561-1626) was the first author to recommend scientific inquiry regarding diet and longevity.[4] He advocated a frugal diet and encouraged study of people in various climates and living situations to determine those characteristics which influence life span. In his opinion, diet was the most important component in prolonging life. Unfortunately, Bacon's recommendation for evaluating relationships between diet, life-style, and mortality is only beginning to receive attention.

Early writings also stress a prudent diet for the aged. A physician living in 1000 A.D. urged eating only small amounts of food at a time and avoiding foods leading to digestive upset, such as spiced and pickled items.[82] A treatise on geriatric medicine appearing in 1796 advised older people to avoid sugar and confectionary foods, consume liberal amounts of vegetables, limit intake of meat, and eat only sparingly at night.[4] A paper entitled "Food and Hygiene of Old Age" appearing in the *Journal of the American Medical Association* in 1892 suggested that errors in food selection are less serious in the young who can recover from such mistakes.[5]

Within this century Metchnikoff,[48] a Russian physiologist, proposed the theory of autointoxication, suggesting that death occurred as a result of toxins produced in the large intestine by fecal wastes and then absorbed into the body. Current fears relating to the dangers of constipation are no doubt rooted in these writings. Fermented milk products, such as yogurt, containing lactic acid–producing bacilli were recommended to destroy the intestinal microbes responsible for the poisonous waste.[48]

Swanson[73] proposed that alterations in the internal environment brought about by inappropriate levels of nutrients may initiate age-related changes in the cell. Conversely, a suitable diet might delay or slow the occurrence of such changes.

CALORIC RESTRICTION AND THE AGING PROCESS

Length of Life

Studies[8-9,44,47,56] over the past 40 years with a variety of animal models and experimental designs have confirmed that caloric restriction increases the life span. The classic studies of McCay and coworkers[47] in the 1930s demonstrated that caloric intake controls not only the rate of growth but also the rate of development and aging. Rats, following weaning at three weeks of age, were given either (1) unlimited access to food (fed ad libitum) or (2) only sufficient calories to maintain their weaning weight (diets were adequate in protein, vitamins, and minerals). Animals provided with unlimited calories grew and matured normally. In the restricted group all maturation ceased. Restricted animals were held at weaning weight for 300 to 1000 days; when calories were increased, growth and development progressed. While the animals held at weaning weight maintained their youthful appearance, the ad libitum fed rats progressively aged.

It is difficult to believe that both animals pictured in Fig. 2-1 are identical in age. The rat on the right died several days after the photograph was taken. The animal held at weaning weight was given sufficient calories to commence growth at 1000 days of age and lived nearly a year following this photograph. Half of the ad libitum fed animals survived less than 700 days; animals held at weaning weight for 300 or 1000 days lived an additional 535 and 138 days, respectively, after completing growth. Restricted animals never achieved normal body size or body weight but were 10% to 20% smaller than nonrestricted. This work established that (1) level of calorie intake significantly influences life span; (2) reduced calorie intake and body weight increases life span; and (3) level of calorie intake controls the rate of maturation and aging.

Incidence of Degenerative Disease

Calorie restriction may increase the life span by retarding development of degenerative disease. Berg and coworkers[8-9] fed their restricted rats about half that consumed by ad libitum fed controls. The

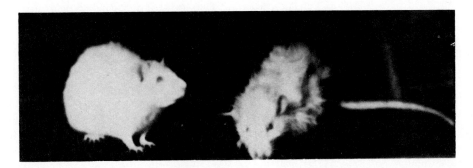

Fig. 2-1. Rats at 964 days of age. (From McCay, C.M., and others: Retarded growth, life span, ultimate body size and age changes in the albino rat after feeding diets restricted in calories, J. Nutr. **18**:1, 1939. Photograph courtesy Department of Manuscripts and Archives, Cornell University Libraries.)

Table 2-1. Disease incidence in older rats (800 days of age)

	Restricted		Unrestricted	
	M	F	M	F
Kidney lesions	0%	0%	100%	57%
Vascular lesions	3%	0%	63%	24%
Myocardial lesions	24%	0%	96%	23%

Modified from Berg, B.N., and Simms, H.S.: Nutrition and longevity in the rat. 2. Longevity and onset of disease with different levels of food intake, J. Nutr. **71**:255, 1960.

unrestricted animals grew and matured normally but by 800 days of age had developed chronic disease (Table 2-1). Although disease was frequent (63% to 100%) among ad libitum fed males, restricted males were for the most part free of chronic problems. No restricted females had any specified lesion, and even among ad libitum fed females, disease incidence was half or less that of males. A striking difference between the restricted and ad libitum fed was the lack of body fat in those given less food; histologically, they appeared younger. Those authors[8-9] concluded that a high degree of body fat, even within normal range, enhances the development of degenerative disease.

Current work indicates that the aging process itself *in the absence of infectious disease* leads to degenerative changes, although food restriction delays the appearance of lesions.[44,81] Among animals maintained in a barrier facility excluding all pathogenic microbes, median life span was 1047 days in restricted as compared to 714 days in nonrestricted animals.[44,81] More than 60% of the restricted animals were still alive when the oldest ad libitum fed rat died at age 963 days. Chronic kidney disease, testicular tumors, and fatty changes in the liver appeared 6 to 12 months earlier and were more severe in the ad libitum fed animals.[81] Renal disease was the cause of death for most on unlimited feeding; in contrast, end stage renal disease was not observed in any restricted animal.

In contrast to the conclusions of Berg and coworkers,[8-9] Bertrand and coworkers[10] suggested that absence of body fat was not responsible for the observed differences in life span and physical disease. Although the restricted animals had both lower body weights and less body fat, both the number of fat cells and total adipose tissue continued to increase in all animals throughout most of adulthood.[10] Calorie restriction therefore exerts an influence on longevity by some means other than, or in addition to, reducing body fat.

Biochemical Alterations

A delay in cellular changes as a result of calorie restriction is evident in many tissues.[39,41,44,46,79] In skeletal muscle resting oxygen consumption falls more rapidly in ad libitum versus restricted feeding.[46] Loss of neural dopamine receptors is slowed under conditions of calorie restriction.[39] Immune response, evaluated by quantitative antibody response to antigen stimulation, retains youthful qualities for a longer period when animals are food restricted.[79] The thymus of restricted animals continues to increase in size when that of ad libitum fed animals has undergone involution. Decreased calorie intake also suppresses production of autoimmune antibody complexes that contribute to tissue degeneration.[23]

Food restriction appears to delay age-related alterations in serum lipids.[41] In both humans and animals serum cholesterol increases with advancing age, reaching a peak at about age 60 in humans, and at age 24 months in laboratory rats. In restricted animals serum cholesterol levels increase only moderately between the ages of 12 and 24 months (Fig. 2-2) and at age 30 months are still below usual levels. Because serum lipids represent the balance between absorption and synthesis, and storage and utilization, Liepa and coworkers[41] consider these age-related changes to reflect alterations at the tissue level.

Although experimental findings from animal models are not necessarily applicable to human

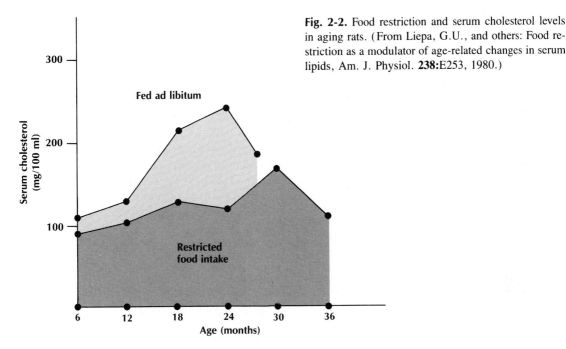

Fig. 2-2. Food restriction and serum cholesterol levels in aging rats. (From Liepa, G.U., and others: Food restriction as a modulator of age-related changes in serum lipids, Am. J. Physiol. **238**:E253, 1980.)

populations, limiting calorie intake does appear to exert an influence on the rate of aging. Masoro and coworkers[44] propose that diet restriction alters the environment at the cellular level and thus delays pathologic changes. Identification of the mechanism involved would allow development of preventive health measures.

DIET COMPOSITION

Relative proportions of dietary protein, fat, and carbohydrate influence the appearance of degenerative changes and length of life. It is difficult, however, to evaluate findings because a change in level of one dietary component results in a change in at least one other. A diet high in caloric density can accelerate weight gain and alter body composition; consequently, the influence of the nutrient itself is less easily recognized. Influences of both protein and fat upon the life span will be examined in the following sections.

Protein/Calorie Ratio

Length of Life. Ross and coworkers[56-62] evaluated the effect of diets characterized as high or low in protein and carbohydrate (sucrose), fed on a restricted or nonrestricted basis, on the life span and rate of growth in laboratory rats. With the exception of the diet low in protein and high in carbohydrate, life span increased when diets were fed on a restricted basis.[56] Animals fed a low protein diet self-restrict food intake; therefore food consumption was not appreciably different from the restricted animals.

A diet advantageous in early life may be deleterious in later life. Although more deaths occurred early in life among those on the low protein, low carbohydrate regimen, this diet was conducive to extended adult life. No deaths occurred over the first year among animals receiving a diet high in protein and low in carbohydrate, but mortality increased rapidly beyond that point.[56]

During early life and active growth, dietary protein is the most important influence on survival. When growth is complete total calories also become important.[61-62] Animals consuming high protein early in life and low protein with moderate calories thereafter had the longest life spans. The shortest life spans occurred in those with low protein intakes initially and increased protein thereafter. The composition of the diet consumed up to 100 days of age (rats reach puberty at 50 days of age) successfully predicted the length of life. For the mature animal a protein/calorie ratio of 1:5 was most beneficial.[59]

The level of protein and calories consumed influences both rate of growth and weight gain.[61-62] Animals who grow slowly are more likely to have extended life spans than those who gain weight rapidly and reach their maximum weight early in adulthood. Among mice having a growth rate double that of normal controls, total life span is about half that expected.[22] Duration of growth is more important than maximum body weight.[25] Among obese mice of similar body weight, those who required 16 months to reach their maximum weight had a mean life span of 22 months; when maximum weight was reached in 8 months, mean life span dropped to 13 months. Rapid growth and increased body weight are also associated with incidence of both benign and malignant tumors, although tumor incidence in all groups increases with age.[60]

Enzyme Induction. Hepatic enzymes such as ATPase, sensitive to dietary intake, are also influenced by rate of growth.[57] Enzyme levels are low in the young animal and gradually increase in later life. This increase is directly proportional to both calorie intake and body weight. Diets high in protein and carbohydrate result in more rapid increases and higher absolute enzyme levels than diets low in calories.[57] Life expectancy is inversely related to enzyme activity; lower enzyme levels typical of a young animal are associated with increased life span. Ross[57] suggests that the rise in enzyme levels accompanying rapid growth is a homeostatic response to larger body size. At the same time dietary

patterns that bring about this rapid rate of change are most detrimental, leading to early onset and increased severity of disease.

The suggestion that rapid growth and increased body weight accelerate the aging process has serious implications for current growth patterns in children. Children are both taller and heavier and reach puberty at earlier ages as compared with previous generations. Stini[71] notes that males appear to be more susceptible to environmental influences on growth than females and suggests that more rapid attainment of maximum size may, in part, be responsible for the mortality differential existing between males and females.

Dietary Restriction in Maturity. Restricting protein and calories in early life is inappropriate for humans. It is possible, however, to consider reducing calorie intake in early adulthood after growth and maturation are complete. Animals provided with unlimited calories prior to sexual maturity and then restricted[58-59] had a death rate only one third that of animals given free access to food throughout life. When restriction was begun at midlife there was still a significant improvement in life span, if the imposed limitation was moderate. If the food allotment was reduced to one third the accustomed level, mortality was three times that expected. When restriction was less severe, about half the former level, gains in life span were significant. Stuchlikova and coworkers[72] reported a 40% increase in survival time among rats fed ad libitum throughout their first year of life and then restricted.

The benefit of calorie restriction at older ages could relate to body weight. Ross[59] reported that a 10% increase in body weight following maturity resulted in a 13% decrease in life expectancy in laboratory animals.

High Fat Diets

Several factors including weight gain,[64] genetic characteristics,[66] and toxic components present in fat[33] have been cited as contributing to the injurious effect of a high fat diet. A metabolic consequence of a high fat diet is increased feed efficiency resulting in increased weight gain per number of calories consumed. Increased utilization of calories is directly related to the decrease in life span; females and genetic strains having reduced feed efficiency, regardless of diet, have a longer life span even when fed the high fat ration.[66] Body weight per se does not completely explain the negative effects.

Efforts to define chemical properties of fat responsible for the deleterious effect have not been successful. Kaunitz and coworkers,[33] comparing fats on the basis of melting point, linoleic acid content, or degree of unsaturation, suggest that substances present in fats, rather than characteristics of the triglyceride, induce degenerative disease, as neither mortality nor pathologic lesions (i.e., cardiac fatty infiltration, tumors) was consistently related to the properties evaluated. Survival time of animals fed vegetable oils processed for human consumption[32] was improved when fats were subjected to mild heating (60° C) and aeration. Those investigators concluded that such treatment inactivated toxic antioxidants responsible for the degenerative effects.

Current animal work suggests that a high fat diet promotes the development of tumors; polyunsaturated fats appear to be most detrimental although cholesterol and saturated fats as well as their metabolic products may be involved.[49-50] Newberne[49] postulates that dietary fat acts on the immune system, thereby increasing susceptibility to tumors.

Although this discussion has focused on animal studies, it is appropriate to mention an epidemiologic report evaluating cause of death among men consuming above average levels of polyunsaturated fat. In an eight year double-blind clinical trial of a diet containing 40% fat (10% or 40% from polyunsaturates), fatalities from atherosclerotic heart disease were reduced among those consuming the diet high in polyunsaturated fat.[54] An unexpected outcome, however, was the increased number of deaths from cancer. Although 70 in the control

versus 48 in the experimental group died from atherosclerotic heart disease, 17 versus 31 died of cancer. Total mortality was similar in both groups (178 versus 174). A fact to be considered, however, is the age of the men involved. Most were above 65 years of age and urogenital cancer, common among this age group, represented 28% of the cancers reported in the experimental group.

Increased cancer risk was not observed in five clinical trials of serum cholesterol–lowering diets conducted with nearly 2500 men varying in age.[21] As suggested by Pearce and Dayton,[54] older men protected from heart disease may eventually develop cancer, the second leading cause of death in the aging population. Nevertheless, the Food and Nutrition Board[24] recommends that polyunsaturated fat provide 8% to 10% of total calories.

Energy Balance

Body weight, metabolic efficiency, and physical exercise continue to be important issues for discussion when considering the mechanism by which diet influences longevity. Level of food intake during the first 3 months of life has, in animals on self-selected feeding, been shown to explain 50% of the variation in life span.[61-62] Body weight at 150 days of age can predict the months of life. Heavier animals appear to be more efficient, gaining more weight than would have been anticipated on the basis of food intake alone.[61] It may be that animals consuming more calories become more efficient as a result of greater food intake. Alternatively, the heavier animals may experience greater weight gain because they are genetically more efficient.

In animals regular physical exercise brings about an increase in metabolic rate (oxygen consumption per unit body weight) that continues throughout life.[26] Animals provided with an exercise wheel allowing voluntary physical activity also had slower growth rates, lower body weights, and longer life spans than nonexercised controls.[26] Although body fat was not measured, the higher oxygen consumption in the exercised group would point to increased lean body mass and decreased body fat.

The influence of food restriction on fuel efficiency and metabolic rate is still unresolved. One reviewer evaluating calorie intake and length of life concluded that food restriction prolonged life by reducing the metabolic rate.[63] Masoro and co-workers[43] on the basis of measured food intakes, maintain that caloric intake per gram of body weight does not differ in restricted versus ad libitum fed animals. It is likely that energy utilization plays an important role in the life-prolonging effect of food restriction although the mechanism is not defined.

Antioxidant Compounds

Because oxidation reactions producing free radicals are involved in many degenerative processes, dietary supplementation with antioxidants has been explored as a means of increasing the life span.[12,28,36,74-75] Both synthetic (butylated hydroxytoluene, mercaptoethylamine hydrochloride)[36] and biologic (vitamin E, vitamin C, methionine)[12,74-75] antioxidants increase the average life span in some species, particularly those susceptible to tumors; however, maximum life span is unchanged. Apparently, antioxidants inhibit toxic environmental substances but do not alter aging processes.[12] Recent work with humans exposed to ozone and animals treated with carbon tetrachloride or excessive iron suggests that dietary vitamin E does reduce lipid peroxidation.[74] Adequate vitamin E status may therefore offer some protection; however, further study is needed.

NUTRIENT INTAKE AND HUMAN LIFE SPAN

Scope of Problem

Little information is now available to evaluate the influence of lifelong dietary habits on health and longevity. Longitudinal studies now in progress at government and university research centers have not included dietary habits as a major focus. The few studies that have collected detailed nutrition information did not follow subjects at regularly scheduled intervals, nor did they continue throughout the life span. Life-style and health habits, degree of physical exercise, occupational stress, and smoking habits or use of drugs should be included in a longitudinal evaluation of nutrition and physical health. Watkin[78] points out that a longitudinal approach, following the same individual over time, provides information on both the rate of change and the periods when changes occur. Such an evaluation of the influence of diet on physiologic and biochemical aging is urgently needed. Data obtained could provide the basis for dietary recommendations.

Obesity and Mortality

The negative aspects of a liberal amount of body fat have only in recent times become a concern. Historically, the individual who could store reserves of body fat when food was abundant was most likely to survive periods of famine.[42] When food is plentiful all year round, a person highly efficient in laying down body fat is at a disadvantage. Although excessive body fat is believed to contribute to development of degenerative disease and increase risk of mortality,[11,68-69] this suggestion is based primarily on measurements of body weight, not body fat.

Life Insurance Statistics. Records of life insurance companies are the primary sources of statistics concerning body weight and length of life.[11,68-69] Since 1887 records have been compiled on the height, weight, and subsequent mortality of policyholders. It is important to the company to be able to predict how long a particular individual can be expected to live or, conversely, when the company should anticipate paying the insurance claim.

Based on the records of past policyholders who lived the longest, insurance companies have derived tables of standard weights for persons of a particular sex and height. Although these tables are widely used by both insurance companies and health professionals, they have many inherent limitations. An increase in body weight does not presume an increase in body fat; a change in weight can reflect increase in muscle mass (see Chapter 3). Body weight tables do not always allow for variations in body build. Finally, standard weights are not representative of the general population because middle and upper socioeconomic groups are more likely to purchase life insurance than low income or minority groups. Despite these problems the general conclusion drawn from statistics collected over nearly 100 years is the greater the deviation between actual body weight and standard weight, the greater the mortality risk.[11,68-69]

The most recent compilation of life insurance data is the Build Study, 1979, tracing the mortality experience of 4.2 million policyholders between 1954 and 1972.[69] These individuals were considered to be in good health although about 10% were over- or underweight to some extent. In general mortality ratios were below 100 for persons about average or somewhat below average in weight, and increased at higher degrees of over- or underweight (Table 2-2). Overweight, even when 55% to 65%

Table 2-2. Mortality risk according to body weight

| Classification | Mortality Risk* (Ratio of actual to expected mortality) | |
	Men	Women
25%-35% under-weight	117	128
5%-15% underweight	95	93
Within 5% of average	95	97
5%-15% overweight	106	100
25%-35% overweight	130	103
55%-65% overweight	186	140

*Standard risk = 100.

Modified from Society of Actuaries: Build study, 1979, Chicago, 1980, Society of Actuaries.

above standard, carries less additional risk for women than men (40% versus 86%). In females as much as one third above average weight, risk increases by only 3%; in males of this class, risk increases by 30%. Extreme underweight (25% to 35%) carries greater risk for females.

Mortality patterns at various levels of over- and underweight also differ according to age.[69] Underweight carries greater risk for those ages 40 to 69, whereas weight gain is more serious at younger ages (15 to 39 years). Body weight 30% above average decreases the life expectancy of men by 3 years at age 30; this drops to 2 years at age 60.[69] Even for the morbidly obese (50% to 150% above standard weight),[20] mortality risk decreases with advancing age. Among 200 morbidly obese men evaluated over a 7-year period, probability of death was 12 times that of the general population for those between ages 25 and 34; between ages 65 and 74, mortality risk was only about twice that of the general population.

Mortality risk associated with overweight is reduced following weight loss.[11] Persons more than 30% overweight benefit more than those less overweight, and men benefit more than women. Mortality risk in markedly overweight (≥30%) males decreased from 179 to 109 on return to standard weight. Among women risk declined by less than half (161 versus 135).[11] Why the impairment resulting from overweight is less reversible in women is not understood.

The physiologic explanation for the influence of obesity on mortality is unclear although overweight individuals have greater risk of developing diabetes, cardiovascular and renal diseases, and disorders of the liver or gallbladder. However, risk of death from these disorders decreases among overweights after age 60.[40] Cancer risk increases substantially only at weights 40% above standard. Whether increased mortality results from a direct effect of overweight on physiologic function or the association of obesity with other risk factors such as elevated blood pressure and serum cholesterol is still being debated. (For a review of this topic see reference 35.) Regardless of the relationship, risk decreases significantly with advancing age.

Obesity in the Aged

Incidence of Overweight. Although life insurance data point to increased mortality in the overweight, the fact remains that there are people both old and obese.[52] A national survey of over 13,000 persons revealed that the percent overweight did not differ significantly among age groups (Table 2-3).[69] At least one fourth of all individuals above age 60 were 10% or more above average weight, and the highest incidence of overweight (30%) was found among women age 60 to 69.

It is difficult to compare one study with another as standards used to evaluate body weight or body fat are not consistent; however, of particular interest is the number of older persons identified as 30% or more above desirable weight. In a study of over 1300 persons in a London suburb 17% of the women and 5% of the men above age 50 were more than 30% overweight.[3] Among 200 older persons above age 65, living in the community and attending an outpatient clinic, over one fifth were 30% to 115% overweight.[67] Twelve of the 42 were more than 50% overweight. In a New Zealand community, 14% of the women above age 70 were more than 40% above ideal weight.[7] Why some individuals in the community survive to a relatively

old age despite excessive body weight or body fat while others suffer morbidity leading to premature death is a question requiring further study.

History of Body Weight. One factor influencing the long term effect of overweight may be the time interval when weight gain occurred. Individuals who become overweight as children tend to remain overweight as adults. In a 40-year follow-up of men first evaluated when they were 9 to 13 years of age, 41% of those moderately overweight (relative weight = 105 to 119) as children were in the same category as adults, although 20% had become markedly overweight (relative weight ≥120).[1] Of those markedly overweight as children, 63% remained in that category while 21% were only moderately overweight as adults.

Overweight appeared to be more detrimental to those who gained weight rapidly in adulthood as compared to those overweight since childhood.[1] The incidences of hypertensive vascular disease and cardiovascular renal disease were 23% and 36%, respectively, among persons who continued to be moderately overweight. In contrast, those underweight as children who had become moderately overweight in adulthood were twice as likely to have either hypertension or cardiovascular problems (incidence of 47% and 63%, respectively).

The lowest incidence of chronic disease was found among individuals moderately overweight as children who reduced to below average weight as adults. None had hypertensive vascular disease and only 25% had cardiovascular renal disease. However, individuals with static, moderate overweight were not disadvantaged, as prevalence of both hypertensive and cardiovascular disease was similar in the moderate overweights and average weights. This evaluation, however, did not differentiate between overweight related to increased bone or muscle mass and that caused by excessive body fat.

When obese aged were questioned regarding their weight histories, the majority recalled being obese as children.[55] In those families overweight was associated with good health and weight loss

Table 2-3. Percent of overweight persons according to age

Age	At Least 10% Overweight		At Least 20% Overweight	
	Men	Women	Men	Women
20-29	24	20	11	15
40-49	23	24	12	16
60-69	24	30	11	15

Modified from Society of Actuaries: Build study 1979, Chicago, 1980, Society of Actuaries.

associated with illness. Frequently, other family members such as parents, brothers, or sisters were also decidedly overweight.

Ill-advised attempts at weight loss, using imbalanced or starvation diets, can lead to dramatic losses in weight but also depletion of vitamins, protein, and electrolytes. Such recurrent episodes, common among those who regularly lose and regain substantial amounts of weight, may be more detrimental to continued good health than static obesity. Other problems, such as hypertension, can be further aggravated by the mental anxiety related to unsuccessful attempts at weight loss.

Body weight does decline in some older individuals making no conscious effort at weight reduction. In one group of 681 persons at least 65 years of age, 25% of men and 31% of women within 20% of average weight had at some time been more than 20% overweight and 7% of the total had been more than 40% above average weight.[29] At the same time 35% of men between ages 75 and 84, 31% of women between ages 75 and 84, and 40% of women between ages 85 and 94 remained at least 30% above average weight.[29] Gains in relative weight among people over age 60 may result from actual weight gain or from the decrease in average weight in older age cohorts. Weight loss in advanced age has been associated with deteriorating physical condition and chronic disease.

Lack of Agreement in Mortality Statistics. The disparity between life insurance data suggesting a relationship between overweight and premature death, and surveys revealing significant numbers of overweights in older age groups has not been resolved. One reviewer pointed out several inherent problems with life insurance statistics: (1) the additional premium charged overweight policyholders limits the number who apply; (2) overweight policyholders may not admit to other existing health problems; and (3) heights and weights recorded on applications are often estimates rather than actual measurements.[27] Although about 90%

of applicants in the Build Study (1979) were weighed and measured, recorded values were not corrected for street clothing and shoes, which vary according to geographical location and season.[69] Heights were evaluated to the nearest inch and weights recorded with the last digit as 0 or 5. Because the incidence of overweight among insurance policyholders is less than that of the general population, the mortality relationships suggested are not necessarily applicable to all groups.

An evaluation of 16 long term studies of men and women in the United States and the United Kingdom found a lack of correlation between body weight, obesity, and mortality.[2] In general, survivors were no less obese than nonsurvivors. In a recent 6-year follow-up of the 12,000 residents of Framingham, Massachusetts,[70] mortality was generally lower among average weights and higher among underweights. Moreover, average weights were actually 20% above "desirable" weights, or those considered to present the lowest risk. In men, age-adjusted mortality was 8.8% among underweights, 4.5% among average weights, and 5.7% and 3.9% in the moderate and marked overweight groups. In women, age-adjusted mortality formed a U-shaped curve with rates of 3.7%, 2.7%, and 4.1% in underweights, average weights, and overweights, respectively.

According to Sorlie and associates,[70] individuals who are losing weight without consciously dieting can have above average mortality. This could reflect diminished appetite or a side effect of disease as men who died over the 6-year period had caloric intakes of 2416 kcal as compared to 2626 kcal among survivors. The ages of the two groups were not given. Neither known debilitating disease nor smoking significantly influenced the higher mortality observed among underweights, although, in general, mortality was increased among smokers in all categories.

Although excessive body weight is associated with chronic diseases that can shorten the life span, it does not exert a similar effect on overall mortality. Andres[2] has speculated that overweight persons, recognizing their increased risk, may seek medical check-ups regularly and make a greater effort toward preventive health. These people may be more likely to stop smoking, for example, although such information is not available. On the other hand, an individual with fat stores could have a better chance of recovery from serious illness.

For whatever reason, there appears to be some advantage to being average or somewhat above average in weight, at least in the absence of chronic problems such as diabetes or hypertension. Several practitioners have questioned the advantage of weight loss in the healthy individual of average weight or only moderate overweight, although those in higher weight categories may benefit.[2,27] Strenuous weight reduction in the healthy individual of average or near average weight appears to be of no benefit, at least in terms of adding years to life.

Cardiovascular Disease and Mortality. Risk of circulatory disorders differs in younger and older age groups. Although coronary artery disease is common in all adult groups, cerebral thrombosis (stroke) and cardiac failure seldom occur before age 60.[31] Smoking does not influence cardiovascular risk after age 65, although risk is reduced by half among those who give up smoking prior to age 65. Age itself, with accompanying cardiovascular changes, is a factor as risk increases sharply with advancing age in the absence of other risk factors. Diabetes and elevated serum cholesterol levels carry less risk at older than younger ages. High density lipoproteins (HDL) are higher in those older persons with decreased incidence of coronary heart disease, whereas elevated low density lipoproteins (LDL) increase risk. General lowering of blood lipid levels, of therapeutic value at younger ages, has little effect at advanced ages.

Elevated blood pressure continues to be a major risk factor for the aged.[31] Even borderline hypertension about doubles the incidence of cardiovascular incidents in men age 65 to 74 (17 versus 33/

1000) and nearly triples the incidence in women of that age (9 versus 22/1000).

Overweight per se does not appear to increase risk of cardiovascular and renal, coronary artery, or cerebrovascular disease past age 65. In a long term evaluation of 3000 urban aged mortality was highest in the leanest group; the most obese had the lowest percent of deaths.[52] One explanation for increased deaths among those lowest in weight could be higher incidence of undiagnosed cancer resulting in weight loss. Nevertheless, excessive obesity did not lead to increased deaths from cardiovascular disorders.

There was a U-shaped association between incidence of cerebrovascular attacks and hemoglobin levels in that urban group.[52] Those with hemoglobin below 12.0 gm/100 ml or above 14.5 gm/100 ml were more likely to have a stroke. Ostfeld[52] suggests that treatment of anemia could lower stroke incidence among persons age 65 and above.

Evaluation of Long-Lived Populations

Actual Life Span. In the last decade attention has been directed toward populations who appear to enjoy exceptionally long lives with a minimum of chronic disease. Three isolated locations thought to have above average numbers of older residents were (1) the village of Vilcabamba located high in the Andes Mountains of Ecuador;[19,37-38] (2) the Hunza, a small territory in the Himalayas of Pakistan;[37-38,76] and (3) the Georgian province in the Caucasus Mountains of the Soviet Union.[37-38] Although the number of centenarians in the United States has been estimated to be about 3 per 100,000, the number in the Caucasus Mountains was believed to be 35 to 65 per 100,000.[37] Early reports from these communities described individuals claiming to be 130 years of age and older.[19,37-38]

Recent survey data from Vilcabamba has revealed that residents systematically exaggerated their ages beginning about age 70.[45] The average age of so-called centenarians was actually 86, and of nonagenarians 82. In general, ages were exaggerated by at least one decade and occasionally by two decades. Although it has been suggested that attention from both scientists and the press encouraged this exaggeration, examination of death records confirms that this was a long-standing practice.[45] Extreme age brings status within that community.

Although critical documentation of records has not been carried out in the other two communities studied, it is likely that age exaggeration also occurs. The fact remains, however, that these communities do have large numbers of individuals of advanced age who remain physically active. Therefore examination of their diet and exercise patterns may provide clues of positive health practices.

Dietary Intake. Several researchers have characterized the dietary patterns of these communities (Table 2-4).[19,37-38,76] The Vilcabambians and Hunzas are primarily vegetarians, whereas the Georgians have a mixed diet, generous in meat and dairy foods. In Vilcabamba the preponderance of calories are obtained from carbohydrates, such as soup prepared from grains and vegetables, including corn, beans, and potatoes.[19,38] Fruits, more plentiful in the summer, include oranges and bananas. Meat is consumed less than once per week[19] and total protein from animal sources is estimated to be about 12 gm daily.[38] What little milk is available is made into cheese. Although adults consume only small amounts of unrefined sugar, they drink two to four cups of homemade rum per day, as well as herbal teas.

Hunza is primarily an agrarian society raising grains such as barley, wheat, and millet; vegetables; fruits; and nuts.[37,76] The rough terrain prohibits the raising of livestock; therefore less than 1% of daily calories comes from meat or dairy foods. Meat, usually mutton, is eaten only once or twice a year as part of a festival celebration. Oil derived from apricot seeds is generally used in cooking. In most years there is not enough food to last through the winter, resulting in a period of semistarvation.

In contrast, food is plentiful among the Georgians. Milk, goat cheese, and yogurt are consumed three times a day and provide the main source of protein, although meat (beef or mutton) is served frequently.[37-38] Use of either butter or vegetable oil depends on the community.[38] Bread is the major carbohydrate food, although corn meal mush is made into patties and dipped in spicy sauces or red pepper. It is believed that the appetite and digestion are improved by hot spices, even in the aged. Beverages consist of sour milk diluted with cold water, tea, and homemade wine (two to three glasses daily with meals).[38]

In general, diets in these communities are low to moderate in calories. Although intakes of protein and saturated fats differ considerably, the primary source of calories for all groups is complex carbohydrates, suggesting a generous intake of fiber.

Physical Activity. A general characteristic of these populations is a high degree of physical activity, continuing into advanced age.[38] In a survey of 27,000 persons above age 80 in the Soviet

Table 2-4. Estimated daily nutrient intake of long-lived populations

	Vilcabambians	Hunzas	Georgians
Calories (kcal)	1200-1700	1900	1700-1900
Total protein (gm)	35-38	50	70-90
Animal protein (gm)	About 12	Minimal	(intake predominately animal)
Fat (gm)	12-19	35	40-60

Data from references 19, 37, 38 and 76.

Union, 60% continued to work after the age of 70, and among those involved in farming, 30% were still working beyond age 80.[15] Physical exercise combined with low to moderate caloric intake appears to prevent weight gain. Aged in Vilcabamba and Hunza are usually slim, although obese are observed occasionally in Georgia.[37]

Among seven aged Vilcabambians, systolic blood pressure ranged from 90 to 160 mm Hg, and diastolic pressure from 50 to 70 mm Hg.[37] Among 25 older Hunzas, the highest systolic pressure equalled 150 mm Hg and blood cholesterol ranged from 150 to 180 mg/100 ml.[76]

Various explanations, including genetic strength, lack of pollution, and cardiovascular adaptation to the altitude, have been suggested as contributing to the physical well-being of these groups.[38] Moderate calorie intake, continued physical activity, and avoidance of weight gain may contribute to normal heart function and low serum lipids. Although a pattern in which unsaturated fats predominate is looked on favorably in this country, the Georgians, with liberal intakes of saturated fat, appear to enjoy a healthy old age. One factor may be the relative intake of fat as, among the Georgians, fat provides less than one third of total calories. The Vilcabambians and Hunzas, on the other hand, appear to adapt to low or moderate levels of protein, primarily vegetable in origin.

Nutrient Intake and Life Span

Longitudinal Dietary Studies. Longitudinal studies, evaluating dietary patterns and subsequent morbidity and mortality, indicate that optimum nutrient intake contributes to both continued good health and survival in middle age and beyond.[16-17,34,65] A study of nearly 600 Californians over 50 years of age, pointed to the importance of consuming recommended levels of vitamins.[16-17] Over a 4-year period, more deaths occurred among those with intakes below the RDA (as defined in 1948) for vitamin A, niacin, and ascorbic acid. Mortality was 14% among those consuming less than 5000 IU

vitamin A per day and 5% among those with at least this amount. Differences in mortality were even greater according to intakes of ascorbic acid (18% of those with intakes below 50 mg as compared to 4% of those consuming 50 mg or above). Age may have influenced these findings, however, as vitamin intakes tend to decrease among the very old. Specific ages of deceased and survivors were not reported. Chope[16] urged that no conclusions be drawn from the study, but that it serve as a basis for further research in nutrient-health relationships.

An association between hematologic values and mortality was observed in a 10-year evaluation of 723 older Britons.[77] Twice as many deaths as expected (20 versus 11) occurred among men with hematocrits above 49. (Acceptable hematocrit levels are 44 and above for males.) Survivors were more likely to have normal serum iron levels; nonsurvivors had low or deficient serum iron. This increase in hematocrit might demonstrate a secondary polycythemia resulting from the tissue hypoxia occurring in advanced heart or lung disease. Increased production of red blood cells could deplete iron stores, leading to lowered serum iron. Normal hemoglobin and serum iron levels were associated with survival in a recent 4-year follow-up of 500 aged attending a congregate meals program.[51]

The relationship of hematologic values and serum iron to mortality very likely involves oxygen transport, although impaired erythropoiesis or protein synthesis may also enter into observations involving poor hemoglobin status (see Chapter 8). As noted earlier, both elevated and depressed hemoglobin levels were associated with increased incidence of cerebral hemorrhage.

Diet quality influenced physical well-being and length of life in a longitudinal study of 100 Michigan women over a 24-year period (1948 to 1972).[34,65] Selected on the basis of geographical sectors to represent a socioeconomic cross-section of older women in a midwestern city, subjects ranged in age from 40 to 85 years. Over a 7-year period, mortality was higher in women consuming diets containing less than 40% of the RDA for one or more nutrients.[34] Nutrients most frequently deficient were calcium, vitamin A, and ascorbic acid. As would be expected, more deaths occurred among those above age 65.

Physical well-being was evaluated using common symptoms of chronic disease. Unexplained tiredness, pain in joints, and shortness of breath were the most common complaints.[34] Complaints were more frequent among those with generally poor diets (intakes of one or more nutrients ≤40% RDA) or deficient intakes of vitamins A and C.

In 1972 (24 years after the first interview) 28 of the women ranging in age from 64 to 90 years were located and reinterviewed.[65] Mean age was 75 years. It was apparent that survivors reduced the quantity but not the quality of food consumed. Calories, fat, and carbohydrate decreased by 25% although mean intakes of protein, vitamins, and minerals (with the exception of calcium) met or exceeded 67% of the RDA.

Calories declined from 1683 to 1297 over the interim, and fat from 74 to 51 gm. Protein intake was 58 and 59 gm, respectively, in 1948 and 1972. Foods high in carbohydrate and fat but providing few other nutrients had been deleted from the diet. Fruits, vegetables, milk products, and bread and cereals were emphasized.

Nutrient intake of survivors at the time of the first survey was compared with those who died sometime between 1948 and 1972.[65] Although the nonsurvivors were older in 1948 (67 versus 52 years), they also had lower intakes of protein (51 versus 58 gm) and ascorbic acid (51 versus 73 mg). Both groups had equal intakes of vegetable protein, but the survivors consumed more animal protein. This difference in intake of animal protein could reflect financial status, as the older women were living on retirement incomes. Increased intakes of ascorbic acid among survivors could relate to income or the food selection patterns of a younger group of women.

Although evidence is limited, there does appear to be a relationship between intake of nutrients, physical well-being, and survival. Adequate intakes of vitamins, in particular, have been associated with continued health in both the Michigan and California surveys. Whether this relates to particular vitamins or is evidence of the overall quality of the diet is not known. The change in food intake observed among the Michigan survivors could provide a model for transition from middle to advanced age.[65] Protein, fat, and carbohydrate provided 18%, 35%, and 47% of calories, respectively. A decrease in calories to prevent weight gain, with continued emphasis on protein, vitamins, and minerals, is an appropriate goal.

Effects of Vitamin Supplementation. Relationships between nutrient intake and survival are especially complicated in aged with severe chronic disease. In a study of 209 hospitalized English aged with deficient leukocyte ascorbic acid levels who were supplemented with 200 mg of ascorbic acid daily, individuals were grouped according to their biochemical response to supplementation (increase or lack of increase in leukocyte ascorbic acid levels).[80] Mortality over 4 weeks was significantly higher among those not responding to the added vitamin (50% versus 11% in men; 28% versus 7% in women). The trend of enhanced survival among responders was still evident after 6 months. Although all nutrients were not evaluated, it is likely that these patients had other deficiencies in addition to ascorbic acid.

The association between poor vitamin status and mortality in the chronically ill may have its basis in the ability of the individual to *absorb* or *metabolize* nutrients effectively. When this is no longer possible, vital biochemical processes deteriorate and survival is threatened regardless of nutrient intake.

Health Practices and Mortality

A longitudinal study of about 7000 adults in Alameda, California, examined the influence of a cluster of health practices—adequate sleep, eating regular meals (including breakfast), desirable body weight, not smoking, limited use of alcohol, and regular physical activity—on mortality.[6,14] After 5 years it was evident that poor health practices resulted in earlier death, whereas good health habits led to longer life. Men who followed six or seven health practices had a life expectancy 11 years longer than men who followed three or less health practices. For women the comparable difference was 7 years. Improvement in life expectancy with positive health habits occurred in both low and high income groups and in persons rated on entry as being in poor or good health. Between ages 65 and 74, mortality rates were more than doubled among those following zero to three as compared to six good health habits. Because this effect continued over a period of 9 years, it cannot be attributed to the earlier death of those in poor health when the study began.[14] Positive health practices appear to have an additive effect in contributing to physical well-being.[53]

Poor health itself, however, may hinder the practice of positive health habits.[53] Increasing physical disability can interfere with meal preparation or reduce physical activity leading to weight gain. Breslow[13] emphasized the need to identify personal habits as risk factors and develop community education programs for successful intervention. Improvement in health practices has a positive effect even among those in poor health status at the time, preventing further decline and possibly bettering the situation. Nutrition education should be an integral part of such a program.

Need for Continued Research

Although optimum nutrient intake, regular physical activity, and weight control appear to extend physical well-being and delay physiologic deterioration, the mechanisms by which this is accomplished are not understood. Furthermore, the literature on which these conclusions are based is fragmentary, involving only small numbers of persons observed over short periods of time. When longitudinal studies were extended for several decades, data were collected at sporadic intervals making it impossible to construct the food pattern of an individual on a year-to-year basis.

Howell and Loeb[30] consider the evaluation of the lifelong food intake of individuals in relation to their physical health in later years to be essential. Such a study should begin in infancy, as animal work suggests that food habits early in life influence biochemical processes, development of chronic disease, and ultimate life span. Obviously, such an evaluation is a mammoth undertaking from the standpoint of funding and organization required.

A starting point could be expansion of the nutritional component of longitudinal studies now being carried on by the Gerontology Research Center of the National Institute on Aging and the Duke University Gerontology Center. Although these programs have focused on the stages of life beyond adolescence, younger individuals might be added to the ongoing age cohorts. Only by such a strategy will we learn what diet patterns are necessary at one stage to ensure optimal health at a later stage in the life cycle.

SUMMARY

Both qualitative and quantitative aspects of the diet influence physical well-being and length of life. A nutritionally adequate diet, restricted only in calories, increases the life span and delays the appearance of degenerative disease in experimental animals. Biochemical changes at the cellular level delayed by food restriction include loss of neural receptors and normal immune response, as well as increases in serum lipid levels. Diets high in fat significantly decrease the life span; toxic contaminants, alterations in metabolic efficiency, and increased body weight may contribute to this effect.

High protein and calorie intakes throughout life lead to rapid growth, exaggerated displacement of enzyme levels, and rapid deterioration and death in animal models. Limiting protein and calories following maturity results in a significant extension of life and has application to human populations.

Evaluation of human populations based on life insurance statistics suggests that body weight above average is detrimental to health. This conclusion is controversial as others have found that extreme underweight significantly increases mortality; average or somewhat above average weight is most favorable for life expectancy. Many overweight individuals do survive to advanced ages.

Although longitudinal studies of humans have been limited, evidence suggests that individuals consuming recommended levels of nutrients, including vitamins, have reduced mortality and incidence of chronic complaints. A reduction in calories, carbohydrates, and fat between middle and old age, with emphasis on foods high in nutrient density, was observed among healthy older women. Positive health habits such as regular meals and exercise, maintaining an appropriate weight, and avoidance of smoking improve life expectancy.

REVIEW QUESTIONS

1. How does caloric restriction influence (a) life span, (b) incidence of degenerative disease, and (c) biochemical measurements in animal models? Discuss possible mechanisms by which changes may occur.
2. What are potential benefits of caloric restriction after growth is complete? What cautions are necessary?
3. How are rate of growth, weight gain, and life span related? Discuss the implications for diet and preferred growth patterns of children.
4. What evidence exists to suggest that body weight above average shortens life? What evidence exists to refute this presumption? Would you advise weight loss for a healthy aged client who has been overweight throughout adult life? Justify your decision.
5. Using available evidence from both animal studies and evaluations of human populations, develop recommendations for dietary intake and health patterns in both middle and advanced age to achieve optimum health and longevity.

REFERENCES

1. Abraham, S., Collins, G., and Nordsieck, M.: Relationship of childhood weight status to morbidity in adults, Public Health Rep. **86:**273, 1971.
2. Andres, R.: Effect of obesity on total mortality, Int. J. Obes. **4:**381, 1980.
3. Baird, I.M., and others: Prevalence of obesity in a London borough, Practitioner **212:**706, 1974.
4. Beeuwkes, A.M.: Early speculations on diet and longevity. 1, J. Am. Diet. Assoc. **28:**628, 1952.
5. Beeuwkes, A.M.: Early speculations on diet and longevity. 2, J. Am. Diet. Assoc. **28:**707, 1952.
6. Belloc, N.: Relationship of health practices and mortality, Prev. Med. **2:**67, 1973.
7. Benson-Cooper, D., and others: Obesity in a New Zealand community, N.Z. Med. J. **82:**115, 1975.
8. Berg, B.N.: Nutrition and longevity in the rat. 1. Food intake in relation to size, health and fertility, J. Nutr. **71:**242, 1960.
9. Berg, B.N., and Simms, H.S.: Nutrition and longevity in the rat. 2. Longevity and onset of disease with different levels of food intake, J. Nutr. **71:**255, 1960.
10. Bertrand, H.A., and others: Changes in adipose mass and cellularity through the adult life of rats fed ad libitum or a life-prolonging restricted diet, J. Gerontol. **35:**827, 1980.
11. Blackburn, H., and Parlin, R.W.: Antecedents of disease. Insurance mortality experience, Ann. N.Y. Acad. Sci. **134:**965, 1966.
12. Blackett, A.D., and Hall, D.A.: The effects of vitamin E on mouse fitness and survival, Gerontology **27:**133, 1981.
13. Breslow, L.: Prospects for improving health through reducing risk factors, Prev. Med. **7:**449, 1978.
14. Breslow, L., and Enstrom, J.E.: Persistence of health habits and their relationship to mortality, Prev. Med. **9:**469, 1980.
15. Chebotaryov, D.F., and Sachuk, N.N.: Sociomedical examination of longevous people in the U.S.S.R., J. Gerontol. **19:**435, 1964.
16. Chope, H.D.: Relation of nutrition to health in aging persons. A four-year follow-up of a study in San Mateo County, California Med. **81:**335, 1954.
17. Chope, H.D., and Dray, S.: The nutritional status of the aging: Public health aspects, California Med. **74:**105, 1951.
18. Cornaro, L.: How to live one hundred years: The famous treatise written four hundred years ago on health and longevity, Surrey, England, 1951, Health For All Publishing Co.
19. Davies, D.: A Shangri-la in Ecuador, New Scient. **57:**236, 1973.
20. Drenick, E.J., and others: Excessive mortality and causes of death in morbidly obese men, JAMA **243:**443, 1980.
21. Ederer, F. and others: Cancer among men on cholesterol-lowering diets: Experience from five clinical trials, Lancet **2:**203, 1971.
22. Eklund, J., and Bradford, G.E.: Longevity and lifetime body weight in mice selected for rapid growth, Nature **265:**48, 1977.

23. Fernandes, G., Yunis, E.J., and Good, R.A.: Influence of diet on survival of mice, Proc. Natl. Acad. Sci. USA **73**:1279, 1976.

24. Food and Nutrition Board: Recommended dietary allowances, ed. 9, Washington, D.C., 1980, National Academy of Sciences.

25. Goodrick, C.L.: Body weight change over the life span and longevity for C57BL/6J mice and mutations which differ in maximal body weight, Gerontology **23**:405, 1977.

26. Goodrick, C.L.: Effects of long-term voluntary wheel exercise on male and female Wistar rats. 1. Longevity, body weight, and metabolic rate, Gerontology **26**:22, 1980.

27. Gunby, P.: A little (body) fat may not hasten death, JAMA **244**:1660, 1980.

28. Harmon, D.: Free radical theory of aging: Dietary implications, Am. J. Clin. Nutr. **25**:839, 1972.

29. Hollifield, G., and Parson, W.: Overweight in the aged, Am. J. Clin. Nutr. **7**:127, 1959.

30. Howell, S.C., and Loeb, M.B.: Nutrition and aging: A monograph for practitioners, Gerontologist **9**(suppl.):1, 1969.

31. Kannel, W.B., and Gordon, T.: Cardiovascular risk factors in the aged: The Framingham study. In Haynes, S., and Feinleib, M., eds.: Epidemiology of aging, DHHS Publication No. (NIH) No. 80-969, Bethesda, 1980, U.S. Government Printing Office.

32. Kaunitz, H., Johnson, R.E., and Pegus, L.: Longer survival time of rats fed oxidized vegetable oils, Proc. Soc. Exp. Biol. Med. **123**:204, 1966.

33. Kaunitz, H., Johnson, R.E., and Pegus, L.: Differences in effects of dietary fats on survival rate and development of neoplastic and other diseases in rats, Z. Ernaehrungswiss **10**:61, 1970.

34. Kelley, L., Ohlson, M.A., and Harper, L.J.: Food selection and well-being of aging women, J. Am. Diet. Assoc. **33**:466, 1957.

35. Keys, A.: W.O. Atwater memorial lecture: Overweight, obesity, coronary heart disease and mortality, Nutr. Rev. **38**:297, 1980.

36. Kohn, R.R.: Effect of antioxidants on life-span of C57BL mice, J. Gerontol. **26**:378, 1971.

37. Leaf, A.: Unusual longevity: The common denominators, Hosp. Prac. **8**(10):75, 1973.

38. Leaf, A.: Youth in old age, New York, 1975, McGraw-Hill Book Co.

39. Levin, P., and others: Dietary restriction retards the age-associated loss of rat striatal dopaminergic receptors, Science **214**:561, 1981.

40. Lew, E.A., and Garfinkel, L.: Variations in mortality by weight among 750,000 men and women, J. Chronic Dis. **32**:563, 1979.

41. Liepa, G.U., and others: Food restriction as a modulator of age-related changes in serum lipids, Am. J. Physiol. **238**:E253, 1980.

42. Mann, G.V.: The influence of obesity on health, N. Engl. J. Med. **291**:178, 1974.

43. Masoro, E.J., Yu, B.P., and Bertrand, H.A.: Action of food restriction in delaying the aging process, Proc. Natl. Acad. Sci. USA **79**:4239, 1982.

44. Masoro, E.J., and others: Nutritional probe of the aging process, Fed. Proc. **39**:3178, 1980.

45. Mazess, R.B., and Forman, S.H.: Longevity and age exaggeration in Vilcabamba, Ecuador, J. Gerontol. **34**:94, 1979.

46. McCarter, R.J., Masoro, E.J., and Yu, B.P.: Rat muscle structure and metabolism in relation to age and food intake, Am. J. Physiol. **242**:R89, 1982.

47. McCay, C.M., and others: Retarded growth, life span, ultimate body size and age changes in the albino rat after feeding diets restricted in calories, J. Nutr. **18**:1, 1939.

48. Metchnikoff, E.: The prolongation of life, English translation, Mitchell, P.C., ed., New York, 1977, Arno Press.

49. Newberne, P.M.: Dietary fat, immunological response, and cancer in rats, Cancer Res. **41**:3783, 1981.

50. Nigro, N.D.: Animal studies implicating fat and fecal steroids in intestinal cancer, Cancer Res. **41**:3769, 1981.

51. Nordstrom, J.W.: Trace mineral nutrition in the elderly, Am. J. Clin. Nutr. **36**(suppl.):788, 1982.

52. Ostfeld, A.: Nutrition and aging. In Ostfeld, A.M., and Gibson, D.C., eds.: Epidemiology of aging, DHEW Publication No. (NIH) 75-711, Bethesda, Md., 1975, U.S. Dept. of Health, Education and Welfare.

53. Palmore, E.: Health practices and illness among the aged, Gerontologist **10**:313, 1970.

54. Pearce, M.L., and Dayton, S.: Incidence of cancer in men on a diet high in polyunsaturated fat, Lancet **1**:464, 1971.

55. Pomeranze, J.: Obesity as a health factor in geriatric patients, Geriatrics **12**:481, 1957.

56. Ross, M.H.: Length of life and nutrition in the rat, J. Nutr. **75**:197, 1961.

57. Ross, M.H.: Aging, nutrition and hepatic enzyme activity patterns in the rat, J. Nutr. **97**(suppl.):565, 1969.

58. Ross, M.H.: Life expectancy modification by change in dietary regimen of the mature rat, Proceedings of the Seventh International Congress of Nutrition, Vol. 5, Braunschweig, West Germany, 1966, Verlag Friedr. Vieweg & Sohn.

59. Ross, M.H.: Length of life and caloric intake, Am. J. Clin. Nutr. **25**:834, 1972.

60. Ross, M.H., and Bras, G.: Lasting influence of early caloric restriction on prevalence of neoplasms in the rat, J. Natl. Cancer Inst. **47**:1095, 1971.

61. Ross, M.H., and Bras, G.: Food preference and length of life, Science **190**:165, 1975.

62. Ross, M.H., Bras, G., and Lustbader, E.: Dietary practices and growth responses as predictors of longevity, Nature **262**:548, 1976.

63. Sacher, G.A.: Life table modification and life prolongation. In Finch, C.E., and Hayflick, L., eds.: Handbook of the biology of aging, New York, 1977, Van Nostrand Reinhold Co., Inc.

64. Schemmel, R., Mickelsen, O., and Motawi, K.: Conversion of dietary to body energy in rats as affected by strain, sex and ration, J. Nutr. **102**:1187, 1972.

65. Schlenker, E.D.: Nutritional status of older women, Ph. D. thesis, Michigan State University, East Lansing, 1976.

66. Silberberg, M., and Silberberg, R.: Factors modifying the life-span of mice, Am. J. Physiol. **177**:23, 1954.

67. Skillman, T.G., Hamwi, G.J., and May, C.: Nutrition in the aged, Geriatrics **15**:464, 1960.

68. Society of Actuaries: Build and blood pressure study, vol. 1, Chicago, 1959, Society of Actuaries.

69. Society of Actuaries: Build study, 1979, Chicago, 1980, Society of Actuaries.

70. Sorlie, P., Gordon, T., and Kannel, W.B.: Body build and mortality: The Framingham study, JAMA **243**:1828, 1980.

71. Stini, W.A.: Association of early growth patterns with the process of aging, Fed. Proc. **40**:2588, 1981.

72. Stuchlikova, E., Juricova-Horakova, M., and Deyl, Z.: New aspects of the dietary effect of life prolongation in rodents: What is the role of obesity in aging? Exp. Gerontol. **10**:141, 1975.

73. Swanson, P.: Adequacy in old age. 1. Role of nutrition, J. Home Econ. **56**:651, 1964.

74. Tappel, A.L., and Dillard, C.J.: In vivo lipid peroxidation: Measurement via exhaled pentane and protection by vitamin E, Fed. Proc. **40**:174, 1981.

75. Tappel, A., Fletcher, B., and Deamer, D.: Effect of antioxidants and nutrients on lipid peroxidation fluorescent products and aging parameters in the mouse, J. Gerontol. **28**:415, 1973.

76. Toomey, E.G., and White, P.D.: A brief survey of the health of aged Hunzas, Am. Heart J. **68**:841, 1964.

77. Waters, W.E., and others: Ten-year haematological follow-up: Mortality and haematological changes, Br. Med. J. **4**:761, 1969.

78. Watkin, D.M.: The physiology of aging, Am. J. Clin. Nutr. **36**(suppl.):750, 1982.

79. Weindruch, R.H., and others: Influence of controlled dietary restriction on immunologic function and aging, Fed. Proc. **38**:2007, 1979.

80. Wilson, T.S., and others: Relation of vitamin C levels to mortality in a geriatric hospital: A study of the effect of vitamin C administration, Age Ageing **2**:163, 1973.

81. Yu, B.P., and others: Life span study of SPF Fischer 344 male rats fed ad libitum or restricted diets: Longevity, growth, lean body mass and disease, J. Gerontol. **37**:130, 1982.

82. Zeman, F.D.: Fundamental considerations, old and new, in nutrition of the elderly, Fed. Proc. **11**:794, 1952.

Chapter 3

Body Composition, Calories, and Physical Activity

According to Hippocrates,[52] the constituents of the human body were blood, yellow bile, black bile, and phlegm. Although the biochemical compartments of the body have been identified, the relative proportion of particular tissues is still of concern. Body fat increases gradually throughout adult life at the expense of lean tissue; even in the absence of weight gain, the older individual is relatively obese. Whether this process is a natural consequence of aging or results from a sedentary life-style and excessive calorie intake is still a matter of controversy. Age-related changes in body composition contribute to a decrease in caloric requirements. Energy balance in the older individual is usually complicated further by a decline in physical activity. These relationships are important clinically in helping the older individual achieve weight control.

BODY COMPARTMENTS

Definitions

The body is composed of muscle, organs, skeleton, fat, and fluid. On a biochemical basis these compartments are classified as (1) water, (2) lean body mass, (3) fat, and (4) mineral.[13,51] Precise definition is difficult as compartments overlap. Both the absolute and relative sizes of body compartments are influenced by the aging process as well as pathologic conditions.

Total Body Water (TBW). On a weight basis water is the most abundant constituent in the body, comprising about 60% of body weight in young adult males.[34] Water is both intracellular (55% TBW) and extracellular (45% TBW).[65] Extracellular water consists of plasma, lymph, and the interstitial fluid bathing the cells. Muscle and organ cells are about 72% water, adipose cells only 15% to 22%.[40,52] Body water decreases in men from about 60% to 50% of body weight between ages 20 and 60,[65] as intracellular water is lost.[4,89] Body water can increase proportionately as a result of cardiac failure or sodium retention, with elevated plasma and tissue fluid.[65] Generalized edema or fluid retention in the lower extremities is sometimes observed in the older person with hypertension and heart disease. Sodium is the primary extracellular and potassium the primary intracellular cation. Eighty-five percent of body sodium is found in the extracellular compartment; 98% of body potassium is in the cell.[71]

Lean Body Mass. Muscle, organs, and skeleton comprise the lean body mass, about 80% of body weight.[71] Biochemical constituents include water, cell protein, minerals, and "essential" fat. The percentage of fat is very low (2%-3%) including only structural fatty acids found in the brain, nervous system, and cell membranes.[6] *Fat-free body* is a term used to describe lean body mass with essential fat tissue removed. A basic characteristic of the lean tissue is the high potassium content (68.1 mEq/kg), often used to quantify the size of this compartment.[31-33] Lean body mass is about 73% water.

Mineral and Ash. This compartment includes both bone mineral and the electrolytes distributed throughout the intracellular and extracellular fluids. Approximately 85% of body mineral is found in the skeleton.[72]

Body Fat. Body fat is found primarily in the adipose tissue although, as noted previously, a small percentage exists in the lean tissues. Although body fat comprises about 14% of the reference male, this compartment is unlimited in size.[37] Ingested calories above those required to meet energy needs will be stored as body fat.[52]

Body compartments are constantly subject to change as a result of internal (i.e., maturation, aging) or external (i.e., calorie intake, physical exercise) influences.[13] A shift in the size of one compartment will consequently bring about changes in another.[65] Total body water will be altered according to the proportion of lean body mass versus body fat. Since adipose tissue contains less water, an increase in fat at the expense of lean tissue will decrease total body water. These relationships are useful in developing methods for determining body composition in both health and disease.

METHODS OF DETERMINING BODY COMPOSITION

Early researchers studied body composition by analyzing human cadavers for water, fat, nitrogen, and specific minerals.[30] Highly specialized methods have since been developed to evaluate body composition as a function of age, sex, or level of nutrition.[5,32,65,68] Unfortunately, methods are based on assumptions regarding fluid-electrolyte relationships, which although constant in young healthy individuals may differ in older persons as a result of normal aging or chronic disease. Methods based on physical measurements do not always take into account the age-related movement of body fat from one location to another, nor may external dimensions accurately reflect internal changes in tissue

composition. Methods to assess body composition that are reasonably accurate, inexpensive, and non-invasive are urgently needed for evaluation of older persons. Those now used for research or assessment of clients all have serious limitations with older populations.

Isotope Dilution Method

Stable isotope tracers such as K^{42}, Br^{82}, Na^{24}, tritium (H^3), and O^{18} administered intravenously and allowed to reach equilibrium with existing ions can, by a series of equations, provide an estimate of total body water.[65,83] Because body water is assumed to be a constant proportion (73%) of lean body mass, the weight of body water has been used to calculate the relative size of body compartments.[65] However, Garrow[40] pointed out that fat-free tissues vary in water content. Although fat-free lean tissue is considered to be 73% water, adipose tissue when all fat is removed is 88% water. Therefore as body fat and adipose tissue increase, the water content of fat-free tissue (which includes the fat-free adipose tissue) also increases. If the water content of fat-free tissue is assumed to remain constant, the percent of body fat is underestimated. This is especially pertinent to the evaluation of older individuals who in comparison to younger people have greater adipose tissue. Another problem with isotope dilution methods is general fluid balance, because older people with clinical disease can retain both water and sodium.[104]

Whole Body Counting

The naturally occurring potassium in the body contains a known percentage (0.012%) of the radioactive isotope K^{40}.[30-31] Therefore whole body scintillation counters measuring radioactivity have been used to evaluate body composition. It is assumed that the potassium content of the lean body is constant (68.1 mEq/kg) and closely proportional to total body water[32]; however, the potassium level in lean body mass varies on the basis of both age and type of tissue. Potassium concentration is highest in muscle (134 mEq/kg), somewhat lower in heart and kidney (70 to 80 mEq/kg), and lowest in skin and connective tissue (34 mEq/kg).[104] This has important implications when using potassium concentration as an indicator of lean body mass. The aging process results in loss of muscle and an increase in connective tissues. Since the relative sizes of muscle and organ tissues cannot be estimated, calculations based upon usual assumptions can lead to overestimation of body fat.[31,33,68] Lye[55] reported the whole body potassium content of older persons to be about 10% lower than expected based on height and weight.

Increased body fat in older people can also lead to inaccuracies in whole body counting; body fat absorbs radiation rays, decreasing the potassium count and underestimating lean body mass (overestimating body fat). Garrow[40] suggests using both total body water and body potassium methods, as the errors in opposite directions (underestimate versus overestimate of body fat), when combined, may provide a more reliable value.

Density Measurement

Using the principle of Archimedes, body density can be determined by weighing the individual first in air and then completely submerged in water, obtaining an estimate of water displacement.[51-52,106,108-109] Keys[51] established that the specific gravity of body fat (0.9 gm/cc) differs from lean tissue (1.1 gm/cc), which is higher in water content. Therefore a series of equations were developed for computing percentage of body fat. Such calculations, however, assume reference values for body water, influenced by a variety of clinical conditions, and for bone mineral, known to decrease with advancing age. Although providing a reasonable estimate of body compartments, underwater weighing requires specialized equipment and is impractical with frail older persons. A recent modification of this method eliminates the need for complete submersion of the subject.[40]

Excretion of Muscle Metabolites

Both 3-methylhistidine[104] (see Chapter 5) and creatinine,[63] products of muscle metabolism, have been used to estimate lean body mass. Urinary creatinine, derived from creatine phosphate, is a valid index of lean body mass in young adults using height as a standard for body size; however, the creatinine height index (CHI),[63] used to identify protein-calorie malnutrition, appears to be of limited usefulness in identifying malnourished older people, particularly women. Both older well-fed controls and patients with severe protein-calorie malnutrition had creatinine excretion values suggesting below average levels of lean body mass. Age-related changes in height and alterations in kidney function influence this measurement. Furthermore, most older people regardless of nutritional status have decreased muscle mass as compared to younger people of similar age, sex, and body build. Substitution of arm length for height offers potential for refinement of this tool.

Excretion of 3-methylhistidine, a product of muscle catabolism, has been verified as a valid estimate of muscle mass using animal models. This compound has also been used successfully under research conditions for estimating lean body mass in humans.

Both methods, however, require considerable cooperation on the part of the client, who should avoid eating meat for 2 days prior to the evaluation period and be willing to assume the inconvenience of a 24-hour urine collection.[40] Although this may be accomplished with hospitalized or institutionalized individuals, it is not generally possible in large surveys.

Body Electrical Conductivity

Lean body tissue is a better conductor of electrical current than adipose tissue.[46] Instruments based on this principle are currently used for evaluating the leanness/fatness of meat samples.[46,104] Although still in the developmental stage, this method holds considerable promise for use with older clients, as it requires little time (a few seconds for actual measurement after the individual has been positioned) and the person need not disrobe. The initial cost of such a device will influence the extent of use.

Although dilution, density, and whole body counting methods provide reasonable estimates of body fat, they require sophisticated equipment, highly trained personnel, and extensive cooperation by the subject. These methods have provided information regarding age-related changes in body composition and are useful for validation of more simple methods to be used with clients or in large-scale nutrition surveys.[13,30,71]

Anthropometric Measurements

Body measurements to evaluate relative leanness or obesity are usually included in physical examinations and nutrition assessments; body weight, height, circumferences, and skinfold thicknesses are most commonly used (see Chapter 10). Unfortunately, these measurements, although simple and inexpensive to perform, have limited value for estimating body fatness.[60,84-86]

Body Weight. Measurement of body weight is one of the least reliable methods of estimating body fat, even when corrected for height, sex, and age.[54] Desirable or relative weights, often used as standards of evaluation, were developed by life insurance companies based on the mortality experience of policyholders. The limitations of these standards were discussed in Chapter 2. Because body weights are not normally distributed about the mean but skew to the right (more persons are heavier in weight), the average weight is usually above the median weight of the population.[95,103]

The greatest error associated with body weight measurements is oversimplification of the obesity question.[84-86] Although excessive fatness is inferred when an individual is overweight, the extra weight could represent bone, fluid, muscle, or a combination of these. Nevertheless, the two terms are related as an obese individual will very likely be overweight; the overweight person, however, may not be obese. All aged are somewhat obese relative to younger individuals of similar height and weight. Fluid retention or dehydration will result in significant fluctuations in body weight. (Two cups of water equal 1 pound.)

Body build, or proportion of muscle to fat, differs among older individuals as well as between older and younger individuals. The aged man who engaged in hard physical labor prior to retirement differs in body composition from the retired executive who sat most of his working day.[60,84-85] Seltzer and coworkers[21,86] evaluated relative body weight and obesity (determined by skinfold thickness) in over 1700 healthy men age 25 to 64 years. Of those 15% above average weight (relative weight = 115) only one third were obese. Among men 25% above average weight, about half were obese. In those overweight men who were not obese, overweight consisted of large body frame (skeletal mass) and heavy muscular development.

The reliability of height-weight measurements in assessing relative fatness is strengthened by use of the body mass index of weight/height^2, originally developed by Quetelet. Any index of relative weight should be equally reliable with tall or short individuals and provide a reasonable estimate of body fat. According to Keys and coworkers[54] the body mass index has a stronger correlation with body density and K^{40} measurements and thus provides a better estimate of body fat than relative weight derived from height-weight tables.[54] Unfortunately, there are at present no body mass index standards developed for evaluation of people above age 60.

Skinfold Thickness. About half of all body fat is subcutaneous, lying directly under the skin.[85] Standard methods of measurement have been developed using Lange skinfold calipers at constant pressure (10 gm/mm^2).[15] Estimations of body fat based on skinfold measurements at various anatomical sites compare favorably with values obtained by body density, K[40], and dilution techniques, although these conclusions were based on work with young adults.[106] Estimations of body fat based on several skinfold measurements are more closely related to density measurements than those based on a single skinfold thickness.[26,66] Skinfold thicknesses provide better estimates of total body fat in women than men and in younger versus older men.[106]

Skinfold Measurements. The most common skinfold measurements are the triceps and biceps (upper arm), subscapular (upper back), and abdomen. The triceps skinfold is most widely used since the individual does not have to disrobe. The circumference of the upper arm should be measured at the same location as the skinfold thickness to allow calculation of total arm muscle area (cm^2) and total fat area (cm^2). A nomogram for the rapid calculation of these areas is given in Fig. 3-1.[44] Although cross-sectional fat areas do not provide a better estimate of the relative proportion or percentage of body fat than does the corresponding skinfold thickness, they are more appropriate for estimating the absolute amount of body fat.[48] Although triceps skinfold thicknesses may be equal, more fat would be required to cover a large arm circumference than a small arm circumference.[36] Therefore fat areas provide a better estimate of total fat than skinfold thickness alone. Evaluating corresponding arm muscle area provides an indication of protein status as well.

Calculation of upper arm fat and muscle areas has been proposed as a simple yet effective method to determine severe protein-calorie malnutrition or excessive body fatness in routine nutritional evaluation.[36] For an individual with paralysis or atrophy on one side of the body, the opposite arm can be measured. Roche[76] pointed out the usefulness of arm measurements with edematous individuals for whom body weight is not a valid measure of nutritional state. Skinfold thickness and circumference measurements of the thigh or calf might also be investigated as alternative sites for estimation of body fat and muscle.[76]

Limitations of Skinfold Measurements. The triceps skinfold provides an acceptable estimate of obesity in younger persons but is less reliable in older persons.[85] Although subcutaneous fat is proportional to total body fat in younger groups, fat changes location as a function of age. Body fat moves in a centripetal direction, from the limbs to the trunk, as a person grows older.[94] Less fat is deposited in subcutaneous locations with a corresponding increase in internal fat.[94]

Work with healthy women, age 20 to 69, revealed that all skinfold measurements decrease after age 64.[107] Equations that estimate percentage of body fat based on the triceps skinfold thickness alone can be misleading when used with older adults. A healthy woman age 74 and free from edema, weighing 197 pounds (standard weight = 144), was found on the basis of such a calculation to be 27% fat[82]; women of standard weight and similar age are reported to be about 45% fat.[109]

Body circumference provides a more reliable estimate of fatness in older individuals. Among 62 healthy women the abdominal circumference at the umbilicus was highly correlated (r = 0.717) with body density (determined by underwater weighing).[108-109] Circumference or envelope measurements may be an alternative for assessing body fat in research or clinical situations. Unfortunately, circumference measurements of the body trunk requiring the individual to disrobe are not applicable

Fig. 3-1. Nomogram for calculation of upper arm fat and muscle areas. (From Gurney, J.M., and Jelliffe, D.B.: Arm anthropometry in nutritional assessment: Nomogram for rapid calculation of muscle circumference and cross sectional muscle and fat areas, Am. J. Clin. Nutr. **26**:912, 1973.)

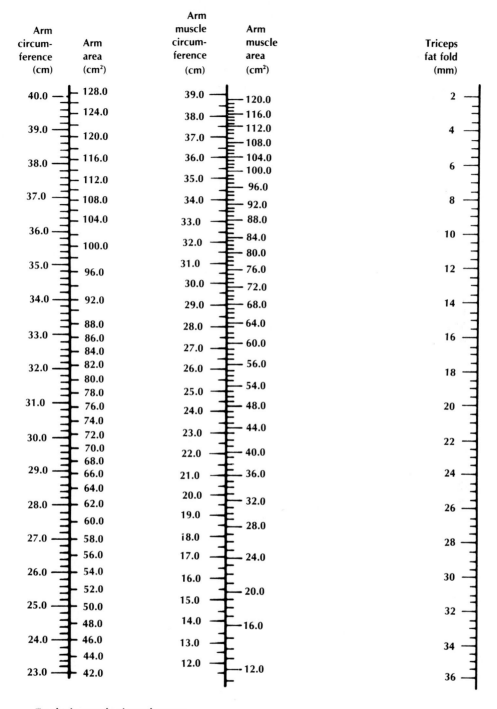

Arm circumference (cm)	Arm area (cm²)	Arm muscle circumference (cm)	Arm muscle area (cm²)	Triceps fat fold (mm)
40.0	128.0	39.0	120.0	2
	124.0	38.0	116.0	
39.0	120.0	37.0	112.0	4
			108.0	
38.0	116.0	36.0	104.0	
	112.0	35.0	100.0	6
			96.0	
37.0	108.0	34.0	92.0	8
	104.0	33.0	88.0	
36.0		32.0	84.0	10
	100.0		80.0	
35.0	96.0	31.0	76.0	12
		30.0	72.0	
34.0	92.0	29.0	68.0	14
	88.0	28.0	64.0	
33.0	86.0			16
	84.0	27.0	60.0	
32.0	82.0	26.0	56.0	18
	80.0			
	78.0	25.0	54.0	
31.0	76.0	24.0	48.0	20
	74.0			
30.0	72.0	23.0	44.0	22
	70.0	22.0	40.0	
	68.0			
29.0	66.0	21.0	36.0	24
	64.0	20.0		
28.0	62.0		32.0	26
	60.0	19.0	28.0	
27.0	58.0	i8.0		28
	56.0	17.0	24.0	
26.0	54.0	16.0		30
	52.0		20.0	
25.0	50.0	15.0		32
	48.0	14.0	16.0	
24.0	46.0	13.0		34
	44.0	12.0		
23.0	42.0		12.0	36

To obtain muscle circumference:
    1. Lay ruler between value of arm circumference and fatfold
    2. Read off muscle circumference on middle line
To obtain tissue areas:
    1. The arm area and muscle area are alongside their respective circumferences
    2. Fat area = arm area − muscle area

Fig. 3-1. For legend see opposite page.

to large scale surveys with limited personnel and facilities, nor have appropriate standards been developed.

The exact location of the skinfold measurement can influence the results obtained.[80] The triceps skinfold is taken at the midpoint between the elbow and acromion tip. Among middle-aged and older men, the triceps skinfold thickness was significantly different 1 inch above and below the midpoint as compared to the thickness at the midpoint.[15] Although general patterns of fat distribution are influenced by sex, age, and nutritional status, relative patterns are a highly individual characteristic. Body fat is not gained or lost equally at all locations on the limbs or trunk.[27,39]

Methods and values for skinfold thicknesses have been standardized using the Lange caliper, which is highly accurate but relatively expensive. A lightweight, inexpensive plastic caliper is now available to health care professionals. When readings of triceps skinfolds obtained with both the Lange and plastic McGaw calipers were compared, the Lange readings were found to be significantly greater.[16] Moreover, the differences between the two readings increased as skinfold thickness increased. Because the maximum scale of the plastic caliper is 40 mm, it is not applicable for use with the extremely obese (relative weight ≥ 150). Although readings from both instruments are highly correlated ($r = 0.97$), individual readings will be lower with the plastic caliper, particularly in fatter individuals. Plastic calipers can provide an approximation of skinfold thickness; however, values obtained cannot be compared with standards derived using a Lange instrument.

Skinfolds change in compressibility as a person ages.[15] Adipose tissue is less compressible in older individuals, leading to higher values in both skinfold thickness and calculated fat area. Decreased compressibility can result from reduced elasticity of skin with increased connective tissue[15] or edema.[27] People who have repeatedly gained and lost weight appear to have increased tissue fluid reten-

tion.[27] Although there are no sex differences in compressibility, there are differences between individuals and between different sites on the same individual.[47] Although there is no way at present to correct for individual differences, it is suggested that this factor be considered when evaluating skinfold measurements.[76]

Standards for Evaluation. Evaluation and interpretation of body measurements usually involves comparing those obtained from the client to a set of standard or reference values. Standards representing ideal values are usually derived from work with younger people and are not always appropriate for older individuals. Measurements of older people should be compared with reference values from

Table 3-1. Desirable body weights for adults

Height* (in)	Weight† (lb)
Men	
62	123 (112-141)
64	130 (118-148)
66	136 (124-156)
68	145 (132-166)
70	153 (140-174)
72	162 (148-184)
74	171 (156-194)
Women	
58	102 (92-119)
60	107 (96-125)
62	113 (102-131)
64	120 (108-138)
66	128 (114-146)
68	136 (122-154)
70	144 (130-163)

*Height measured without shoes.

†Weight measured without clothes.

Modified from Bray, G.A.: Obesity in perspective, vol. 2, Part 1, DHEW Publication No. (NIH) 75-708, Bethesda, Md., 1975, U.S. Government Printing Office.

people of similar age, as distribution of both fat and muscle differs in younger groups.[9,35-36] Because of the limited information available, reference values are usually actual measurements obtained from an older population and may not represent the ideal. The mere survival of these individuals, however, suggests that such values represent normal ranges.

According to the National Research Council, body weight should not increase throughout adult life.[29] Desirable weights for adults of all ages derived from life insurance statistics are given in Table 3-1. A factor limiting the usefulness of these standards is loss of height among older people.[76] Ideally, weight should be based on known height at younger ages, which may not be available. Actual height measurement is difficult in the older person with poor posture or curvature of the spine. Vertebral compression of the spine related to osteoporosis (see Chapter 8) causes age-related losses in height. The loss in stature occurring throughout adulthood has been estimated to be as much as 3 cm (about 1⅜ in). This difference will significantly influence the reference value for desirable weight.[76]

Body weight can also be evaluated on the basis of measurements obtained from participants age 65 to 74 in the Health and Nutrition Examination Survey (HANES), 1971-1974 (Table 3-2). Because these are actual measurements and not derived norms, body weights may decrease slightly from one height to another or remain unchanged. Expressing body weight on the basis of percentile identifies the relative status of the individual as compared to his peer group. Persons in the extreme upper and lower percentiles require further nutritional evaluation.

Age-specific values for upper arm fat and muscle areas have been derived from HANES data (Table 3-3). These norms are appropriately used to evaluate individuals in relation to their peers, not to compare age groups or describe age-related changes in arm fat or muscle areas.[9] Gray and Gray[41] propose that individuals in the lowest percentiles be examined for protein-calorie malnutri-

Table 3-2. Body weight* in pounds of persons age 65 to 74

Height† (in)	Percentile		
	10th	50th	90th
Women			
57	105	133	167
58	105	130	180
59	104	131	179
60	107	136	178
61	112	140	177
62	115	142	183
63	120	144	183
64	121	150	183
65	122	150	189
66	140	147	208
67	145	168	220
68	138	171	190
Men			
62	124	148	172
63	121	144	177
64	121	148	175
65	124	156	181
66	129	159	189
67	135	167	197
68	137	167	204
69	143	168	209
70	149	177	214
71	153	190	218
72	149	185	211

*Weight measured with light clothes (0.2 to 0.6 lb).

†Height measured without shoes.

From United States Department of Health, Education, and Welfare: Weight by height and age for adults 18-74 years: United States, 1971-1974, DHEW Publication No. (PHS) 79-1656, Washington, D.C., 1979, U.S. Government Printing Office.

tion. The lowest 5% of the population might be considered "depleted" and the next 10% "at risk." Follow-up on those persons should include a food intake record of some kind (see Chapter 10) to evaluate their dietary situation. Because of the variability among older individuals the use of percentiles rather than age-sex specific values is strongly recommended.[9,41]

One limitation of available reference values is the lack of data for people age 75 or over. There is no question that body measurements continue to change throughout the life span; average values for those age 65 to 74 are not necessarily appropriate for people 75 to 84 and 85 and over. Future surveys should collect information on cohorts beyond age 74.

At present anthropometric measurements are the only methods for approximating body fat feasible for the health professional with limited resources. Efforts to improve the reliability of these measurements and develop age-sex appropriate reference values must be continued.

FACTORS AFFECTING BODY COMPOSITION

Sex

The relative proportion of body fat is controlled to some extent by genetic factors. Females at all ages have a higher percentage of body fat than males.[33,51-52,68] Differences between the sexes become evident before 1 year of age. Not only do adult women have more body fat but also it accumulates at a more rapid rate. This increase occurs regardless of physical activity, although women characterized as physically fit have less fat.[70] Increases in body fat from youth to middle age were observed in women before the advent of labor-saving devices, when managing a home and family required heavy physical labor.[70,94] In a study conducted 30 years ago, body fat rose from 26% to 39% in women between 18 and 67 years of age.[94]

Body fat increased from 32% to 39% between middle and older age groups despite the fact that body weight was unchanged, suggesting a concomitant loss of nonfat tissue.

Physical Exercise

Physical exercise influences the rate of accumulation of body fat.[14,70,107] As determined by underwater weighing, physically active older men had less body fat (24% versus 27%) and more lean body mass (62 versus 57 kg) than inactive men of similar age and weight.[14] In fact, the physically active older men (including long-distance runners) had a lower percentage of body fat than inactive men who were younger.[14] Older women employed in positions requiring physical labor were more muscular and less fat than sedentary women of equal age.[70] These observations suggest that lack of physical exercise contributes to the age-related increase in fat.

AGE CHANGES IN BODY COMPOSITION

Age changes in the physical body such as accumulation of body fat on the waist and hips are readily observed; accompanying alterations in internal body compartments are less obvious. There is general agreement that body compartments change as a function of age, although the degree of change in a particular individual is extremely variable.[33,37,68]

Cross-sectional evaluation is complicated by secular as well as age-related changes. Each succeeding generation is taller and heavier; therefore older people tend to be shorter and weigh less than younger people regardless of age-related changes.[96] Ideally, alterations in body composition should be evaluated on the basis of longitudinal changes observed in the same individual over time; however, such data are limited.[33] Available information is generally cross-sectional and therefore may not reflect true aging.

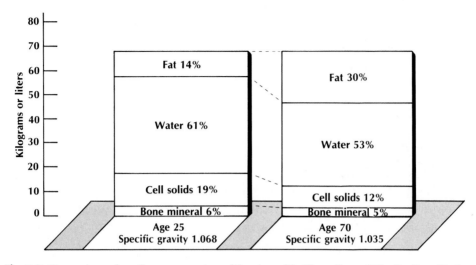

Fig. 3-2. Comparison of a reference man at age 25 and age 70. (From Fryer, J.H.: Studies of body composition in men aged 60 and over. In Shock, N.W., ed.: Biological aspects of aging, New York, 1962, Columbia University Press.)

Table 3-3. Norms for upper arm fat and muscle areas of persons age 65 to 74

	Percentiles for Men			Percentiles for Women		
	10th	**50th**	**90th**	**10th**	**50th**	**90th**
Triceps skinfold (mm)	6	11	19	14	24	34
Arm circumference (mm)	263	307	344	252	299	356
Arm muscle circumference (mm)	235	268	298	195	225	264
Arm muscle area (mm²)	4411	5716	7074	3018	4019	5566
Arm fat area (mm²)	753	1621	2876	1681	3063	4914

Modified from Frisancho, A.R.: New norms of upper limb fat and muscle areas for assessment of nutritional status, Am. J. Clin. Nutr. **34:**2540, 1981.

Proportions of Body Compartments

Fig. 3-2 describes the relative proportions of body compartments in individuals of similar body weight at ages 25 and 70.[37] A general characteristic of the aging process is an increase in body fat at the expense of lean body mass. This influences body water content because adipose tissue contains less water. Bone density also decreases as a result of bone mineral loss (see Chapter 8).

In the general population mean body weight continues to increase through middle age, decreasing only in the oldest age groups.[21,64,102-103] Because an increase in body weight usually results from a gain in fat rather than muscle, percentage of body fat often rises to an even greater extent than suggested in Fig. 3-2.

Loss of Lean Body Mass

Relative changes in lean cell mass have been evaluated by underwater weighing and whole body counting.[13,32,37,68] Loss of lean body mass parallels the age-related decrease in body potassium observed in both men and women (Fig. 3-3).[68] In men total body potassium remains constant until age 44 but decreases in each succeeding decade, with losses most rapid after age 64. Women do not lose body potassium until age 55; they have less body potassium at all ages but lose potassium less rapidly. Men appear to lose 25% of their body potassium between ages 25 and 65; women lose 11%.[68] Forbes and Reina,[33] on the basis of longitudinal studies, estimated that men lose 12 kg and women 5 kg of lean body mass over adult life. This occurred regardless of changes in body weight.

Increase in Body Fat

Both relative and absolute increases in body fat accompany the loss of lean body mass (Table 3-4).[68] Novak[68] evaluated body composition, using whole body counting, in 313 independent-living, healthy individuals ranging from 18 to 85 years of age. Body fat increased as a result of both weight gain and internal changes in body compartments. Women age 46 and over were 43% to 45% fat, whereas men were only 27% to 36% fat. In men body fat increased by about 50% on both an absolute and relative basis between ages 35 and 85, despite an actual loss in body weight beyond age 65. Body fat appeared to stabilize in women by age 65. Forbes and Reina,[33] using whole body counting, found body fat to continue to increase in women up to the age of 70 with total accumulation of body fat equaling 49% of body weight.

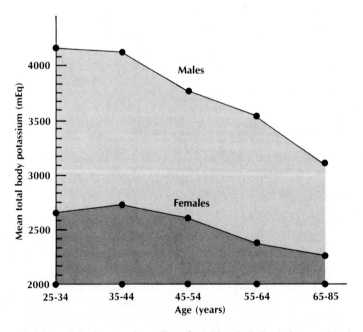

Fig. 3-3. Age-related loss in body potassium. (Data from Novak, L.P.: Aging, total body potassium, fat-free mass, and cell mass in males and females between ages 18 and 85 years, J. Gerontol. **27:**438, 1972.)

The substantial increase in body fat observed among these individuals may have been influenced by the method of evaluation. As noted earlier, in obese individuals whole body counting may underestimate lean body mass and overestimate body fat.[40] Using body density measurements men (mean age = 55)[13] were found to have 25% body fat and women of similar age were found to have 40% body fat.[108] The lower body fat observed in the latter groups also was influenced by their relative weight. Both sexes were standard weight for height whereas Novak's series included general population groups, some of whom could have been above average weight. The higher values therefore are more likely representative of the general population.

Basis for Body Changes

Explanations for the age-related loss of lean body mass have included loss of cells in major organ systems[89] and disuse atrophy of the muscle

Table 3-4. Age changes in body fat and lean body mass (LBM)

Age (yrs)	Weight* (kg)	LBM (kg)	Fat (kg)	Fat (%)
Men (n = 130)				
35-45	78	60	18	23
46-55	76	55	21	27
56-65	76	53	23	30
66-85	73	46	27	36
Women (n = 183)				
35-45	62	39	22	36
46-55	67	38	29	43
56-65	63	35	28	44
66-85	63	34	28	45

*Because of rounding LBM plus fat may not equal body weight.
Modified from Novak, L.P.: Aging, total body potassium, fat-free mass, and cell mass in males and females between ages 18 and 85 years, J. Gerontol. **27:**438, 1972.

mass.[13] Decreasing body potassium implies the loss of potassium-rich tissues and gain in connective and adipose tissues.[68] Loss of body cell mass is confirmed by the age-related decrease in intracellular water.[4]

Diminished creatinine excretion by older adults points to loss of muscle mass.[79] Creatinine excretion in healthy men decreased 30% (1790 mg/24 hr to 1259 mg/24 hr) between groups age 17 to 24 and 75 to 84.[79] Animal experiments indicate that urinary creatinine quantitatively reflects total body water and fat-free body mass and is not influenced by body fat.[105] Creatinine excretion as a predictor of lean body mass has been validated by body density measurements.[62]

Although loss of muscle and gain in body fat may be in part the result of normal aging, patterns of diet and exercise also contribute. Evidence suggests that individuals from regions where intense physical activity is a daily pattern and concentrated sources of calories are less available do not exhibit age-related increases in body weight or body fat. In a comparison of native Cape Verdean Islanders (Cape Verde Islands are 400 miles off the coast of West Africa) with Cape Verdeans who had moved to or been born in New England (Fig. 3-4), all age groups were similar in body height.[2] The body mass index (weight/height[2]) was used as a relative measure of body fat. This index has been validated with body density measurements and is appropriate regardless of height or age.[54] For persons of equal height, the body mass index increases proportionately with body weight and body fat.

As described in Fig. 3-4, not only did the Islanders have less body fat at younger ages but also they gained relatively little fat throughout adulthood. For the New England Cape Verdeans, body mass increased consistently until age 59 and then declined. The Islanders were characterized by extreme leanness, whereas the New England Cape Verdeans resembled United States factory workers in degree of adiposity. As genetic background was similar, life-style and calorie intake appeared to

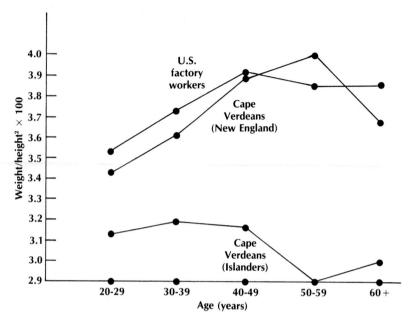

Fig. 3-4. Body mass index according to age and population group. (Data from Albrink, M.J., and Meigs, J.W.: Serum lipids, skin-fold thickness, body bulk and body weight of native Cape Verdeans, New England Cape Verdeans, and United States factory workers, Am. J. Clin. Nutr. **24:**344, 1971.)

influence these differences. The Islanders had a higher degree of physical activity with a general shortage of food. In a study reported by Rossman,[78] skinfold thickness did not increase over adulthood (between ages 25 and 75) in caucasian North Africans living under primitive conditions. By age 45, Parisians had skinfold thicknesses twice that of the North Africans.

A six year longitudinal study of the Tristan da Cunha Islanders (located off the coast of Africa) reported increases in body weight and skinfold thickness with change in life-style.[57] Over this period the island changed from an agrarian to a cash economy based on fishing. Food became more plentiful and physical exercise decreased, particularly among women. Men (age 40 and above) who

combined paid employment with maintenance of their property continued some strenuous physical activity and had a mean weight gain of 4 kg; women of similar age who exercised less had a mean weight gain of 11 kg. Prior to the change in occupation, body weights within age cohorts had been stable, changing by 1 kg or less over a 25-year period.

Evidence presented above strongly suggests that increases in body weight reflecting increases in body fat result from positive calorie balance rather than normal aging. Continued consumption of concentrated sources of calories as energy expenditure declines leads to continued weight gain, not evident in cultures where food is less plentiful. A question still to be answered, however, is whether persons continuing a high level of physical exercise experience age-related loss of lean body mass, observed in more sedentary populations.

Sidney and associates[92] reported a small (4%) but significant increase in body potassium in 38 older persons enrolled in an exercise program over a period of 1 year. Sessions were 4 hours per week and emphasized vigorous walking leading to jogging if possible. Those authors considered this gain in lean tissue to result from muscle building, proceeding at a slow rate. This rate of increase appeared adequate to support an observable improvement in general conditioning.

An on-going longitudinal study of 79 Swedish women, age 44 to 66, may shed light on this question.[66-67] Over a period of 6 years there have been no increases in body fat within these age cohorts, although both body weight and total body fat were highest in the oldest age groups. Total body potassium and total body water actually increased, suggesting a gain in functional tissue. Mean change in body weight over the 6-year period was less than 1 kg in those age 50 to 66.

Differences in these findings as compared with other reports could relate to the limited number of years of observation or the methods used. Body compartments were determined using isotope dilution methods (total body water and exchangeable potassium), less likely to underestimate lean body mass. Other studies relied on whole body counting known to underestimate body potassium and overestimate body fat. An alternative explanation is improved physical fitness based on the diet and exercise programs promoted in that country. Although clinical records did not reveal increased physical exercise among the Swedish women, general interest in diet-health relationships could have been generated by current national health campaigns.

Despite limited data to the contrary it should not be assumed that the appreciable age-related changes in body composition that have been reported are inevitable. Maintaining calorie balance to avoid weight gain and continuing even a moderate level of regular physical activity may slow, if not eliminate, increases in body fat and loss of muscle. A longitudinal evaluation of people with different but consistent levels of physical activity would provide needed information relating to body changes and preventive measures.

CURRENT TRENDS IN BODY MEASUREMENTS

Stature

Although actual loss in height does occur with aging,[70,99] older age cohorts are shorter than younger cohorts as a result of secular changes as well.[21,102-103] The classic work evaluating the relative influence of age-related versus secular changes involved measuring the length of the long bones (femur, tibia and humerus) in 855 cadavers.[99] Bone length does not change with the aging process; therefore any difference between generations is based on secular influences. Age-related losses in height occur from vertical shrinkage and collapse of the vertebrae or from curvature of the spine (lordosis or kyphosis).

In the evaluation described above both secular and age-related factors contributed to differences in stature between age cohorts. Secular differences were found among black males and among females of both races. Age-related changes were observed in all four groups but were most prominent among white females (loss of 7.8 cm as compared with 2.6 to 3.5 cm among the others). Rate of loss across groups was 1.2 cm per 20-year period or 0.6 cm per decade between ages 20 and 90. Changes were not linear, occurring most rapidly after age 50 with only slight losses before age 40.[99] Individuals differ in height loss as a 10-year longitudinal study of 11 women age 48 to 77 revealed no change in 2 of the participants (ages 56 and 77) with losses of 0.5 to 2.0 cm in the other 9.[70]

Recent national surveys (about 21,000 persons examined from 1971 to 1974) demonstrate both

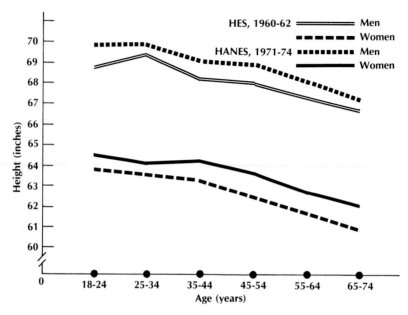

Fig. 3-5. Mean height of adults in 1960-1962 and 1971-1974 by age and sex. (From United States Department of Health, Education, and Welfare: Weight and height of adults 18-74 years of age: United States, 1971-74, DHEW Publication No. [PHS] 79-1659, Washington, D.C., 1979, U.S. Government Printing Office.)

age-related and secular changes in height (Fig. 3-5).[102] Secular influences are responsible for the differences in height between similar age cohorts in 1960-1962 and 1971-1974. Both age-related and secular changes influence the decrease in height between younger and older groups. Among male cohorts measured in 1960-1962, height differences over the age range of 18 to 74 years equaled 1.8 inches; in 1971-1974 it was 2.4 inches.[102] For women of various ages differences in height were greater in 1960-1962 than in 1971-1974 (2.3 versus 2.0 inches). Individuals of all ages were taller in 1971-1974 than their counterparts in 1960-1962; however, differences were greatest among the youngest men (1.0 inch) and oldest women (0.8 inch).

Increases in body height are probably the result of improved diet, living conditions, and health care allowing more individuals to reach their genetic potential. Ohlson and associates[70] pointed to improved vitamin D status as an influence on secular increases in stature among women.

Body Weight

Americans in all adult categories are becoming both larger and heavier (Fig. 3-6).[1,102] In men body weight increases until age 35 to 44 and then declines. In women body weight peaks between ages 35 and 64, declining only in the oldest age group. This is consistent with other reports; as in Table 3-4, the decline in body weight began a decade later in women.[68] Changes in triceps skinfold thickness follow the same trends as body weight.[21,64]

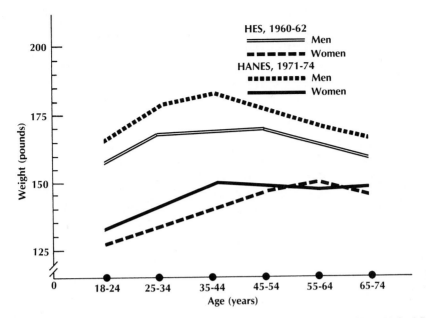

Fig. 3-6. Mean weight of adults in 1960-1962 and 1971-1974 by age and sex. (From United States Department of Health, Education, and Welfare: Weight and height of adults 18-74 years of age: United States, 1971-74, DHEW Publication No. [PHS] 79-1659, Washington, D.C., 1979, U.S. Government Printing Office.)

Decreased body weights in the older age groups[58] could result from actual loss of weight or earlier mortality of those with a higher proportion of body fat. Montoye and coworkers[64] maintain that in either case the survivors are more lean.

Men of all ages and younger women were 4 to 8 pounds heavier in 1971-1974 as compared to 1960-1962, although all were slightly taller.[102] Because, on the average, weight increases 2 to 5 pounds per inch of height, and height increased by less than 1 inch in most age groups, the weight gain observed cannot completely be attributed to the increase in height. Reduced weight gain by older women could relate to greater efforts at weight control or, as suggested by Montoye and coworkers,[64] increased mortality among heavier individuals.

Changes in average weights of life insurance policyholders (published in 1959 and 1980) differ from those of the general population.[95] Men between ages 35 and 55 were only 1 to 3 pounds heavier in 1980; women, on the other hand, were 1 to 5 pounds lighter. Those purchasing life insurance may be more health conscious and, as members of a higher socioeconomic strata, more concerned about their weight on the basis of personal appearance. Health education relating to weight control should be a priority with all age groups.

CALORIE REQUIREMENTS

Energy requirements are determined by both basal metabolism and physical activity.[28-29] Basal metabolism represents the energy required to carry on the involuntary processes of the body such as work of the heart and lungs, and digestive functions. Calories expended in physical exercise vary according to individual activity patterns and play an important role in maintaining calorie balance.

Age-Related Decrease in Basal Metabolism

Basal oxygen consumption (ml/min) is influenced by sex, body size, body composition, and age.[4,8,18,20] Both sex and age differences relate to body composition. Women at all ages have lower basal energy needs per unit of height and weight than men because of their higher proportion of body fat and lower proportion of lean body mass.[4,89] Larger individuals with a greater surface area for heat loss have higher basal needs.

Influence of Cell Loss. Although basal oxygen consumption begins to decline about age 20, the greater changes occur after age 45 and in each decade following and parallel the increase in body fat.[10,53]

Age-related changes in basal metabolism were first described in the 1930s; however, the cause was unclear.[8,10] Decrease in basal needs could represent a decline in number of functioning cells, reduced metabolic activity in existing cells, or a combination of the two. Basal oxygen consumption closely parallels age-related changes in body water (Fig. 3-7).[89] This is consistent with the explanation that aging leads to loss of cells, because total body water and intracellular water are proportional to lean body mass. Basal metabolic rates of men and women do not differ when calculated on the basis

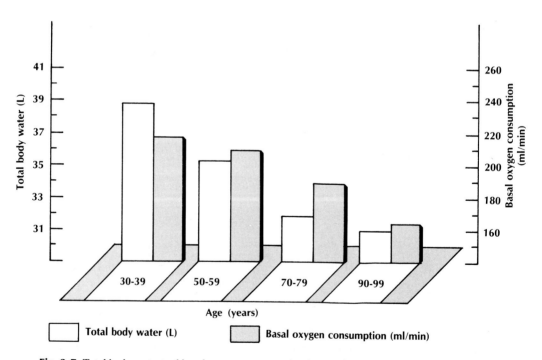

Fig. 3-7. Total body water and basal oxygen consumption by age decade. (Data from Shock, N.W., and others: Age differences in the water content of the body as related to basal oxygen consumption in males, J. Gerontol. **18**:1, 1963.)

of intracellular water.[4,88-89] Measurements of both body composition and basal metabolism in the same group of men over a period of years indicated that losses of skeletal muscle could account for the decrease in basal needs.[100] The metabolic activity of remaining cells appeared unchanged.

Longitudinal studies have identified older persons in whom basal oxygen consumption did not decline.[100-101] A logical question is whether these individuals experienced loss of body cells typical of this age group. It has since been established that the metabolic rate of nonmuscle tissues increased, compensating for reduced muscle mass. Increased oxygen consumption in nonmuscle tissues often reflects elevated metabolic work associated with cardiovascular disorders or malignancy. Basal metabolism can be expected to decline each decade beyond age 40 regardless of sex or total body size.

Influence of Thyroid Hormone. Thyroid hormone controls the metabolic rate in the cell; however, age-related changes in basal metabolism are not caused by lack of thyroxin.[38,42-43] Gregerman and coworkers[43] evaluated thyroid function in 73 euthyroid men age 18 to 91. The observed 50% decrease in thyroxin degradation rate between the youngest and oldest groups was considered to result from reduced tissue utilization and metabolism of the hormone. Decreased secretion of thyroid hormone was interpreted to be a homeostatic response to the altered thyroxine distribution space resulting from loss of lean body mass. In normal older people serum levels of T_4 are not reduced, although T_3 (active form of the hormone) levels are somewhat lower in men over age 60 and women over age 80.[81] This is consistent with the observations of Gregerman and coworkers[43] and known changes in body composition.

Six percent of 344 healthy older persons were found to have elevated serum thyrotropin (TSH) levels, considered to be the most sensitive indicator of primary hypothyroidism.[81] Unfortunately, mild hypothyroidism is not always recognized in older persons because many of the characteristic symptoms such as lethargy, constipation, or limited tolerance to cold are often assumed to be typical of older persons.[93] Hyperthyroidism is equally serious as excessive hormone increases the work of the heart and exacerbates any existing cardiac problems.[77] About 80% of aged with thyrotoxicosis have cardiovascular disturbances.[93] Weight loss is frequent. In contrast to younger hyperthyroid individuals, aged patients do not always have increased appetites, and they may be apathetic or withdrawn. Caloric restriction, stress, and illness can also result in abnormally elevated or lowered thyroxine levels.[69]

Predicting Basal Calorie Needs. Simple prediction equations based on height, weight, and age can overestimate the calorie needs of older individuals.[7,59,74] For overtly obese aged, prediction equations are still less reliable as an even larger proportion of the body is fat.[19-20,59] Early studies suggested the daily basal requirement of women age 65 or above to be about 1000 kcal.[7,59] This estimate, however, was based on work with institutionalized women, not necessarily representative of healthy aged. More recent basal measurements of both independent-living and institutionalized older persons range from 1100 to 1300 kcal for women and 1100 to 1400 for men.[4,20,89] For sedentary aged, the total caloric requirement is very close to the basal requirement.

Physical Activity

Benefits of Physical Activity. Physical fitness is characterized by the ability of the muscular, cardiovascular, and respiratory systems to respond to physical work with rapid recovery and minimal fatigue.[24] Changes in fitness can occur as a result of smoking, lack of exercise, or age-related deterioration.[75] Supervised physical training both improves the response of cardiovascular and respiratory systems and alters body composition in older men and women.[91-92] A year long exercise program consisting of four 1-hour sessions each week, developed for persons age 65 or over, brought about a slow but progressive loss of body fat.[92] Activities included calisthenics and warm-up exercises and walking or jogging. Exercise was designed to require 150 to 200 kcal per session. Skinfold thicknesses (mean of measurements at eight locations) decreased 1.6 mm after 7 weeks, 2.4 mm after 14 weeks, and 3.3 mm after 1 year of training. Loss of body fat was proportional to frequency of attendance (two or more or less than two sessions per week) and intensity of exercise (based on maximum heart rates).

Consistent exercise can lead to improved functional capability equal to that of a sedentary individual 10 to 20 years younger.[87] Walking on a regular basis increases aerobic capacity with decreased fatigue, increases mental alertness and effectiveness, and increases bone strength (see Chapter 8). Improvement in functional capacity enhances the individual's ability to carry on daily activities and remain independent. No strenuous exercise regimen should be undertaken, however, without a medical evaluation beforehand and professional supervision.

Developing an Exercise Pattern. The individual must enjoy the exercise planned if he is to cooperate and continue with the program.[87] For those with muscular or skeletal problems, walking at a comfortable pace is appropriate exercise. Abrupt, overly strenuous activity for those who have been primarily sedentary can be dangerous for both the heart and the locomotor system. Allowing for individual differences and a gradual increase in activity when conducting a group exercise program at a senior center will increase the probability of success. Although some older persons enjoy doing exercises or walking and jogging in a group, others prefer to exercise in privacy. The previously sedentary individual with stiff joints and awkward movements might find group activities embarrassing but attend sessions to hear about exercises that could be carried out at home. Walking outdoors can be both pleasurable and healthful for an older person when weather and neighborhood conditions are favorable.

The cost of equipment must be considered when planning exercise activities. Although pedaling on a stationary bicycle has the advantage of being an indoor activity and people can easily stop and rest when necessary,[17] such a purchase is prohibitive for many. Activities requiring no financial expenditure are more likely to be adopted by older clients.

Arm and hand exercises are possible for individuals no longer able to walk.[87] Flexing the arm and finger muscles can reduce and retard stiffness and promote self-feeding activities and recreational pursuits (arts or crafts; playing a musical instrument). These activities can be presented in the context of nutrition education or as group social activity.

Calorie Intake and Energy Expenditure

Decline in Energy Needs. Increases in body weight throughout adulthood can result from continued consumption of previous calorie levels as both basal metabolism and physical exercise decline. Diaries of food intake and physical activity from 252 independent-living men[61,88] age 30 to 80 have allowed analysis of calorie intake and expenditure at various ages. Total caloric intake declined an average of 12.4 kcal/day/year (Fig. 3-8).[88] Physical activity fell more rapidly than basal requirements (7.8 as compared to 5.2 kcal/day/year). Total energy needs declined by about 800 kcal/day over the 50 years (2811 to 1964), with the steepest drop between age 70 and 80. Energy balance as calculated from total caloric intake (from food records) and total energy expenditure (BMR measurement plus activity records) differed by 7% or less in particular age cohorts. Because these men were physically healthy and they exercised regularly, they most likely experienced a smaller decrease in energy needs than more sedentary individuals.

In younger people energy needs are influenced by occupation, if sedentary or active.[22,25] Unless one is motivated toward physical fitness, leisure activities require little exercise. For retired persons

Table 3-5. Seven-day activity records of older women*

	Employed Women (minutes)	Retired Women (minutes)
Sitting	3004	1941
Standing	872	1344
Walking	864	1213
Driving/riding (car, bus)	295	443
Bathing/dressing/eating	1101	1011
Sleeping	3106	3187
Light physical effort	385	548
Moderate physical effort	427	264
Heavy physical effort	26	129

*Total number of minutes = 10,080.

Modified from Sidney, K.H., and Shephard, R.J.: Activity patterns of elderly men and women, J. Gerontol. **32**:25, 1977.

Table 3-6. Recommended energy intakes

	51-75 Years	76+ Years
Females		
Calories (kcal)	1800	1600
Range	1400-2200	1200-2000
Males		
Calories (kcal)	2400	2050
Range	2000-2800	1650-2450

Modified from Food and Nutrition Board: Recommended dietary allowances, ed. 9, Washington, D.C., 1980, National Academy of Sciences.

leisure activities occupy most of the day and for those lacking the inclination or ability to participate in higher energy-requiring tasks, calorie expenditure can be very low. For those previously employed in hard physical labor, the need to decrease calorie intake is imperative. Even when older people remain employed, occupations are usually sedentary and activity levels not different from those with more leisure time.

Among Canadian women above age 60 (n = 21) full time employment did not result in greater caloric expenditure, although the employed women spent more time in moderate physical effort than the retired women did (Table 3-5).[90] Employed women spent less time in homemaking tasks, although during working hours less than 20% of their time involved any form of physical activity including walking. Retired women appeared to engage in activities about the home such as gardening or home maintenance. Calculated caloric expenditure (including adjustment for basal metabolism) was 2264 and 2212 kcal for the employed and retired women, respectively. Continuing physical activity following retirement may be easier for women than men as household tasks are continued.

Social conditions and patterns of activity since childhood are a factor in the energy expenditure patterns of both obese and nonobese. Obese aged have even less physical activity than those of average weight or moderate overweight.[23]

Recommended Energy Intake. Recommended levels of calories for persons above age 50 assume only light physical activity such as standing, walking, or carrying light loads (Table 3-6).[29] Prior to 1980 the RDAs combined all individuals above age 50 in a single category.[28-29] It has since been recognized that both BMR and activity levels continue to drop throughout later decades and specific age groupings are appropriate. Activity levels declined by about 250 kcal/day between ages 40 and 70 and by about 300 kcal/day beyond that age in the men described in Fig. 3-8.

Surveys of both institutionalized[12,50] and independent-living aged[12,45,73] report mean energy intakes of 1366 to 2166 kcal for men and 1291 to 1633 kcal for women. Psychologic and sociologic factors also influence the quantity of food consumed (see Chapter 11). Efforts at weight control—loss of unwanted weight or prevention of weight gain—lead many older people to severely restrict their caloric intake. The National Research Council reiterates that diets containing less than 1800 to 2000 kcal may not be adequate in required nutrients unless intakes of sugar, fat, and alcohol

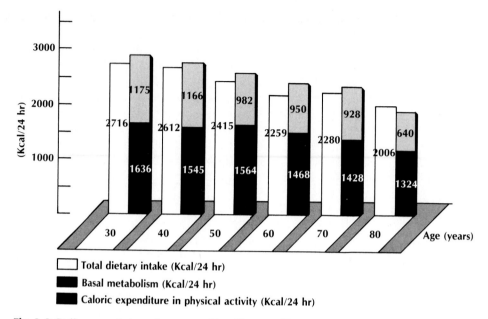

Fig. 3-8. Daily energy balance in men age 30 to 80 years. (From Shock, N.W.: Energy metabolism, caloric intake, and physical activity of the aging. In Carlson, L.A., ed.: Nutrition in old age, Symposia Swedish Nutrition Foundation X, Stockholm, Sweden, 1972, Almqvist and Wiksell.)

are restricted.[29] Older women consuming 1200 to 1600 kcal are particularly vulnerable to poor nutrition.

Energy Metabolism. Critical issues relating to the energy requirement of older people include (1) calorie intake required for optimum rather than maintenance levels, and (2) limitation of calories required for weight loss. In a metabolic evaluation of six healthy men, age 63 to 77, BMR equaled 1622 kcal/day; the calorie intake required to maintain body weight was 2554 kcal or about 1.6 times the BMR.[17] With the exception of 30 minutes of cycling on a stationary bicycle, the men were sedentary; in fact, most reported having higher levels of activity when at home. Therefore calories consumed during the study were believed to represent their minimum requirement for maintenance.

Calloway and Zanni[17] consider the maintenance energy requirement for ambulatory but inactive older people to be 1.5 times the BMR as suggested for other age groups. From their perspective an RDA of 2400 kcal represents minimal rather than optimal intake; active older people will require more than this level. The older men in this study were, however, in good physical condition, which would influence both degree of muscle mass and physical activity. Healthy older men (see Fig. 3-8) are reported to consume 2400 kcal or less. A high level of physical activity would be required to avoid weight gain on intakes above 2400 kcal.

This issue is further clouded by a recent analysis of long term energy balance, which suggests that individuals possess a regulatory mechanism that acts to ensure energy homeostasis.[97] Seldom do caloric intake and energy output balance on a week-to-week basis; shifts in metabolic rate conserve energy when fewer calories are ingested and dissipate unneeded calories as heat when intake exceeds expenditure. This implies that decreasing caloric intake will result in energy conservation with no real benefit to the older individual.

Although this theory requires further study, it raises questions regarding the efficacy of strict calorie limitation to achieve weight reduction in older people for whom a metabolic pattern has developed over a lifetime. Although decreasing calories may be necessary to prevent weight gain, severe restriction may be required to accomplish weight loss. Inappropriately low calorie intake resulting in weakness will further limit activity and decrease calorie expenditure, setting in motion a vicious cycle. For those who are severely arthritic and extremely limited in movement, excess weight can be totally debilitating and weight loss a necessity.[98] A serious health problem such as hypertension or diabetes would under doctor's supervision mandate strict calorie control.[49]

Although older overweight individuals should be encouraged to (1) avoid high calorie items low in nutrient density, (2) limit the number of servings of all foods, and (3) increase physical activity, any attempt to reverse a lifelong weight pattern will probably have only limited success (Chapter 2). Exercise using 150 to 200 kcal per day will help in weight control.[91] In older people weighing 70 kg, a 10-minute walk will cost about 40 kcal.[56]

SUMMARY

Evaluation of body composition in older people is difficult as standards and methods developed for younger individuals are not always appropriate for older clients. Whole body counting, underwater weighing, and dilution techniques provide reasonable estimates of body fat and lean tissue but require expensive equipment, highly trained personnel, and extensive cooperation on the part of the client. Use of the mid-arm skinfold and circumference measurements to calculate fat and muscle areas provides some indication of body fat and protein/calorie status when compared with values obtained from people of similar age.

Advancing age is accompanied by increases in body fat and loss of lean body mass. As this pattern is not evident among individuals with limited calorie intake and continued intense physical exercise, life-style and over-consumption rather than normal aging may be the cause. Loss of lean body mass and decreasing physical activity lead to a decrease in the energy needs of the older individual. Nutrition counseling should stress selection of nutrient-dense foods[3] and when possible, regular exercise.

REVIEW QUESTIONS

1. Define the four body compartments. Describe the changes occurring in each compartment between ages 25 and 65.
2. Is the age-related increase in body fat an inevitable result of the aging process or could it be prevented? Cite evidence to justify your answer.
3. How may anthropometric measurements be used to assess body composition? What are the limitations of such measurements? What standards exist for the evaluation of anthropometric measurements?
4. What factors contribute to the age-related decrease in caloric requirements? Explain the observed alterations in thyroid secretion.
5. Energy needs of older people are a matter of controversy. The average daily intake of many older people is 1600 to 1800 kcal. Do you consider this to be adequate? Justify your answer.

REFERENCES

1. Abraham, S., and Johnson, C.L.: Prevalence of severe obesity in adults in the United States, Am. J. Clin. Nutr. **33**:364, 1980.
2. Albrink, M.J., and Meigs, J.W.: Serum lipids, skin-fold thickness, body bulk and body weight of native Cape Verdeans, New England Cape Verdeans, and United States factory workers, Am. J. Clin. Nutr. **24**:344, 1971.
3. American Dietetic Association, American Diabetes Association: Exchange lists for meal planning, New York, 1976, American Dietetic Association, American Diabetes Association.
4. Baker, S.P., Shock, N.W., and Norris, A.H.: Influence of age and obesity in women on basal oxygen consumption expressed in terms of total body water and intracellular water. In Shock, N.W., ed.: Biological aspects of aging, New York, 1962, Columbia University Press.
5. Barter, J., and Forbes, G.B.: Correlation of potassium-40 data with anthropometric measurements, Ann. N.Y. Acad. Sci. **110**:264, 1963.
6. Behnke, A.R.: Anthropometric evaluation of body com-

position throughout life, Ann. N.Y. Acad. Sci. **110**:450, 1963.

7. Benedict, F.G.: Old age and basal metabolism, N. Engl. J. Med. **212**:1111, 1935.

8. Berkson, J., and Boothby, W.M.: Studies of the energy of metabolism of normal individuals: A comparison of the estimation of basal metabolism from (1) a linear formula and (2) surface area, Am. J. Physiol. **116**:485, 1936.

9. Bishop, C.W., Bowen, P.E., and Ritchey, S.J.: Norms for nutritional assessment of American adults by upper arm anthropometry, Am. J. Clin. Nutr. **34**:2530, 1981.

10. Boothby, W.M., Berkson, J., and Dunn, H.L.: Studies of the energy of metabolism of normal individuals: A standard for basal metabolism, with a nomogram for clinical application, Am. J. Physiol. **116**:468, 1936.

11. Bray, G.A.: Obesity in perspective, vol. 2, Part 1, DHEW Publication No. (NIH) 75-708, Washington, D.C., 1975, U.S. Government Printing Office.

12. Brown, P.T., and others: Dietary status of elderly people: Rural independent-living men and women vs. nursing home residents, J. Am. Diet. Assoc. **71**:41, 1977.

13. Brozek, J.: Changes of body composition in man during maturity and their nutritional implications, Fed. Proc. **11**:784, 1952.

14. Brozek, J., and Keys, A.: Relative body weight, age and fatness, Geriatrics **8**:70, 1953.

15. Brozek, J., and Kinzey, W.: Age changes in skinfold compressibility, J. Gerontol. **15**:45, 1960.

16. Burgert, S.L., and Anderson, C.F.: A comparison of triceps skinfold values as measured by the plastic McGaw caliper and the Lange caliper, Am. J. Clin. Nutr. **32**:1531, 1979.

17. Calloway, D.H., and Zanni, E.: Energy requirements and energy expenditure of elderly men, Am. J. Clin. Nutr. **33**:2088, 1980.

18. Cunningham, J.J.: A reanalysis of the factors influencing basal metabolic rate in normal adults, Am. J. Clin. Nutr. **33**:2372, 1980.

19. Cunningham, J.J.: An individualization of dietary requirements for energy in adults, J. Am. Diet. Assoc. **80**:335, 1982.

20. Dalderup, L.M., Opdam-Stockmann, V.A., and Rechsteiner-de Vos, H.: Basal metabolic rate, anthropometric, electrocardiographic, and dietary data relating to elderly persons, J. Gerontol. **21**:22, 1966.

21. Damon, A., and others: Age and physique in healthy white veterans at Boston, J. Gerontol. **27**:202, 1972.

22. Durnin, J.V.: Intake and expenditure of calories by the elderly, Proc. Nutr. Soc. **19**:140, 1960.

23. Durnin, J.V.: Age, physical activity, and energy expenditure, Proc. Nutr. Soc. **25**:107, 1966.

24. Durnin, J.V.: The influence of nutrition, Can. Med. Assoc. J. **96**:715, 1967.

25. Durnin, J.V.: Energy-requirements, intake, and balance, Proc. Nutr. Soc. **27**:188, 1968.

26. Durnin, J.V., and Womersley, J.: Body fat assessed from total body density and its estimation from skinfold thickness: Measurements on 481 men and women aged from 16 to 72 years, Br. J. Nutr. **32**:77, 1974.

27. Edwards, D.A.W.: Observations on the distribution of subcutaneous fat, Clin. Sci. **9**:259, 1950.

28. Food and Nutrition Board: Recommended dietary allowances, ed. 7, Washington, D.C., 1968, National Academy of Sciences.

29. Food and Nutrition Board: Recommended dietary allowances, ed. 9, Washington, D.C., 1980, National Academy of Sciences.

30. Forbes, G.B.: Methods for determining composition of the human body, Pediatrics **29**:477, 1962.

31. Forbes, G.B., Gallup, J., and Hursh, J.B.: Estimation of total body fat from potassium-40 content, Science **133**:101, 1961.

32. Forbes, G.B., and Hursh, J.B.: Age and sex trends in lean body mass calculated from K^{40} measurements, Ann. N.Y. Acad. Sci. **110**:255, 1963.

33. Forbes, G.B., and Reina, J.C.: Adult lean body mass declines with age: Some longitudinal observations, Metabolism **19**(9):653, 1970.

34. Friis-Hansen, B.: Hydrometry of growth and aging. In Brozek, J., ed.: Human body composition: Approaches and applications, New York, 1965, Pergamon Press, Inc.

35. Frisancho, A.R.: Triceps skin fold and upper arm muscle size norms for assessment of nutritional status, Am. J. Clin. Nutr. **27**:1052, 1974.

36. Frisancho, A.R.: New norms of upper limb fat and muscle areas for assessment of nutritional status, Am. J. Clin. Nutr. **34**:2540, 1981.

37. Fryer, J.H.: Studies of body composition in men aged 60 and over. In Shock, N.W., ed.: Biological aspects of aging, New York, 1962, Columbia University Press.

38. Gaffney, G.W., Gregerman, R.I., and Shock, N.W.: Relationship of age to the thyroidal accumulation, renal excretion and distribution of radioiodide in euthyroid man, J. Clin. Endocrinol. **22**:784, 1962.

39. Garn, S.M.: Relative fat patterning: An individual characteristic, Hum. Biol. **27**:75, 1955.

40. Garrow, J.S.: Overview: New approaches to body composition, Am. J. Clin. Nutr. **35**(suppl.):1152, 1982.

41. Gray, G.E., and Gray, L.K.: Anthropometric measurements and their interpretation: Principles, practices, and problems, J. Am. Diet. Assoc. **77**:534, 1980.

42. Gregerman, R.I.: The age-related alteration of thyroid function and thyroid hormone metabolism in man. In Gitman, L., ed.: Endocrines and aging, Springfield, Ill., 1967, Charles C Thomas Publisher.

43. Gregerman, R.I., Gaffney, G.W., and Shock, N.W.: Thyroxine turnover in euthyroid man with special reference to changes with age, J. Clin. Invest. **41**(11):2065, 1962.

44. Gurney, J.M., and Jelliffe, D.B.: Arm anthropometry in nutritional assessment: Nomogram for rapid calculation of muscle circumference and cross sectional muscle and fat areas, Am. J. Clin. Nutr. **26**:912, 1973.

45. Guthrie, H.A., Black, K., and Madden, J.P.: Nutritional practices of elderly citizens in rural Pennsylvania, Gerontologist **12**:330, 1972.

46. Harrison, G., and Van Itallie, T.B.: Estimation of body composition: A new approach based on electromagnetic principles, Am. J. Clin. Nutr. **35**(suppl):1176, 1982.

47. Himes, J.H., Roche, A.F., and Siervogel, R.M.: Compressibility of skinfolds and the measurement of subcutaneous fatness, Am. J. Clin. Nutr. **32**:1734, 1979.

48. Himes, J.H., Roche, A.F., and Webb, P.: Fat areas as estimates of total body fat, Am. J. Clin. Nutr. **33**:2093, 1980.

49. Jelliffe, N.: Some basic considerations of obesity as a public health problem, Am. J. Public Health **43**:989, 1953.

50. Justice, C.L., Howe, J.M., and Clark, H.E.: Dietary intakes and nutritional status of elderly patients. Study in a private nursing home, J. Am. Diet. Assoc. **65**:639, 1974.

51. Keys, A.: Body composition and its change with age and diet. In Eppright, E.S., Swanson, P., and Iverson, C.A., eds.: Weight control, Ames, 1955, Iowa State College Press.

52. Keys, A., and Brozek, J.: Body fat in adult man, Physiol. Rev. **33**:245, 1953.

53. Keys, A., Taylor, H.L., and Grande, F.: Basal metabolism and age of adult man, Metabolism **22**:579, 1973.

54. Keys, A., and others: Indices of relative weight and obesity, J. Chronic Dis. **25**:329, 1972.

55. Lye, M.: Distribution of body potassium in healthy elderly subjects, Gerontology **27**:286, 1981.

56. Mahadeva, K., Passmore, R., and Woolf, B.: Individual variations in the metabolic cost of standardized exercises: The effects of food, age, sex, and race, J. Physiol. **121**:225, 1953.

57. Marshall, W.A., and others: Anthropometric measurements of the Tristan da Cunha islanders, 1962-68, Hum. Biol. **43**:112, 1971.

58. Master, A.M., Lasser, R.P., and Beckman, G.: Tables of average weight and height of Americans aged 65 to 94 years: Relationship of weight and height to survival, JAMA **172**:658, 1960.

59. Matson, J.R., and Hitchcock, F.A.: Basal metabolism in old age, Am. J. Physiol. **110**:329, 1934.

60. Mayer, J.: Obesity: Diagnosis, Postgrad. Med. **25**:469, 1959.

61. McGandy, R.B., and others: Nutrient intakes and energy expenditure in men of different ages, J. Gerontol. **21**:581, 1966.

62. Miller, A.T., and Blyth, C.S.: Estimation of lean body mass and body fat from basal oxygen consumption and creatinine excretion, J. Appl. Physiol. **5**:73, 1952.

63. Mitchell, C.O., and Lipschitz, D.A.: Creatinine height index in the elderly. In Assessing the nutritional status of the elderly, state of the art, Report of the Third Ross Roundtable on Medical Issues, Columbus, Ohio, 1982, Ross Laboratories.

64. Montoye, H.J., Epstein, F.H., and Kjelsberg, M.O.: The measurement of body fatness. A study in a total community, Am. J. Clin. Nutr. **16**:417, 1965.

65. Moore, F.D., and others: The body cell mass and its supporting environment, Philadelphia, 1963, W.B. Saunders Co.

66. Noppa, H., and others: Body composition in middle-aged women with special reference to the correlation between body fat mass and anthropometric data, Am. J. Clin. Nutr. **32**:1388, 1979.

67. Noppa, H., and others: Longitudinal studies of anthropometric data and body composition. The population study of women in Göteborg, Sweden, Am. J. Clin. Nutr. **33**:155, 1980.

68. Novak, L.P.: Aging, total body potassium, fat-free mass, and cell mass in males and females between ages 18 and 85 years, J. Gerontol. **27**:438, 1972.

69. Nusynowitz, M.L., and Young, R.L.: Thyroid dysfunction in the ailing, aging, and aberrant, JAMA **242**(3):275, 1979.

70. Ohlson, M.A. and others: Anthropometry and nutritional status of adult women, Hum. Biol. **28**:189, 1956.

71. Olesen, K.H.: Body composition in normal adults. In Brozek, J., ed.: Human body composition: Approaches and applications, New York, 1965, Pergamon Press, Inc.

72. Passmore, R.: Stores in the human body. In Brozek, J., ed.: Human body composition: Approaches and applications, New York, 1965, Pergamon Press, Inc.

73. Rawson, I.G., and others: Nutrition of rural elderly in southwestern Pennsylvania, Gerontologist **18**:24, 1978.

74. Robertson, J.D.: Basal metabolic rate in old men, Lancet **1**:296, 1958.

75. Robinson, S., and others: Training and physiological aging in man, Fed. Proc. **32**(5):1628, 1973.

76. Roche, A.F.: Anthropometric variables: Effectiveness and limitations. In Assessing the nutritional status of the elderly, state of the art, Report of the Third Ross Roundtable on Medical Issues, Columbus, Ohio, 1982, Ross Laboratories.

77. Rosenbaum, R.L., and Barzel, U.S.: Clinical hypothyroidism in the elderly: A preventable disorder? J. Am. Geriatr. Soc. **29**(5):221, 1981.

78. Rossman, I.: Anatomic and body composition changes with aging. In Finch, C.E., and Hayflick, L., eds.: Handbook of the biology of aging, New York, 1977, Van Nostrand Reinhold Co, Inc.

79. Rowe, J.W., and others: The effect of age on creatinine clearance in men: A cross-sectional and longitudinal study, J. Gerontol. 31(2):155, 1976.

80. Ruiz, L., Colley, J.R.T., and Hamilton, P.J.S.: Measurement of triceps skinfold thickness: An investigation of sources of variation, Br. J. Prev. Soc. Med. 25:165, 1971.

81. Sawin, C.T., and others: The aging thyroid. Increased prevalence of elevated serum thyrotropin levels in the elderly, JAMA 242(3):247, 1979.

82. Schlenker, E.D.: Nutritional status of older women, Ph.D. Thesis, E. Lansing, 1976, Michigan State University.

83. Schoeller, D.A., and others: Total body water measurement in humans with ^{18}0 and ^{2}H labeled water, Am. J. Clin. Nutr. 33:2686, 1980.

84. Seltzer, C.C.: Limitation of height-weight standards, N. Engl. J. Med. 272:1132, 1965.

85. Seltzer, C.C., and Mayer, J.: A simple criterion of obesity, Postgrad. Med. 38:A-101, 1965.

86. Seltzer, C.C., and others: Reliability of relative body weight as a criterion of obesity, Am. J. Epidemiol. 92(6):339, 1970.

87. Shephard, R.J.: Physical activity and aging, Chicago, 1978, Year Book Medical Publishers, Inc.

88. Shock, N.W.: Energy metabolism, caloric intake and physical activity of the aging. In Carlson, L.A., ed.: Nutrition in old age, Symposia Swedish Nutrition Foundation X, Stockholm, 1972, Almqvist & Wiksell.

89. Shock, N.W., and others: Age differences in the water content of the body as related to basal oxygen consumption in males, J. Gerontol. 18:1, 1963.

90. Sidney, K.H., and Shephard, R.J.: Activity patterns of elderly men and women, J. Gerontol. 32:25, 1977.

91. Sidney, K.H., and Shephard, R.J.: Frequency and intensity of exercise training for elderly subjects, Med. Sci. Sports 10(2):125, 1978.

92. Sidney, K.H., Shephard, R.J., and Harrison, J.E.: Endurance training and body composition of the elderly, Am. J. Clin. Nutr. 30:326, 1977.

93. Sirota, D.K.: Thyroid function and dysfunction in the elderly: A brief review, Mt. Sinai J. Med. 47(2):126, 1980.

94. Skerlj, B., and others: Subcutaneous fat and age changes in body build and form in women, Am. J. Phys. Anthropol. 11:577, 1953.

95. Society of Actuaries: Build study 1979, Chicago, 1980, Society of Actuaries.

96. Stoudt, H.W.: The anthropometry of the elderly, Hum. Factors 23(1):29, 1981.

97. Sukhatme, P.V., and Margen, S.: Autoregulatory homeostatic nature of energy balance, Am. J. Clin. Nutr. 35:355, 1982.

98. Traut, E.F., and Thrift, C.B.: Obesity in arthritis: Related factors: Dietary therapy, J. Am. Geriatr. Soc. 17:710, 1969.

99. Trotter, M., and Gleser, G.: The effect of ageing on stature, Am. J. Phys. Anthropol. 9:311, 1951.

100. Tzankoff, S.P., and Norris, A.H.: Effect of muscle mass decrease on age-related BMR changes, J. Appl. Physiol. 43(6):1001, 1977.

101. Tzankoff, S.P., and Norris, A.H.: Longitudinal changes in basal metabolism in man, J. Appl. Physiol. 45(4):536, 1978.

102. United States Department of Health, Education and Welfare: Weight and height of adults 18-74 years of age, United States, 1971-74, DHEW Publication No. (PHS) 79-1659, Washington, D.C., 1979, U.S. Government Printing Office.

103. United States Department of Health, Education and Welfare: Weight by height and age for adults 18-74 years: United States, 1971-74, DHEW Publication No. (PHS) 79-1656, Washington, D.C., 1979, U.S. Government Printing Office.

104. Van Itallie, T.B.: Other body composition studies that could be applied. In Assessing the nutritional status of the elderly, state of the art, Report of the Third Ross Roundtable on Medical Issues, Columbus, Oh., 1982, Ross Laboratories.

105. Van Niekerk, B.D., and others: Urinary creatinine as an index of body composition, J. Nutr. 79:463, 1963.

106. Ward, G.M., and others: Relationship of anthropometric measurements to body fat as determined by densitometry, potassium-40, and body water, Am. J. Clin. Nutr. 28:162, 1975.

107. Wessel, J.A., and others: Age trends of various components of body composition and functional characteristics in women aged 20-69 years, Ann. N.Y. Acad. Sci. 110:608, 1963.

108. Young, C.M.: Predicting specific gravity and body fatness in older women, J. Am. Diet. Assoc. 45:333, 1964.

109. Young, C.M, and others: Body composition of older women, J. Am. Diet. Assoc. 43:344, 1963.

Chapter 4

Nutrient Digestion and Absorption

Possible changes in the gastrointestinal tract affecting the rate or completeness of digestion and absorption have not been defined. Such alterations would have important implications for the nutritional status of older people. Incomplete digestion with consequent reduced nutrient absorption could precipitate nutrient deficiencies regardless of the adequacy of intake. Altered functional capacity of the gastrointestinal tract resulting in abdominal discomfort may lead to a reduction in general food intake increasing the likelihood of nutrient deficiency. For these reasons complaints from older clients regarding gastrointestinal upset require careful evaluation.

CHANGES IN THE GASTROINTESTINAL TRACT

Functional Disorders

Basis of Concern. Of all organ systems, the gastrointestinal tract is the most common source of chronic discomfort in older people.[48] Physical distress may be intensified by mental anxiety resulting in less pleasure in eating or, worse yet, a reduction in the quantity or quality of food consumed. In some instances gastrointestinal upset is related to organic disease, although in about half of all cases there is no apparent anatomic cause.[45] Symptoms may include nausea, vomiting, diarrhea, constipation, heartburn, or pain and bloating sensations. According to Sklar,[45] functional complaints are frequently related to poor eating and bowel habits,

as well as an exaggerated concern regarding disease.

Gastrointestinal distress is not necessarily indicative of malabsorption; persons with no discomfort may absorb nutrients poorly whereas others with constant gastric upsets may absorb nutrients normally.[35] Because of the potential impact of gastrointestinal problems on nutritional status, and the fact that such symptoms may signal organic disease, all should be investigated carefully.[45,48]

Incidence of Problems. Changes in gastrointestinal function seem to occur before age 50 (Fig. 4-1). In a study of nearly 1200 in Uppsala, Sweden, symptoms were rare among young persons; however, incidence did not differ between those of middle age and those above age 67.[51] The number of symptoms reported in middle age is rather surprising in view of the fact that these individuals had no known diseases. Moreover, frequency of symptoms did not increase between ages 70 and 80. All persons age 67 and over (n = 742) were considered to be in good health.

Among outpatients over age 65 (number not given) seeking help for digestive problems 56% had no demonstrable disease, 10% had a malignancy, 8% gallbladder disease, 9% an ulcer, and 3% diverticulosis.[45] The remainder (14%) had a variety of other disorders. About 10% were intolerant to fat. Although not mentioned in this study, a wide variety of commonly used drugs including aspirin, digitalis, anticonvulsants, and diuretics can cause abdominal distress.[41] In summary, gastrointestinal

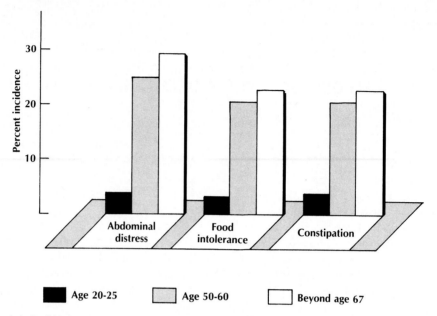

Percent incidence

Age 20-25   Age 50-60   Beyond age 67

Fig. 4-1. Incidence of gastrointestinal symptoms according to age. (Data from Werner, I., and Hambraeus, L.: The digestive capacity of elderly people. In Carlson, L.A., ed.: Nutrition in old age, Symposia Swedish Nutrition Foundation X, Stockholm, 1972, Almqvist & Wiksell.)

problems among older people do not in many cases reflect clinical disease. The nonspecific nature of the problems adds to difficulty in treatment.

Food Avoidance. Discomfort following eating will significantly influence nutrient intake if a particular food group is consistently avoided. Among 28 Michigan women, age 64 to 90, 64% avoided legumes, cabbage, and similar vegetables, 57% avoided fats, 18% avoided whole grains or fruits, and 14% avoided milk.[44] In those women avoidance of fat was frequently related to lowering calorie intake. Those avoiding acid fruits had intakes below 67% the RDA for vitamin A and ascorbic acid.[44] Eliminating whole grains reduces intake of trace minerals and exacerbates constipation problems as well. In some instances the women were encouraged to follow bland, low-fiber diets to alleviate symptoms associated with diverticulosis. Avoidance of milk was based on personal taste; no

one reported abdominal distress or the belief that milk leads to constipation.

Because bloating or distention is a common complaint, vegetables such as cabbage or onions may be limited in the diet; however, these vegetables usually provide only a small portion of the fiber intake. Major sources are bread, fruit, cereal, and other vegetables.[26] Fat avoidance, if extreme, limits intake of linoleic acid and hinders absorption of the fat soluble vitamins.[17]

The greater the number of foods avoided, the greater the likelihood of a diet deficient in one or more nutrients. One Michigan woman was avoiding fats, whole grains, acid and fibrous fruits and vegetables, and milk.[44] The only fruits consumed were canned peaches and pears and fresh bananas. Although she did eat cooked carrots, the limited fat in her diet coupled with known gallbladder disease likely reduced absorption of the available carotene as her serum vitamin A was deficient (<20 μg/100 ml). Although most older people enjoy a reasonably varied diet, the individual with high food avoidance is at risk and should receive dietary counseling.

Dysphagia

Problems in swallowing can result from changes in esophageal motility and decreased secretion of saliva.[1,30,48] If the problem is severe, food may be rejected as swallowing becomes more difficult. Normally, the swallowing reflex initiates a peristaltic wave in the esophagus that moves food along the passageway.[7,18] As the peristaltic wave nears the stomach, it is preceded by a wave of relaxation that acts on the esophageal sphincter and allows food to move on into the stomach. Studies in older people suggest that in some individuals normal peristaltic waves do not always occur or are decreased in amplitude, resulting in delayed esophageal emptying and dilation of the esophagus as food accumulates.[22,46] This results in muscle contractions that can be painful and ineffective in propelling the food bolus. Although the individual attempts to swallow, food may still be regurgitated a few minutes later. Fluids are usually more easily swallowed. Changes in innervation are believed to cause the problem; the muscle is able to contract but coordinated responses are lost.[18] Heartburn from backflow of stomach acid into the esophagus is more frequent when the esophageal sphincter has lost normal control.[48]

Dry mouth resulting from reduced secretion of saliva or general dehydration adds to difficulty in swallowing.[19,48] Certain drugs such as antidepressants, anticonvulsants, and amphetamines can cause dry mouth,[41] as can dentures, anxiety, or breathing through the mouth. Alterations in the thirst mechanism reducing water intake can contribute to general dehydration.[48] Some older people consciously restrict their fluid intake to limit trips to the bathroom, particularly if this involves going up a flight of stairs.[1] Increasing intake of fluids or use of lozenges can provide some relief.

Problems in swallowing can lead to fear of choking and reduced food intake. Older people should eat only when seated in an upright position so gravity can aid in the swallowing motion. Being fed in a supine position increases risk of food aspiration and pneumonia.[18-19,30]

Stomach-Intestinal Dysfunction

Stomach Motility. There is little substantiating evidence to support the generally held concept of age-related degenerative changes in the musculature or physiologic capability of the stomach, small intestine, and large bowel.[4,7-8,18] As suggested in one review, problems more frequently relate to disease, poor general health, lack of physical activity, or use of drugs.[7] Van Liere and Northup[50] examined gastric emptying following a high carbohydrate meal (tagged with barium sulfate) in younger versus older (mean age = 71 years) men. Mean emptying time was 1.9 hours (range 1.3 to 2.8) in the older men as compared to 2.1 hours (range 1.0 to 3.1) in the younger. This meal, however, did consist of farina, an easily digested food; subjects were also allowed to move about, which could have enhanced gastric motility.

Gastric emptying has since been studied in relation to drugs requiring rapid assimilation.[15] Passage of a labeled test substance dissolved in 300 ml of orange juice was followed by a gamma scintillation camera.[15] The rate of emptying, expressed as the time required for half of the test dose to move into the duodenum, was 123 minutes in the older (mean age = 77 years) as compared to 50 minutes in the younger (mean age = 26 years) people tested. Although motility is enhanced by the presence of food in the stomach (this test was performed following an overnight fast), the fact remains that movement of food out of the stomach seems to be less rapid in older people. The clinical significance of this change is not clear.

Smaller, more frequent meals may be appropriate for the older person with abdominal distress. Large quantities of food remaining in the stomach for an extended period, particularly after a high fat meal, could add to feelings of distention and discomfort.

Intestinal Motility. Although it is assumed that decreased peristalsis and muscle tone are the cause of constipation in older people, evidence is lacking to confirm this idea.[8,19,47] Associated conditions such as hypothyroidism and hypokalemia can weaken muscle tone and propulsive contractions.[6] Pulmonary disease or general weakness in the frail individual contributes to colonic problems, although diet and drugs may be primary.[6]

It was believed that weakness and deterioration of the colonic muscle was responsible for the increased incidence of diverticulosis in older people. Further investigation, however, has revealed actual thickening of the musculature in some areas, suggesting that loss of neural control may prevent the colon from elongating normally despite the ability of the muscle to contract.[18,30] Deterioration of the neural ganglia can result in muscle spasms or uncoordinated contractions.

Colon dysfunction over a long period of time precipitated by poor bowel and dietary habits no doubt contributes to the development of diverticular disease; age-related factors may also be involved.

Constipation

General Considerations. It is estimated that constipation is a problem for at least 25% of older people.[30] Incidence is five times more frequent in the old than in the young.[36] Low intake of fluids, diets low in fiber and bulk, and various medications (i.e., diuretics, sedatives, antacids of aluminum hydroxide or calcium carbonate) can produce constipation.[6,11,30] Lack of exercise, reducing general muscle tone, contributes to the problem as does excessive intake of foods that harden the stool such as milk or processed cheese.[11,36]

Constipation is often more perception than fact as many older people have an exaggerated concern with bowel habits and the belief that a daily bowel movement is essential for good health. True constipation is characterized by (1) fewer than two bowel movements per week, (2) difficulty passing stools, (3) bleeding, or (4) pain with bowel movements.[36] Any bleeding from the rectum, persistent pain, or difficulty passing stools should be reported to a physician immediately. Chronic constipation requires medical evaluation.

Individuals with normal bowel function who do not have a bowel movement daily sometimes turn to laxatives in an effort to relieve the perceived problem. After the purging effect of the laxative, normal bowel movements may not resume the following day. This reinforces the idea that they are constipated and leads to a vicious cycle. Older people are among the most frequent abusers of laxatives.[11,30] Use of laxatives or enemas over a prolonged period results in loss of natural bowel function and can lead to chronic diarrhea. (Nutrient problems related to laxative abuse are discussed in Chapter 9.)

Fiber Intake. Increasing dietary fiber, fluid intake, and physical exercise can prevent constipation.[6,11-12] Diets generous in fiber produce large, soft stools and more frequent bowel movements. Fiber constituents act as a gel in holding water and increasing bulk. Adequate intake of fluids (1500 to 2000 ml daily) also contributes to formation of a soft stool.

Both physiologic and psychologic factors contribute to fiber-poor diets in older persons. Physical disability or lack of interest in cooking can increase the use of canned soups or prepared items often low in fiber. Abdominal distress may lead to avoidance of high fiber foods. Edentulous aged may depend on soft, highly processed items from which most of the fiber has been removed.

Fiber supplementation in a long term care facility eliminated any need for laxatives in 270 of the 300 residents.[24] Addition of bran to the hot breakfast cereal, increasing the crude fiber content from 4 to 6 gm to 6 to 8 gm, restored normal bowel function in 60% of the residents, most of whom had previously required laxatives. For those still troubled by constipation a blended supplement was developed composed of bran buds and prune juice with unsweetened applesauce to improve flavor and texture, providing 0.56 gm crude fiber per ounce. The supplement was given in 1-ounce increments until bowel habits approached normal. A third supplement of bran buds and prune juice was developed for those receiving tube feedings. Not only were patients more comfortable once the program was in place but cost savings for laxatives equaled $44,000 for the year.

Hull and coworkers[24] emphasize that initiation of such a program requires the cooperation of the dietary, nursing, and medical staffs as well as the patients themselves. During adaptation to the fiber diet (about 2 weeks) residents experienced flatulence, abdominal distress, and in some cases, more irregular bowel habits than when dependent on laxatives. Therefore all must be aware of potential difficulties and be prepared for the initial problems. Before initiating dietary treatment it is imperative that organic causes of constipation (i.e., bowel obstruction) be eliminated as contributing factors.

The older person living at home can alter food patterns to increase dietary fiber and fluid intake. Suggestions for avoiding or alleviating constipation are given below.[6,36]

1. Use whole grain breads and cereals.
2. Use liberal amounts of vegetables and fruits, either raw or cooked.
3. Limit highly processed foods and foods high in fat.
4. Use dried fruits such as prunes or figs, or prune juice, as often as possible. (Cost of dried fruits may prohibit their use.)
5. Drink plenty of fluids (6 to 8 glasses each day) unless advised otherwise by a physician because of renal or circulatory problems.
6. Try to go for a walk every day.
7. Limit use of antacids.
8. Develop regular bowel habits.

Gastrointestinal Distress

Abdominal discomfort following food ingestion can have many causes. Drugs such as digitalis, levodopa, or aspirin may be at fault.[41,48] Overconsumption of food or alcohol can produce gastrointestinal distress. Discomfort resulting from burning sensations caused by irritation of the stomach mucosa or distention often leads to constant swallowing in an effort to relieve the distress. Swallowing of air, however, results in belching and more discomfort.

Flatulence and intestinal gas can be a source of both annoyance and embarrassment.[48] Gas-forming vegetables such as cabbage and legumes, swallowing air, and chronic constipation add to the problem. People with chronic flatulence may have only a normal volume of gas; however, it passes back into the stomach causing distress.

Following are intake patterns that may relieve functional distress.

1. Divide food evenly among all meals rather than having one or two very heavy meals.
2. Avoid alcohol and highly seasoned foods.
3. Limit the amount of fat at any one meal and eat slowly.
4. Chew foods thoroughly; if edentulous, select foods that are soft enough to be handled easily.[48]

Anorexia or gastrointestinal complaints such as bloating, constipation, and heartburn can create emotional distress in the aged who often associate such problems with cancer or other serious disorders.[45,48] Conversely, psychologic stress or tension can itself lead to stomach and intestinal disorders. Client concerns should not be dismissed lightly. Evaluation for presence of organic disease is indicated.

ENZYME SECRETION AND DIGESTION

Problems in Evaluation

Studies evaluating digestive enzyme secretion in older people have been limited and results inconsistent. In some cases findings may have been influenced by the selection of institutionalized or hospitalized aged who may differ from independent-living older people in state of health and degree of chronic disease. Previous diet influences observed

Table 4-1. Age-related changes in digestive secretions

Secretion	Digestive Function	Level of Secretion (on stimulation)
Salivary amylase	Moistens food and aids in mastication and swallowing; breaks down starch to maltose	Decreased
HCl	Activates pepsin for protein digestion; some breakdown of sucrose to glucose and fructose	Decreased
Pepsin	Breaks down complex proteins to peptides and peptones	Decreased
Pancreatic juice	Contains pancreatic amylase, pancreatic lipase, and trypsin for digestion of carbohydrates, lipids, and proteins, respectively; neutralizes the acidity of chyme	No change
Pancreatic amylase	Breaks down most carbohydrates except cellulose to disaccharides	No change
Trypsin	Splits peptide bonds to form small polypeptides and amino acids	No change
Pancreatic lipase	Hydrolyses lipids to fatty acids and glycerol	Decreased
Bile	Emulsifies lipids to smaller fat particles for digestion; combines with lipids and fatty acids for absorption	No change

levels of digestive enzymes. Age-related changes also vary according to measurement under basal or stimulated conditions.

Although several digestive secretions decrease in older adults (Table 4-1) the functional significance of these changes is not understood. It is believed that enzyme levels (although sometimes reduced) are sufficient to adequately digest the food consumed.[4,19,51] This relates to the fact that digestive enzymes are normally secreted at levels substantially above that required, allowing a margin of safety. Bayless[4] notes that fat malabsorption does not become evident until pancreatic lipase secretion is decreased by 90%.

Degree of malabsorption caused by changes in digestive secretions is also influenced by the dietary habits of the individual. Consuming one or two very large meals rather than several smaller meals may result in some degree of malabsorption if enzyme levels are significantly reduced.[51] The form in which a nutrient is consumed (i.e., heme versus inorganic iron) may influence the digestive secretions required. Alkaline drugs that raise the pH of the stomach may exceed the capacity of parietal cells to maintain an acid pH. Therefore older people must be evaluated on an individual basis. At this time, however, there is no convincing evidence that lack of digestive secretions impairs nutrient absorption in healthy older people.

Digestion in the Mouth

Secretion of Salivary Amylase. Although both the level and ptyalin content of salivary amylase is reduced in older people, this has little significance as far as nutrient absorption is concerned.[34] Of greater importance is the reduction in fluid, which no doubt contributes to dry tongue, dry mouth, or problems in swallowing. In one report fluid secretion following stimulation by chewing was 14 ml versus 6 ml in younger and older persons, respectively.[34] That older group, however, ranged in age from 69 to 100 years and included an individual with very low (1.5 ml) secretion.

Digestion in the Stomach

Secretion of Gastric Juice. Both the total volume and hydrochloric acid concentration of gastric juice at basal and stimulated (by histamine injection) levels are reduced in older people.[16,34] Although the volume of gastric juice secreted at maximal levels differed by only 10% between older people (ages 60 to 75 years) and young controls (ages not given), the hydrochloric acid content was 25% lower in the older group.[16] Pepsin activity was also reduced by about one fourth in those beyond age 60. None of the individuals studied, despite significant decreases in digestive enzymes, reported abdominal discomfort after eating.

When calculated on the basis of body potassium content, gastric acid production does not change with age.[28] Sex differences in hydrochloric acid secretion (higher in males at younger ages) are also less obvious in older groups. Decreased acid production does not result from less stimulation by gastrointestinal hormones as serum gastrin levels did not differ between persons 18 to 45, or 46 to 71 years of age.[3] Fasting serum gastrin levels were actually higher in persons above 60 years of age. This was suggested to be a response to the lower stomach acid production in older individuals.

Changes in acid secretion and stomach pH can interfere with the conversion of inorganic iron from the ferric to ferrous form required for absorption. The possible influence of reduced pepsin on the effective breakdown of proteins has not been evaluated.

Change in Stomach Mucosa. Fikry[16] concluded that reduced gastric secretion was the result of both a loss in parietal cells as well as a decrease in the secretory capacity of existing cells. Atrophy or thinning of the stomach mucosa increases in both incidence and severity with advancing age.[9] Secretory cells are lost and in extreme cases the stomach lining takes on the appearance of the duodenum with simple epithelial cells.[9] When severe, atrophic gastritis can cause reduced secretion of intrinsic factor and subsequent vitamin B_{12} deficiency.

Digestion in the Small Intestine

Secretion of Pancreatic Enzymes. Available information regarding pancreatic secretions in older persons is sparse. Although Rosenberg and coworkers[43] compared individuals over and under 50 years of age they observed no age-related effect on either total pancreatic secretion or bicarbonate content following stimulation with secretin. Meyer and Necheles[34] comparing young controls with people age 69 and above reported a decline in basal but not stimulated secretions of pancreatic amylase and trypsin in the older group. Lipase was reduced by 20% under both fasting and stimulated conditions.

Bile salts appear to be secreted at normal levels in healthy older people although definitive evidence is lacking.[4] Gallbladder dysfunction does increase with age. Evaluation at autopsy of over 1000 persons above age 70 revealed that 35% had gallbladder problems at some point in their lives.[2] Nearly 6% had cholecystectomies whereas 29% had gallstones with no gallbladder surgery. Amberg and Zboralske[2] concluded that gallstones do not necessarily cause acute symptoms.

Evidence of a decrease in pancreatic lipase and the incidence of gallbladder abnormalities implies less efficient digestion of dietary fat. Impaired fat digestion may contribute to the fat intolerance among older people suggested earlier.

NUTRIENT ABSORPTION

Factors Influencing Absorption

Absorption is dependent on various factors including completeness of digestion, integrity of the intestinal mucosa, and blood supply to the absorption site.[18] Digestion is assumed to be reasonably complete, placing nutrients in the molecular or ionic form necessary. There appears to be a decrease in the number of follicles on the mucosal surface of the small intestine, but little is known regarding possible morphologic changes.[9] Physical alterations in the cell membrane are known to cause an age-related decline in the transport capacity of other organ cells, and this may be true for intestinal cells as well.[40]

Decreased blood perfusion might influence the rate if not degree of nutrient absorption. Reduced blood flow lowers the concentration gradient between the mucosal cell and the blood, slowing absorption.[40] Evidence for this concept comes from animal work evaluating drug absorption.[40] Compounds affected most by blood flow were those with the highest absorption rates. Sorbose absorption (occurring by passive diffusion) did not change when blood flow was only 10% the normal level. Rate of uptake of lipid soluble compounds decreased by half when blood flow fell by 35%. In light of the fact that blood perfusion to the intestinal region drops by 40% to 50% in older age groups, the influence of flow rate on absorption of specific nutrients should be examined.

Carbohydrate Absorption

Glucose Absorption. D-Xylose is customarily used to test absorption of sugars as the mechanism of active transport is similar to that of both glucose and galactose.[27,33] As digestion is not required, it serves as a test of intestinal mucosal function and adequacy of blood supply. Since D-xylose is not metabolized, rate and completeness of absorption have been determined by renal excretion. Because of the age-related decrease in blood flow to the kidneys and the subsequent reduction in glomerular filtration, reduced excretion of a test substance relates to renal impairment as well as possible changes in absorption.[33]

Several investigators evaluated the time course of appearance of xylose in the blood and reported no differences between young controls and older persons up to age 80.[20,27] After 1 hour blood xylose levels in those above age 80 were about half those in young controls.[20] Peak blood levels were also delayed in that group, occurring at 180 versus 120 minutes, and decreased more slowly.

The conclusion that xylose is easily absorbed although at a slower rate is further supported by the observation that excretion over a 5-hour period was similar in all age groups following an intra-venous or oral dose.[20] Although absorption is slowed in the older individual, there is no evidence to suggest that absorption is incomplete.

Animal work suggests that rate of absorption may be slowed as a result of a decrease in the height of the intestinal villi.[25] Also, glucose transport molecules have a lower affinity for substrate in older versus younger animals.[25] These findings have not been confirmed in humans.

Lactose Absorption. Reduced lactase levels and consequent lactose intolerance have been implicated in the low milk consumption of many older persons. In some individuals lactase activity in adulthood is very similar to that in infancy, while in others it drops to low levels.[29] Comparison of various age groups suggested that lactase activity (measured by intestinal biopsy) changed little before age 5.[29] Beyond that, one group (25%) developed low lactase activity while the others maintained their previous level. The low lactase group consumed little milk and when tested was clinically lactose intolerant. Those with normal lactase averaged about 1 quart of milk per day with no discomfort and were clinically normal.

The relationship between demonstrated lactase deficiency and symptoms following a glass of milk consumed with a meal has been one of controversy. An evaluation of milk drinking habits at a Title III-C congregate meal program revealed differences among racial and ethnic groups (Table 4-2).[31] Although a higher percentage of Mexican-Americans

Table 4-2. Percentage of Title III-C congregate meal participants not drinking milk

	Digestive Symptoms	General Dislike	Total
Mexican-Americans	6	9	15
Blacks	1	5	6
Whites	3	3	6

Modified from Marrs, D.C.: Milk drinking by the elderly of three races, J. Am. Diet. Assoc. **72:**495, 1978.

refused milk, other groups also indicated a dislike for milk or reported symptoms of intolerance. The type of milk available may be a critical factor, as a higher proportion of blacks chose buttermilk whereas relatively few of the Mexican-Americans chose that milk. Since buttermilk contains only about 0.5% less lactose than whole milk, it is questionable whether this would significantly influence acceptability. Marrs[31] suggests the cultural acceptance of milk may be as important as lactose tolerance in determining consumption.

An evaluation of 87 healthy Boston aged (mean age = 77 years)[42] confirmed that psychologic attitudes toward milk are as important, or more important, than physiologic factors in lactose intolerance. All persons were tested for lactose intolerance using hydrogen expiration following a 25 gm-lactose load. On subsequent days each was given in a double blind design 240 ml of a chocolate drink either lactose free or containing 4.5% (11 gm) lactose. Twenty-three subjects (26%) malabsorbed lactose on the basis of hydrogen expiration; however, none complained of symptoms during the actual test. The incidence of malabsorption was 70% to 75% among black, Jewish, and Italian subgroups, compared to 12% among Northern Europeans.

Malabsorption, however, was not related to incidence of digestive symptoms following ingestion of the two test beverages. About equal numbers (28% and 30% of absorbers and malabsorbers) reported symptoms after the lactose-containing drink. About one fifth of the malabsorbers complained of distress after both the lactose-containing and lactose-free chocolate drink, suggesting that a component other than lactose was causing the problem. Over half of the malabsorbers (based on hydrogen expiration) reported drinking more than one glass of milk per day.

Lactose malabsorption does not in itself appear to be a deterrent to milk consumption in most older people, particularly at the moderate levels of intake usually followed by this age group. Expectation of discomfort, whether based on known lactose intolerance or previous distress following milk drinking regardless of the cause, is an important consideration.

Fat Absorption

Human Studies. Both the rate and the absolute amount of fat absorbed appear to decrease with age.[5,32,37,51] The appearance of fat in the blood is both time-[32] and enzyme-dependent.[5] A peak in plasma lipids occurs about 2 hours later in aged as compared to young controls (5 versus 3 hours) following a test meal.[32] Labeled chylomicrons appeared at the same rate in both young and old when lipase was administered with the test fat.[5]

Screening older people with or without digestive symptoms reveals a significant number with incomplete fat digestion. Among 41 aged (62 to 96 years), institutionalized but generally free of organic disease, nearly 40% exhibited steatorrhea (fat was 20% to 56% dried fecal weight).[37] In 10 of the 17 the greater proportion of stool fat was neutral fat, indicating a failure of digestion. Normally, neutral fat comprises only a minor portion of fecal fat with fatty acids the predominate form. There was no indication, however, of the level of fat included in the normal diet of these individuals.

In practice, the level of fat fed at one meal influences the degree of both digestion and absorption. When older Swedes, age 67 to 72 years, were fed 115 gm fat daily, fecal fat ranged from 5 to 16 gm compared to 3 to 9 gm for young controls.[51] The excess fat excreted was predominately neutral fat. This does represent, however, a fat intake higher than is usually consumed by older people. Among older Michigan women daily fat intake ranged from 22 to 111 gm with a mean of 51 gm.[44]

In a subsequent evaluation the same level of fat (115 gm) was distributed across all meals and snacks; 10 to 40 gm were fed at one time.[51] Fecal fat dropped to 5 to 7 gm, equal to young controls. In general older people are able to tolerate and digest normal amounts of dietary fat if it is distributed over several meals. The amount of pancreatic lipase present appears to be the limiting factor.

Animal Studies. Work with animal models proposes that changes at the mucosal level also contribute to altered fat absorption.[23] There appears to be a decrease in mucosal surface area in older animals. In addition, fat is less efficiently incorporated into chylomicrons and released into the lymph. Whether similar cellular alterations contribute to age-related changes in fat absorption in humans is unknown.

Protein Absorption

Dietary Protein. Despite the importance of this nutrient to general health, evaluation of protein absorption in older people has been limited. Rate of digestion and degree of absorption do not, however, seem to differ in old and young adults at normal levels of intake. When Chinn and associates[14] fed a test meal of I[131] labeled albumin to 12 older people (72 to 88 years) and young controls, no differences were observed in the rate of appearance or level of isotope in the blood.

At protein levels of 1.5 gm/kg body weight or above, however, nitrogen excretion in the feces of older subjects exceeded young controls.[51] In seven older people fecal nitrogen ranged from 1.9 to 4.4 gm as compared to 1.9 to 2.2 gm for five young controls. On protein intakes of 1.0 gm/kg body weight fecal nitrogen in the older group did not exceed 2 gm (1 to 2 gm/24 hr is considered within normal range). With the exception of people undergoing rehabilitation, protein intake would generally not exceed 1.0 gm/kg body weight. Balance studies conducted with older persons using animal[49,53] or vegetable[13] protein have not reported problems in protein digestion and absorption as characterized by excessive levels of fecal nitrogen.

Amino Acid Absorption. Absorption of amino acids has been explored using animal models. Changes in amino acid uptake appear to be based

on body need. Arginine (an essential amino acid for young animals) was absorbed more rapidly by younger versus older animals, whereas lysine, essential throughout the life span, was absorbed and utilized equally well in animals of all ages.[38-39] Penzes[38] proposed that young animals may have more active carriers for amino acid transport than older animals.

In light of the current controversy regarding the protein needs of older individuals in general[17] and the apparent elevated requirement of some older people (see Chapter 5), possible changes in amino acid absorption need to be clarified.

Absorption of Vitamins and Minerals

Age-related alterations in absorption of vitamins and minerals are poorly understood. For the most part these nutrients have been studied in a clinical context considering age-related changes in nutritional status or incidence of deficiency disorders. For this reason absorption of minerals and the water soluble vitamins will be discussed in Chapters 6 and 7. Basic research focusing on molecular aspects of absorption has concentrated on the fat soluble vitamins.

Absorption of Vitamin A. The absorption of fat soluble vitamins, like the absorption of fat, is slowed in older individuals (Fig. 4-2).[52] Two hours following administration of 100,000 IU of vitamin A, serum vitamin levels were highest in men between ages 40 and 59 and lowest in those ages 80 to 89.[52] Not only did serum vitamin levels peak earlier in the youngest group but also they returned to basal levels more rapidly. Clearance of vitamins from the blood by the liver and other tissues occurred more rapidly in the young. Yiengst and Shock[52] suggest that both uptake and clearance rates are influenced by the increased blood flow and organ perfusion in younger versus older individuals.

Absorption in Animal Models. Work with animal models indicates that net absorption of fat soluble vitamins does not decrease with age.[21] In fact per-

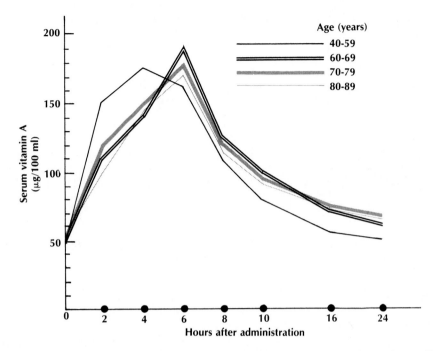

Fig. 4-2. Age-related differences in serum levels following administration of vitamin A. (From Yiengst, M.J., and Shock, N.W.: Effect of oral administration of vitamin A on plasma levels of vitamin A and carotene in aged males, J. Gerontol. **4:**205, 1949. Reprinted by permission of *The Gerontologist/The Journal of Gerontology.*)

cent absorption of a test dose was higher in the older group, a finding that Hollander and Morgan[21] attributed to increased body mass and vitamin need in the older larger animals. Although little is known regarding net absorption of vitamin A in older humans, reduced net absorption of vitamin D has been observed in older people (see Chapters 6 and 8).

SUMMARY

Disturbances of the gastrointestinal tract including dysphagia and constipation increase in number and severity in older age as a result of changes in muscle or neural control, dietary habits, and use of drugs. It has been established that secretion of several digestive enzymes is reduced in older versus younger individuals, although the functional significance of this finding is unknown.

Digestion and absorption of carbohydrate appear to be complete, although the rate of absorption is slowed in older individuals. Fat and protein absorption appear to be normal at usual levels of intake or when intake is spread over several meals throughout the day. The presence of neutral fat in the feces suggests that pancreatic lipase is limiting in some older individuals. Although it has been suggested that net absorption of vitamin A is not reduced in advanced age, further evaluation in human subjects is required.

REVIEW QUESTIONS

1. Describe the following gastrointestinal disorders: (a) gastrointestinal distress, (b) dysphagia, and (c) constipation. What are the nutritional implications of each?
2. Outline the age-related changes in secretion of digestive enzymes. What digestive problems could result from these changes?
3. It has been suggested that lactose intolerance is a major factor in the low milk consumption of many older persons. Do you agree? Cite experimental evidence to justify your conclusion.
4. Does the presence of neutral fat in the feces indicate a problem in digestion, absorption, or both? Explain.

REFERENCES

1. Agate, J.: Common symptoms and complaints. In Rossman, I., ed.: Clinical geriatrics, ed. 2, Philadelphia, 1979, J.B. Lippincott Co.
2. Amberg, J.R., and Zboralske, F.F.: Gallstones after 70, Geriatrics **20:**539, 1965.
3. Archimandritis, A., and others: Serum gastrin concentrations in healthy males and females of various ages, Acta Hepatogastroenterol. **26:**58, 1979.
4. Bayless, T.M.: Malabsorption in the elderly, Hosp. Pract. **14:**57, 1979.
5. Becker, G.H., Meyer, J., and Necheles, H.: Fat absorption in young and old age, Gastroenterology **14:**80, 1950.
6. Benson, J.A.: Simple chronic constipation: Pathophysiology and management, Postgrad. Med. **57:**55, 1975.
7. Berman, P.M, and Kirsner, J.B.: The aging gut. I. Diseases of the esophagus, small intestine, and appendix, Geriatrics **27:**84, 1972.
8. Berman, P.M., and Kirsner, J.B.: The aging gut. II. Diseases of the colon, pancreas, liver and gallbladder, functional bowel disease, and iatrogenic disease, Geriatrics **27:**117, 1972.
9. Bhanthumnavin, K., and Shuster, M.M.: Aging and gastrointestinal function. In Finch, C.E., and Hayflick, L., eds.: Handbook of the biology of aging, New York, 1977, Van Nostrand Reinhold Co., Inc.
10. Brandt, L., and others: Colitis in the elderly, Am. J. Gastroenterol. **76:**239, 1981.
11. Bulmash, J.M.: Confronting the three most common medical problems of long-term illness, Geriatrics **36:**79, 1981.
12. Burkitt, D.P., and Meisner, P.: How to manage constipation with high-fiber diet, Geriatrics **34:**33, 1979.
13. Cheng, A.H., and others: Comparative nitrogen balance study between young and aged adults using three levels of protein intake from a combination wheat-soy-milk mixture, Am. J. Clin. Nutr. **31:**12, 1978.
14. Chinn, A.B., Lavik, P.S., and Cameron, D.B.: Measurement of protein digestion and absorption in aged persons by test meal of I^{131} labeled protein, J. Gerontol. **11:**151, 1956.
15. Evans, M.A., and others: Gastric emptying rate in the elderly: Implications for drug therapy, J. Am. Geriatr. Soc. **29:**201, 1981.
16. Fikry, M.E.: Gastric secretory functions in the aged, Gerontol. Clin. **1:**216, 1965.
17. Food and Nutrition Board: Recommended dietary allowances, ed. 9, Washington, D.C., 1980, National Academy of Sciences.
18. Geokas, M.C., and Haverback, B.J.: The aging gastrointestinal tract, Am. J. Surg. **117:**881, 1969.
19. Goldman, R.: Decline in organ function with aging. In Rossman, I., ed.: Clinical geriatrics, ed. 2, Philadelphia, 1979, J.B. Lippincott Co.
20. Guth, P.H.: Physiologic alterations in small bowel function with age: The absorption of D-xylose, Am. J. Dig. Dis. **13:**565, 1968.
21. Hollander, D., and Morgan, D.: Aging: Its influence on vitamin A intestinal absorption in vivo by the rat, Exp. Gerontol. **14:**301, 1979.
22. Hollis, J.B., and Castell, D.O.: Esophageal function in elderly men: A new look at presbyesophagus, Ann. Intern. Med. **80:**371, 1974.
23. Holt, P.R., and Dominguez, A.A.: Intestinal absorption of triglyceride and vitamin D_3 in aged and young rats, Dig. Dis. Sci. **26:**1109, 1981.
24. Hull, C., Greco, R.S., and Brooks, D.L.: Alleviation of constipation in the elderly by dietary fiber supplementation, J. Am. Geriatr. Soc. **28:**410, 1980.
25. Jakab, L., and Penzes, L.: Relationship between glucose absorption and villus height in ageing, Experientia **37:**740, 1981.
26. Johnson, C.K., and others: Health, laxation, and food habit influences on fiber intake of older women, J. Am. Diet. Assoc. **77:**551, 1980.
27. Kendall, M.J.: The influence of age on the xylose absorption test, Gut **11:**498, 1970.
28. Kenney, R.A.: Physiology of aging, Chicago, 1982, Year Book Medical Publishers, Inc.
29. Leventhal, E., Antonowicz, I., and Shwachman, H.: Correlation of lactose activity, lactose tolerance, and milk consumption in different age groups, Am. J. Clin. Nutr. **28:**595, 1975.
30. Libow, L.S., and Sherman, F.T.: The core of geriatric medicine, St. Louis, 1981, The C.V. Mosby Co.
31. Marrs, D.C.: Milk drinking by the elderly of three races, J. Am. Diet. Assoc. **72:**495, 1978.
32. Matsumoto, S.: Studies on an in vivo fate of triglyceride of the old aged. I. Studies on digestion and absorption of

[131]I-triolein, J. Osaka City Med. Center **17**:29, 1968. (English summary.)

33. Mayersohn, M.: The "xylose test" to assess gastrointestinal absorption in the elderly: A pharmacokinetic evaluation of the literature, J. Gerontol. **37**:300, 1982.

34. Meyer, J., and Necheles, H.: Studies in old age. IV. The clinical significance of salivary, gastric and pancreatic secretion in the aged, JAMA **115**:2050, 1940.

35. Montgomery, R.D., and others: The ageing gut: A study of intestinal absorption in relation to nutrition in the elderly, Q. J. Med. **48**:197, 1978.

36. National Institute on Aging: Age page, Constipation, Washington, D.C., 1982, U.S. Department of Health and Human Services.

37. Pelz, K.S., Gottfried, S.P., and Soos, E.: Intestinal absorption studies in the aged, Geriatrics **23**:149, 1968.

38. Penzes, L.: Effect of concentration on the intestinal absorption of l-lysine in aging rats, Exp. Gerontol. **4**:223, 1969.

39. Penzes, L.: Intestinal transfer of l-arginine in relation to age, Exp. Gerontol. **5**:193, 1970.

40. Richey, D.P.: Effects of human aging on drug absorption and metabolism. In Goldman, R., and Rockstein, M., eds: Physiology and pathology of human aging, New York, 1975, Academic Press, Inc.

41. Roe, D.A.: Handbook: Interactions of selected drugs and nutrients in patients, Chicago, 1982, American Dietetic Association.

42. Rorick, M.H., and Scrimshaw, N.S.: Comparative tolerance of elderly from differing ethnic backgrounds to lactose-containing and lactose-free dairy drinks: A double-blind study, J. Gerontol. **34**:191, 1979.

43. Rosenberg, I.R., and others: The effect of age and sex upon human pancreatic secretion of fluid and bicarbonate, Gastroenterology **50**:191, 1966.

44. Schlenker, E.D.: Nutritional status of older women, Ph. D. thesis, E. Lansing, 1976, Michigan State University.

45. Sklar, M.: The gastrointestinal system. In Chinn, A.B., ed.: Working with older people, vol. IV., Clinical aspects of aging, Rockville, Md., 1971, U.S. Department of Health, Education, and Welfare.

46. Soergel, K.H., Zboralske, F.F., and Amberg, J.R.: Presbyesophagus: Esophageal motility in nonagenarians, J. Clin. Invest. **43**:1472, 1964.

47. Steinheber, F.V.: Interpretation of gastrointestinal symptoms in the elderly, Med. Clin. North Am. **60**:1141, 1976.

48. Straus, B.: Disorders of the digestive system. In Rossman, I., ed.: Clinical geriatrics, ed. 2, Philadelphia, 1979, J.B. Lippincott Co.

49. Uauy, R., Scrimshaw, N.S., and Young, V.R.: Human protein requirements: Nitrogen balance response to graded levels of egg protein in elderly men and women, Am. J. Clin. Nutr. **31**:779, 1978.

50. Van Liere, E.J., and Northrup, D.W.: The emptying time of the stomach of old people, Am. J. Physiol. **134**:719, 1941.

51. Werner, I., and Hambraeus, L.: The digestive capacity of elderly people. In Carlson, L.A., ed.: Nutrition in old age, Symposia Swedish Nutrition Foundation X, Stockholm, 1972, Almqvist & Wiksell.

52. Yiengst, M.J., and Shock, N.W.: Effect of oral administration of vitamin A on plasma levels of vitamin A and carotene in aged males, J. Gerontol. **4**:205, 1949.

53. Zanni, E., Callaway, D.H., and Zezulka, A.Y.: Protein requirements of elderly men, J. Nutr. **109**:513, 1979.

Chapter 5

Nutrient Requirements and Metabolism

The influence of age on the requirements and metabolism of the macronutrients is unclear. Dietary and serum lipid levels have received attention based on possible relationships with development of cardiovascular disorders. Most work examining protein and amino acid requirements utilized the balance technique, which is both laborious and subject to error. Methodology allowing estimation of protein turnover in various body compartments has contributed to present understanding of protein needs in both health and disease. Determination of protein requirements may be particularly important in older individuals whose protein intake can be limited by cost.

RECOMMENDED DIETARY ALLOWANCES

The Recommended Dietary Allowances (RDAs) are designed to provide an estimate of the nutrient needs of all healthy people (Table 5-1). For younger age groups considerable evidence is available on which to base recommendations. Because studies of older adults have been limited, the RDAs for those above age 50 have been extrapolated from those developed for younger adults.[37] For the majority of nutrients including protein and most vitamins and minerals recommended intakes are the same for younger (ages 23 to 50) and older (age 51 and above) adults.[11] Exceptions include the iron allowance for women, which decreases from 18 to 10 mg daily reflecting discontinued menstrual loss, and the thiamin, riboflavin, and niacin allowances

for men, which decline in response to lowered energy intake. Calories are the only nutrient for which there are adjustments beyond age 51, recognizing reduced energy needs after age 75 (see Chapter 3).

The existing RDAs, when applied to older adults, have many limitations. People age 51 differ

Table 5-1. Recommended daily dietary allowances (adults age 51 +)

	Males	Females
Protein (gm)	56	44
Vitamin A (μg retinol equivalents)	1000	800
Vitamin D (μg)	5	5
Vitamin E (mg α-tocopherol equivalents)	10	8
Vitamin C (mg)	60	60
Thiamin (mg)	1.2	1.0
Riboflavin (mg)	1.4	1.2
Niacin (mg niacin equivalents)	16	13
Vitamin B$_6$ (mg)	2.2	2.0
Folacin (μg)	400	400
Vitamin B$_{12}$ (μg)	3.0	3.0
Calcium (mg)	800	800
Phosphorus (mg)	800	800
Magnesium (mg)	350	300
Iron (mg)	10	10
Zinc (mg)	15	15
Iodine (μg)	150	150

Modified from Food and Nutrition Board: Recommended dietary allowances, ed. 9, Washington, D.C., 1980, National Academy of Sciences.

from those age 85 (and those age 23) in body composition, physiologic function, and metabolic adaptation (see Chapters 1 and 3). Munro[36-37] maintains it is therefore unrealistic to assume that all have similar nutrient requirements. Physiologic changes in efficiency of digestion or absorption (e.g., reduced secretion of intrinsic factor) may increase the need for a particular nutrient. Estrogen withdrawal following menopause alters calcium absorption and metabolism. At the same time reduced effectiveness of the renal system in excreting nitrogenous or other waste products contraindicates excessive intakes of protein or water soluble vitamins.

Another concern is the interrelation between particular nutrients and degenerative disease.[19] Chronic disease influences requirements both as a result of the disease process itself and in relation to drugs prescribed for therapeutic management. Impaired gallbladder function resulting in less efficient absorption of fat increases requirements for the fat soluble vitamins. Diuretics prescribed in the management of hypertension can lead to depletion of potassium, magnesium, zinc, pyridoxine, or folate depending on the particular drug.[45] For the older individual receiving constant drug therapy, the RDAs may not provide a realistic estimate of nutrient needs. Based on this premise Munro[36] has advanced the idea of developing recommendations for both healthy aged and those with chronic disease.

Harper[19] stresses the importance of evaluating each older client as an individual, considering general health, level of physical activity, and presence of chronic disease. Appropriate goals are (1) to prevent nutrient depletion and (2) to avoid providing excessive levels of nutrients that cannot be utilized and must therefore be excreted.[19] Either situation is undesirable for optimum health and wellbeing. At the same time there is a continuing need for detailed study of the nutrient requirements of older people. Special areas for emphasis might include nutrient requirements (1) beyond age 75 when physiologic limitations increase, (2) as influenced by long term drug use, and (3) in relation to disease processes.

CARBOHYDRATE REQUIREMENTS

Foods high in carbohydrate such as fruits, vegetables, and whole grain breads and cereals contribute energy, fiber, iron and trace minerals, and important vitamins including A, C, and folic acid to the diet. An unfortunate trend has been the substitution of high sucrose carbohydrate foods for complex carbohydrates containing fiber and other nutrients.[11] For older individuals consuming only limited calories, complex carbohydrates high in nutrient density should provide the major portion of carbohydrates consumed. Although there is no specific requirement for carbohydrate, as glucose can be obtained from the metabolic conversion of amino acids or glycerol, current guidelines suggest that about half of all calories be supplied by carbohydrate.[11]

Low carbohydrate diets advocated for weight loss in the popular press can result in ketosis as well as loss of potassium, sodium, body protein, and fluid. Diets that substitute protein for carbohydrate with a consequent increase in nitrogenous waste put a serious stress on the less efficient aged kidney. Fluid and electrolyte balance, already precarious in older persons with advanced cardiac or renal disease, can be further distorted. Clients seeking to lose weight should be made aware of the dangers of such regimens. Although the minimum level of digestible carbohydrate required for normal metabolic function is considered to be 50 to 100 gm per day (200 to 400 kcal),[11] older people should be encouraged to consume intakes above this level.

LIPID REQUIREMENTS AND METABOLISM
Essential Fatty Acid Requirements

Essential fatty acid deficiency in adults is virtually unknown under normal conditions, although it has been described in patients maintained on parenteral feedings not containing fat.[11] The minimum recommended intake for linoleic acid, the essential fatty acid, is expressed as 3% of total calories.[11] This recommendation assumes that less than 25% of total calories are provided by fat. When fat intake rises to 35% of total calories, an essential fatty acid intake that equals 8% to 10% of total calories is desirable. It is recommended that fat intake not exceed 35% of total calories. In light of the suggested association between dietary fat and cardiovascular disease, plus efforts at weight control, many older people are limiting both fat and calorie intakes. For an individual consuming 1800 kcal daily, linoleic acid intake calculated as 3% of total calories would equal 6 gm.

In a Michigan survey older women with fat intolerance were consuming diets low in both calories (1200 to 1600 kcal) and fat (30% of total calories); linoleic acid intakes were as low as 1 to 2 gm daily.[46] Hyperkeratosis of the skin on the elbows and knees was more frequent among those consuming less than 6 gm linoleic acid per day.

In a survey of 70 women[20] both independent-living and institutionalized, linoleic acid intakes were 6.4, 6.7, and 5.8 gm in those 62 to 75, 76 to 85, and 86 to 99 years of age, respectively. Energy intake over this age span decreased from 1434 to 1283 kcal; linoleic acid represented about 4% of total calories. Although linoleic acid intake decreased with age in the total group, this was not true for the institutionalized who had a mean intake of 6.8 gm as compared to 5.6 gm for those living in the community. Although no information was given regarding food served in the nursing home, the higher content of linoleic acid may reflect an effort to increase polyunsaturated fats and decrease saturated fats. Total fat intake was about the same for both institutionalized and those at home (52 versus 55 gm). Fat provided 36% of total calories in both groups.

Age-related changes in the epidermal and dermal skin layers and atrophy of the sebaceous glands

contribute to the skin problems commonly observed among the aged; however, limited intake of linoleic acid could aggravate such conditions. In an evaluation of fatty acid content of serum lipids in nearly 200 people ranging in age from infancy to 90 years, linoleic acid derivatives decreased in both sexes as a function of age.[24] Although the changes observed were not as great as those found in essential fatty acid deficiency, Holman and associates[24] considered them suggestive of declining status.

The Dietary Guide presented in Chapter 10 recommends 1 tablespoon of vegetable oil or the equivalent each day as a source of vitamin E and linoleic acid. This provides about 7 gm of linoleic acid at a cost of 125 kcal easily within the limitations of a low calorie diet. In view of the variation in calorie and fat intakes, however, consideration should be given to presenting the linoleic acid requirement as an absolute amount, as is the custom with other required nutrients.

Lipid Metabolism

Age-related alterations in lipid metabolism and their possible consequences are poorly understood. Available information relating to lipid synthesis and the excretion of bile acids has, for the most part, come from animal studies.[30] The focus of lipid research in humans has been measurement of serum cholesterol and lipoprotein fractions. As pointed out in Chapter 2, serum lipids have less association with coronary incidents after age 60 than before. Nevertheless, hyperlipidemia may still contribute to coronary risk in the eighth and ninth decades.[69]

Serum Cholesterol Levels. Although there is some evidence that serum cholesterol tends to increase until age 60 and then decline, such findings are not consistent.[6,23,64,69] Recent data from HANES (n = 13,671)[64] suggest that serum cholesterol continues to increase in women beyond age 64, although not in men (Fig. 5-1). Men have higher serum cholesterol levels than women until the fifth decade, at which time the situation is reversed. The

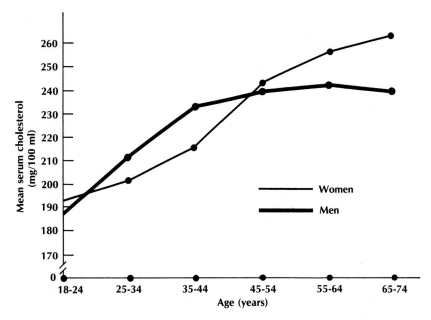

Fig. 5-1. Mean serum cholesterol levels by age and sex. (From United States Department of Health, Education, and Welfare: Total serum cholesterol levels of adults 18-74 years. United States, 1971-1974, DHEW Publication No. [PHS] 78-1652, Washington, D.C., 1978, U.S. Government Printing Office.)

increase in serum cholesterol among women above age 50 may be associated with estrogen withdrawal, as women of that age taking sex hormones have serum levels similar to men of equivalent age.[23]

Woldow,[69] observing 195 residents in a geriatric facility, reported that serum cholesterol levels continued to rise until age 70 and then stabilized (mean = 278 mg/100 ml), with a marked decline beyond age 80 (mean = 244 mg/100 ml). Thirty percent of the residents over age 75 were hyperlipidemic (cholesterol levels above 300 mg/100 ml), which may explain the somewhat higher serum levels of this group as compared with the general population age 65 to 74. According to Fig. 5-1, women of that age had serum cholesterol levels of 262 mg/100 ml, and men, 236 mg/100 ml.

Serum cholesterol also decreased in 70 older women ranging in age from 62 to 99. Values were 238, 226, and 217 mg/100 ml for age groups 62 to 75, 76 to 85, and 86 to 99, respectively.[20] These women had rather moderate intakes of fat (36% of total calories) and may have been receiving drug therapy to lower serum cholesterol levels. Even the youngest group (age 62 to 75) had a mean cholesterol level below that of the older women in the HANES report (238 versus 262 mg/100 ml).

Shock[50] reported a decrease in serum cholesterol levels beyond the sixth decade, based on repeated measurements on the same individuals. Therefore the age-related decline observed in population groups cannot be totally explained on the basis of higher mortality among hyperlipidemic individuals.

Differences in serum cholesterol can relate to genetic influences,[69] diet,[3] or degree of exercise.[17] Women seem to tolerate higher serum cholesterol levels than men at older ages. In the HANES report,[64] 29% of men age 65 to 74 had elevated serum cholesterol (>260 mg/100 ml), as compared to 49% of women. Further evidence for genetic involvement is the observation that adult children of hypercholesterolemic aged have higher serum cholesterol levels than offspring of normal cholesterolemic aged (304 versus 260 mg/100 ml).[69]

Physical exercise appears to play a role in reducing serum cholesterol. Swiss farmers in a mountain village consuming an average of 102 gm fat per day with 86 gm from animal origin had serum cholesterol levels in the range of 160 mg/100 ml at age 60 and beyond.[17] Sedentary individuals from a nonfarm area with similar diets, body weights, and smoking habits had serum cholesterol levels 20 to 30 mg higher than the farmers.

Albanese and coworkers[3] evaluated the effect of diet upon serum cholesterol in 136 institutionalized older women (age range = 68 to 100 years) over a 10-year period. Mean caloric intake was 1560 kcal with about 40% derived from fat. Substitution of vegetable oil for animal fat in food preparation resulted in a change in P/S (polyunsaturated to saturated) ratio from about 0.1 to 0.7. Although serum cholesterol levels fell markedly during the first 2 years on the diets with higher P/S ratios, they slowly returned to former levels during the subsequent 2 years. Women with elevated serum cholesterol levels demonstrated both a greater decline than those with normal levels and a more rapid return to original levels. One factor that could have influenced these findings is the relatively high intake of total fat (40% of calories). Nevertheless, these results suggest that dietary manipulation will have only limited success in reducing serum cholesterol in older people.

Serum Triglyceride Levels. Serum triglyceride levels follow the same general pattern as serum cholesterol, a gradual age-related increase with a decline beyond age 70.[16,20,69] Among 167 men and women from 18 to 77 years of age, fasting triglyceride levels increased an average of 16 mg/100 ml/decade until age 60 to 69 and then declined (peak mean value was about 130 mg/100 ml).[16] In another report serum levels declined only slightly in women between ages 62 and 99 (171 versus 162 mg/100 ml).[20] That group included both institutionalized and independent-living individuals.

In contrast, Woldow[69] reported a marked decline in serum triglycerides among 195 older residents of a geriatric facility. Mean levels were 155, 129, and 102 mg/100 ml in persons age 61 to 70, 71 to 80, and 81 and above, respectively. Woldow considered the lower levels observed in the older age groups to reflect, at least in part, the earlier death of hyperlipidemic individuals, as the death rate from coronary heart disease and myocardial infarction was higher in the hyperlipidemic group.

The association of HDL (alpha-lipoprotein) with lowered susceptibility to coronary heart disease has led to evaluation of age-related changes in this fraction.[14] HDL changes little between ages 20 and 60 in both sexes,[23] although it is always higher in women[23] and in men with lowered incidence of peripheral vascular disease.[47] A relationship between the HDL fraction and longevity is suggested by the high levels of HDL observed among octogenarians.[14] Life expectancy among those kindred groups was 9 to 11 years higher than for the general population, suggesting a genetic component.

Lipid Deposition in Tissues. Lipid deposition leads to arterial disease, which is commonly associated with aging. Crouse and associates,[9] evaluating cholesterol content of human tissues obtained at autopsy from persons age 23 to 78, found less increase (22% to 28%) in muscle, skin, and adipose tissue, as compared to connective tissue, in which cholesterol increased from 130% to 460% over the age range described, with major increases occurring after age 40.

Age-related changes include not only total accumulation but also type of lipid deposited. In the human aorta (observations based on 41 samples), total lipid increased from 4.4 to 10.9 mg/100 mg dry tissue between ages 15 and 65.[51] Cholesterol ester increased by a factor of 10 (0.55 to 5.11 mg/ 100 mg), and in the oldest age group comprised 47% of total lipid, as compared to 12% in the teenage group. Phospholipid on an absolute basis increased by about 40% over the age range studied, but it decreased as a proportion of total lipid (42% versus 24%).

Lipid accumulation may result from a decrease in enzymes required for hydrolysis of cholesterol esters. In animal species that are relatively resistant to atherosclerosis, lipolytic enzyme activity increases with age.[29] Comparable data are not available for humans.

Aspects for Future Consideration

Although all species appear to increase body cholesterol as a consequence of age, animal studies suggest that genetic influences control the rate of cholesterol synthesis at younger ages and therefore the total body pool at older ages.[30] This implies that human populations also differ in their vulnerability to hyperlipidemia. Kindred similarities in HDL levels and longer life expectancy lend credence to this idea and should continue to be explored.[14] Another area for study is the role of the phospholipid sphingomyelin in the prevention of lipid accumulation.[29] Found in rat plasma, this compound may be the basis of rats' resistance to arterial disease. Sphingomyelin prevents the uptake of cholesterol by cells in culture.

On a practical basis increasing physical exercise can decrease age-related lipid accumulation. Animals subjected to strenuous physical activity had significantly less lipid accumulation in the muscle than sedentary animals.[6-7] What effect exercise may have on lipid accumulation in connective and vascular tissue, the site of most concern in humans, is not known. In the Swiss farmers intense physical exercise was associated with decreased serum cholesterol, suggesting a positive effect.[17] At present increasing energy expenditure appears to be an appropriate alternative by which an individual might modify age-related changes in lipid metabolism.

EVALUATION OF PROTEIN REQUIREMENTS

Uncertainties in Protein Requirements

Evaluating protein requirements is tedious, time-consuming, and imprecise. Although information exists regarding the protein needs of young adults, relatively little is known regarding changes, if any, that occur over adult life. Because protein requirements are related to protein synthesis and lean body mass, changes in body composition can influence needs. Emotional and physical stress, known to increase protein requirements is common among older persons with chronic disease and personal losses. Finally, the relatively low caloric intake of many aged (see Chapter 3) could influence the utilization of ingested protein. Such factors make the older individual more vulnerable to protein inadequacy.

Body Need for Protein

Protein Needs of Adults. Protein metabolism continues as a dynamic process throughout adult life.[18] Although growth has ceased, sufficient protein must be consumed to replace body nitrogen losses in the form of desquamated cells, body secretions, and metabolic end products. In the older individual positive nitrogen balance is associated with repletion of body protein stores following illness, malnutrition, or stress. When nitrogen excretion exceeds intake, as occurs following surgery, in debilitating illness, or in adrenal corticosteroid therapy, protein depletion ensues. Although nitrogen balance reflects the sum total of nitrogen gain or loss, it does not provide answers as to the relative gain or loss of individual tissues.[18] Hegsted[22] pointed out that an adult is seldom in nitrogen equilibrium but rather has fluctuating periods of positive and negative balance that on the average produce net balance.

Loss of Body Nitrogen. Even well-nourished adults appear to lose body nitrogen as a function of age. As described in Chapter 3 lean body mass decreases beyond middle age. It has been estimated that body nitrogen decreases from 1320 gm in the young adult to 1070 gm in the aged adult.[73] Although age-related losses in specific tissues are poorly defined, skeletal muscle contributes a major portion of the protein lost as compared with vital organs such as heart or liver.[38] Muscle comprises 25% of body weight in the newborn, increases to 45% in the young adult, and declines to 27% beyond age 70, the last value close to that of infants. Liver, which comprises 4% of body weight in newborns, declines consistently from 3% in the young adult to 2% in the aged adult.[38]

Changes in body nitrogen content have led to different interpretations regarding the protein requirements of older people.[73] First, a decrease in active metabolic tissue and protein synthesis could reduce the need for protein or amino acids. An alternate point of view is that inadequate intake of nitrogen or protein over adulthood ultimately leads to the observed loss in body nitrogen. Evaluations of protein metabolism and nitrogen requirements have not resolved this question.

Changes in Protein Metabolism

Measuring Protein Turnover. Research methods utilizing 3-methylhistidine, a nonmetabolizable amino acid reflecting muscle mass, have made possible the quantification of protein synthesis and degradation in various body compartments.[31,72] Released as a breakdown product of the muscle proteins actin and myosin, 3-methylhistidine is quantitatively excreted in the urine in proportion to total muscle protein turnover. Animal studies have confirmed the validity of 3-methylhistidine excretion as a reliable measure of muscle protein turnover[72]; however, valid interpretation of such data in older age groups requires urinary creatinine as a standard

to quantify total muscle mass. Reduced excretion of 3-methylhistidine in an older versus a younger adult could be interpreted as reflecting decreased protein turnover when in fact it is related to decreased muscle mass.

This method also has application for assessing muscle protein metabolism in pathologic conditions such as protein-calorie malnutrition, infection, or chronic disease.[72] In that situation total nitrogen excretion is also a useful measure. Normally, protein breakdown and protein synthesis are linked, with no net gain or loss in muscle protein. Following an uncomplicated physical injury 3-methylhistidine levels may not change, suggesting no increase in tissue breakdown. Urinary nitrogen, however, will increase, indicating a decrease in subsequent protein synthesis. Under severe physical stress such as infection, 3-methylhistidine levels will increase, indicating accelerated breakdown of muscle protein. Use of this method with appropriate interpretation can provide needed information regarding protein losses and requirements during prolonged therapy with corticosteroids or in those confined to bed or immobilized for long periods of time.

Rate of Protein Synthesis. Comparisons of older and younger adults reveal that total muscle protein turnover as measured by 3-methylhistidine decreases by about 30% in older men and 50% in older women when calculated on the basis of body weight; however, when protein synthesis is related to total muscle mass and calculated per gram urinary creatinine, there are no significant age differences.[63] Rate of muscle protein breakdown is 30.2 gm protein/gm creatinine in young men as compared to 31.9 gm in older men. Therefore the reduction in protein turnover reflects the loss of muscle mass; protein breakdown and synthesis in remaining muscle continue at the same rate as before.

N^{15}-Glycine has been used to estimate total body protein turnover.[63] This value when combined with estimates of muscle protein turnover obtained using 3-methylhistidine provides an indication of the relative contribution of muscle and visceral compartments to total protein turnover. The decrease in muscle mass results in a shift in protein synthesis toward the visceral compartment. In the young adult muscle accounts for 27% of total body protein turnover; in the aged adult it accounts for only 20%. Conversely, visceral organs make a greater contribution to protein metabolism in the older individual. This is the opposite of what occurs during the period of growth, when muscle assumes a greater proportion of total body protein turnover.

Because the rate of protein turnover is believed to be higher in visceral organs (i.e., liver or heart) than in muscle, the rate of protein synthesis when calculated per kilogram body cell mass (muscle + viscera) is actually higher in older than younger men (8.8 versus 7.5 gm/day).[68] Young and others[73] suggest that the proportionate increase in protein synthesis in visceral organs allows more efficient utilization of amino acids which are usually transported first to the liver.

The skeletal muscle serves as a pool of amino acids during adaptation to changes in protein intake, physical injury, or stress. The age-associated decrease in this compartment may increase the vulnerability of the older person to the nutritional environment.[63]

PROTEIN REQUIREMENTS IN THE AGED

Obligatory Nitrogen Loss

Despite the general assumption that older people are less able to adapt to a change in nutrient intake, their nitrogen excretion is reduced on a protein-free diet. In a comparison of young men (mean age = 21), older men (mean age = 71), and older women (mean age = 76)[49,62] neither the time required for urinary nitrogen to reach minimum levels nor the rate of decrease in urinary nitrogen differed among groups. Number of days required to reach stabilization was 4.6 in the young men, 5.0 in the older men, and 4.5 in the older women. Daily obligatory urinary nitrogen losses (following stabilization) were 2.74 and 2.37 gm in the young and older men and 1.54 gm in the older women. Differences in nitrogen excretion between the

Table 5-2. Daily obligatory nitrogen loss according to age and sex

	Young Men	Older Men	Older Women
Urinary nitrogen loss			
mg/kg body weight	37.2	34.5	24.4
mg/mg creatinine excretion	1.6	2.2	2.1
mg/kg body cell mass	77	98	90
Total obligatory nitrogen loss (mg/kg body weight, adjusted for fecal, skin, and other losses)	54	52	39
Safe level of nitrogen intake (mg/kg body weight, increased by 30% to allow for efficiency of nitrogen utilization and an additional 30% to allow for individual variability)	91	87	67
Safe level of protein intake (gm/kg body weight)	0.57	0.55	0.42

younger and older men reflect differences in body composition, as body weight was similar (73.5 versus 71.9 kg).

Obligatory nitrogen losses are influenced by both body composition and age-related changes in protein turnover within various body compartments.[38,49,62] Differences in nitrogen losses per kilogram body weight (Table 5-2) between males and females, regardless of age, relate to the higher proportion of muscle in males (see Chapter 3). Differences in obligatory nitrogen losses calculated on the basis of either creatinine excretion or body cell mass relate to age rather than sex.

It is believed that increased nitrogen excretion per unit of body cell mass in advanced age is the result of the shift in protein turnover from muscle to visceral organs.[49,62] Scrimshaw and coworkers[49] noted that body cell mass is heterogeneous, and the aging process may change not only the proportions of particular tissues but also the metabolic activity within particular tissues. Age-related changes may have a different effect on the rate of protein turnover in muscle as compared to visceral organs, although no human data are presently available. Changes in size of body compartments also contribute to obligatory nitrogen loss, as Zanni and coworkers[74] found no differences in nitrogen losses calculated on the basis of creatinine excretion or body cell mass in older men with preserved muscle mass.

Although data are limited, it appears that total obligatory nitrogen losses do not differ significantly on the basis of age. Mean losses have been estimated to be 54 mg/kg body weight in young males and 52 mg/kg body weight in older males (Table 5-2).[49,62] The influence of age-related changes on tissue protein turnover, however, are poorly understood. Protein requirements per se may still differ between old and young, despite similar nitrogen losses, if dietary protein is less efficiently utilized. Nitrogen balance studies have attempted to examine the issue of protein replacement in the older person.

Nitrogen Balance Studies

Discrepancies Between Balance and Factorial Methods. Estimates of protein requirements from balance studies do not always agree with those from factorial calculations. Factorial estimates of obligatory nitrogen loss, adjusted to allow for efficiency of utilization and individual variability, predict a safe level of protein intake to be 0.42 gm/kg body weight/day for older women and 0.55 gm for older men.[62] These values are lower than those suggested for young adults (0.52 and 0.57 gm/kg body weight/day for women and men, respectively). Older people receiving egg protein, however, were unable to maintain nitrogen equilibrium on the "safe" levels of intake suggested for either young or aged adults.[61]

Nitrogen balance on graded levels of egg protein was evaluated in seven men (age range = 68 to 74 years) and seven women (age range = 70 to 84 years) who, after 1 week of standardization, were randomly placed on three experimental protein levels for a period of 10 days each. As described in Fig. 5-2, neither men nor women were in nitrogen equilibrium on daily intakes below 0.7 gm/kg body weight.[61] Although factorial calculations suggest (Table 5-2) that 67 mg nitrogen/kg body weight is sufficient to allow for individual variability, older women were losing nitrogen at dietary levels above 75 mg nitrogen/kg body weight. Uauy and associates[61] concluded that the inability of many older individuals to maintain a consistent pattern precludes the determination of a minimum protein requirement.

A recent study evaluated, over a 30-day balance period, the adequacy of the current RDA for protein (0.8 gm/kg body weight) fed as egg protein to older men (mean age = 75) and women (mean age = 78).[13] Energy requirements were calculated for each individual. Nitrogen balance was determined over the last 5 days of each 10-day period. After 30 days, four of eight women and three of seven men were still in negative nitrogen balance. Among the men, nitrogen balance ranged from

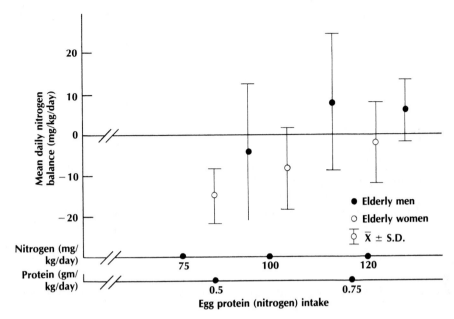

Fig. 5-2. Nitrogen balance in aged subjects on graded levels of egg protein. (From Uauy, R., Scrimshaw, N.S., and Young, V.R.: Human protein requirements: Nitrogen balance response to graded levels of egg protein in elderly men and women, Am. J. Clin. Nutr. **31:**779, 1978.)

+18.6 to −16.1 mg/kg body weight/day; in the women these values were +11.5 to −14.0 mg. Nitrogen balance did improve over the 30-day period in the men, although improvement in the women was slight. At the end of the first 10-day period, all men and six of eight women were losing nitrogen. Hemoglobin values declined slightly over the balance period, although this change was significant only in women (initial level = 13.7 gm/100 ml; final level = 13.0 gm/100 ml).

Increased vulnerability of women to protein loss, as suggested by the decrease in hemoglobin level, could relate to reduced muscle mass.[13] As mentioned earlier, skeletal muscle is vital to nutritional adaptation. Gersovitz and coworkers[13] concluded that the current RDA for protein (even high quality protein) is not sufficient to maintain nitrogen equilibrium in many persons above age 70.

Controversy Regarding Requirement. Other reports have proposed that daily protein intakes above 0.8 gm/kg body weight are required to maintain nitrogen equilibrium in older people.[1-2,28,40-41] Kountz and coworkers,[28] evaluating protein needs over a 6-month period in four previously malnourished men (ages 69 to 76), concluded that intakes of 0.7 gm/kg body weight were not sufficient to replace body protein, and they recommended a level of at least 1.4 gm/kg. Healthy older women, age 52 to 74 years, required protein intakes of 0.7 to 1.3 gm/kg body weight for nitrogen equilibrium.[44] Over a 5-year period, nine healthy institutionalized women with an average protein intake of 0.8 to 1.0 gm/kg had a net gain of 0.7 to 2.4 gm nitrogen.[2]

Zanni and coworkers[74] maintain that older men can achieve nitrogen equilibrium on protein intakes of 0.59 gm/kg body weight, about equal to the FAO/WHO recommendation of 0.57 gm/kg body weight. The discrepancy between these findings and those suggesting protein needs above 0.8 gm/kg body weight could relate to both the individuals evaluated and the experimental protocol.[13] Those fed the lower protein diet (0.59 gm/kg body wt) consumed a protein-free diet immediately prior to the test diet.[74] Prior depletion could have increased nitrogen retention when protein was restored.[13] In addition, the men achieving nitrogen equilibrium on lesser protein were younger; five of six were below age 70.[74] Of the men given 0.8 gm/kg body weight, six of seven were age 72 or above.[13] Moreover, the latter, although ambulatory, had various chronic problems such as heart disease and gastrointestinal disorders for which they were taking medication. Therefore nitrogen absorption and utilization may have been less efficient.

Such individuals, however, are representative of an older population for whom protein requirements appear to be increased. Individuals above age 70 with disease impairments should be encouraged to consume at least the recommended level of protein.

Factors Influencing Protein Requirements

Previous History. According to Horwitt,[25] metabolic response is influenced more by the type and level of protein consumed during the previous months than by current intake. As long as 3 months may be required to adapt to a low protein intake when previous intake has been liberal. This factor could influence results obtained on a balance study when the adaptation period is only a few days. An individual with marginal protein status and limited protein reserves may present strongly positive nitrogen balance when placed on a high protein diet and protein stores are being repleted.[61] Alternatively, a well nourished individual may not demonstrate protein retention regardless of the level and quality of protein fed.

On a self-selected diet, older women were able to maintain positive nitrogen balance at a lower level of protein intake than when fed a test diet with added milk.[44] One individual, age 52, retained 1.5 gm nitrogen/day on a self-selected diet containing 9.3 gm nitrogen. On a test diet containing 10.3 gm nitrogen, she lost 1.1 gm nitrogen daily. Similarly, a 74-year-old retained 1.8 gm nitrogen daily on a self-selected diet of 9.5 gm nitrogen, as compared to 1.0 gm on a test diet of 9.9 gm.

Individuals may, over a lifetime, adapt to a diet actually considered inadequate by general standards. DaCosta and Moorhouse[10] described two older people (man of 76 years; woman of 81 years) who generally consumed about 30 gm protein daily. Their serum albumin levels were 4.8 and 4.1 gm/100 ml, and both were in good health. An individual adapted to a particular type and level of protein appears to retain that accommodation throughout life, if reasonable health is maintained. Previous diet should be considered when developing a therapeutic regimen for an older person.

Individual Variability. Protein requirements vary both among individuals of a particular age and sex group as well as within the same individual from one period to another. In one series healthy, active, normal weight older women had a reduced need for protein as compared to overweight, inactive women with numerous health complaints.[41] Although intakes were moderate (0.6 to 0.8 gm/kg body weight) those in good health had a consistent pattern of intake over many years. The women in poor health had an irregular meal pattern with low intakes of milk, fruits, and vegetables. More than 1.0 gm protein/kg body weight was required to maintain nitrogen equilibrium in the latter, with higher protein intakes producing continued nitrogen retention.

Emotional upset as well as physical stress can result in nitrogen loss and increase protein requirements.[44,53] Inflammation or infection produces negative nitrogen balance and loss of labile body proteins, mediated in part by the stress response of adrenal corticosteroid hormones.[5] Chronic diseases can lead to nitrogen loss over an extended period.

Emotional stress is equally detrimental to nitrogen balance, and even liberal protein intakes may not be sufficient to prevent nitrogen loss if distress is severe. On receiving news that her son was injured an older woman lost 20 gm of nitrogen within 5 days, despite a daily intake of 1800 kcal and 1.0 gm protein/kg body weight. When assured of his safety the following week, she retained nitrogen equal to the amount lost.[66]

Swanson[53] described an older woman living alone who went from negative to positive balance on an equivalent level of protein when a grandson came to live with her and her psychologic outlook improved. As pointed out in Chapter 1, many older people endure constant emotional stress relating to fears concerning their health, financial worries, or loneliness. The long term impact of such distress on nitrogen balance has not been evaluated.

Energy Intake. Classic studies in protein metabolism described the protein-sparing action of carbohydrate and fat and pointed to the need for sufficient calories to promote utilization of protein and amino acids. Balance studies with older people of both sexes indicate that protein and calorie intakes are intimately related[27,40]; when calories are limited, protein metabolism is compromised regardless of protein intake. Older women could not maintain nitrogen equilibrium on protein intakes of 50 to 60 gm daily (0.8 gm/kg body weight) when caloric intake fell below 1500.[40] At least 1800 kcal per day were required to ensure nitrogen retention. Adding 400 kcal to the diet in the form of either carbohydrate or fat increased nitrogen retention in older men to the same extent as adding 5 to 10 gm protein.[27]

Recent work suggests that adults require excessive calories to maintain nitrogen balance when consuming the FAO/WHO standard (0.57 gm egg protein/kg body weight for men).[12] Young adult men required 46 to 50 kcal/kg body weight to avoid nitrogen loss. Current RDA guidelines suggest 33 to 34 kcal/kg body weight for men and women age 51 to 75, and 29 kcal/kg body weight for those age 76 and over.

Differences in energy intake very likely contribute to the conflicting results observed in nitrogen balance studies of older adults. The five older men (ages 60 to 72) studied by Cheng and coworkers[8] who maintained equilibrium (-0.04 to $+0.60$ gm nitrogen/day) on 0.8 gm protein/kg body weight had energy intakes of 40 kcal/kg body weight. The older individuals studied by Gersovitz and coworkers[13] who were apparently unable to achieve nitrogen equilibrium on that level of protein were consuming 29 to 32 kcal/kg body weight. Garza and coworkers[12] maintain that excessive calorie intakes should not be recommended in general practice as a means of promoting efficient use of ingested protein. Intakes approaching 3000 kcal are not feasible for older individuals unable to carry on high levels of physical exercise.

The additional nitrogen retained as a result of increasing calories appears to be handled differently from that retained when protein is increased.[12] Serum albumin and transferrin and other labile protein stores increase when protein is added to a marginal diet. In contrast, nitrogen retained when calories are increased is not as easily lost when energy intake is reduced to former levels. The fact remains, however, that the relatively low caloric intakes of some older people, particularly women, may contribute to poor utilization of ingested protein. In the HANES report[65] median energy intake of women age 65 and over was 1239 kcal. Encouraging physical activity to allow greater flexibility in caloric intake should be a priority in all nutritional counseling.

Recommended Intake of Protein

The question of protein needs of the aged is far from being resolved. Although one report[13] suggests that the RDA of 0.8 gm protein/kg body weight is not sufficient to maintain nitrogen equilibrium, others[74] conclude that 0.59 gm/kg body weight is appropriate for healthy aged. The RDAs of 56 and 44 gm protein for men and women, respectively, which take into account individual variation as well as the efficiency of utilization of a mixed diet, are considered realistic.[11] The Food and Nutrition Board[11] also recommends that protein contribute 12% or more of total calories as, unlike energy needs, protein requirements do not decrease with age.

The relative adequacy of the RDA, however, may be contingent on the health status of the individual evaluated. Munro[38] considers the current allowance to be appropriate for healthy aged with little chronic disease. For those undergoing physiologic or psychologic stress, such levels may not be adequate. This view finds support in the fact that older people with medical problems and high levels of medication appear to require protein levels above those recommended. For those who are physically fit, the current RDA will likely maintain a desirable status.

Individuals with chronic or debilitating disease involving the gastrointestinal tract or those requiring high levels of medication should be monitored closely for signs of protein-calorie malnutrition (i.e., deficient serum albumin). In light of the reduced renal function associated with advanced age, protein intakes above 1.0 gm/kg body weight should not be recommended without medical supervision. For most older people, a protein intake 12% to 14% of total calories is a reasonable goal.[38]

Amino Acid Requirements

Balance Studies with Amino Acids. Protein requirements have been defined on the basis of body need for essential amino acids, supplemented with nonspecific nitrogen. Early efforts to define amino acid requirements used the balance technique. Essential amino acids were fed in synthetic form with nonessential nitrogen provided as glycine, diammonium citrate, or a mixture of nonessential amino acids. Findings, however, have not been consistent.

Tuttle and coworkers,[57-59] in a series of balance studies conducted with men age 52 to 73, suggested that older individuals may have higher requirements for essential amino acids than younger individuals. All five older men fed 44 gm protein with 19 gm supplied as essential amino acids in the proportion found in egg protein were in negative nitrogen balance.[57] Younger men fed similar diets were in nitrogen equilibrium. Caloric intake may have influenced these results; the younger men were given 45 to 50 kcal/kg body weight, whereas energy intake among the older subjects averaged 30 to 41 kcal/kg.

In another evaluation, younger individuals were able to avoid negative nitrogen balance on intakes of 7 gm nitrogen when 1.0 to 1.3 gm were provided by essential amino acids.[59] This level of nitrogen met the requirement of only one of four older men; three of four required 1.8 to 2.4 gm essential amino acid nitrogen to maintain equilibrium. Tuttle and coworkers[59] suggested that individual variability may be greater in older than younger adults.

Both the source and amount of nonessential nitrogen may influence the level of essential amino acids required for nitrogen balance. Nitrogen retention was increased in older men when nonessential nitrogen was supplied as a mixture of nonessential amino acids, rather than totally as glycine.[59] Increasing the nonessential nitrogen fed appears to increase the essential amino acid requirement in older individuals. When total nitrogen intake rose from 7 to 15 gm with no increase in essential amino acids, negative nitrogen balance ensued in seven of eight older subjects (age 59 to 71).[58] This would suggest that older individuals consuming high levels of poor quality protein, low in essential amino acids, may be at risk of essential amino acid deficiency.

Evaluation of specific essential amino acids suggests that older men have higher requirements for methionine and lysine than younger men.[60] Tuttle and coworkers[60] proposed that the apparent increased need for methionine results from a defect in the conversion of methionine to cystine. In contrast Watts and coworkers,[67] feeding essential amino acids in the milk pattern (lower in sulfur-containing amino acids than egg protein) to older men (ages 65 to 84), observed no increase in amino acid requirements in older men. In fact, they found the methionine requirement of their older subjects to be about half that of younger adults. This group of older men was fed nonessential nitrogen in the form of glycine, other amino acids, and diammonium citrate to make a total intake of 10 gm nitrogen. Energy intake ranged from 27 to 43 kcal/kg body weight.

As pointed out by Young and coworkers,[73] differing conclusions may result from the limited numbers of subjects and differences among individuals, as well as errors inherent in the balance method. Studies also differed in the calorie level, total amount of nitrogen, and source of nonessential nitrogen fed.

Plasma Amino Acid Response Curve. Recent work defining amino acid requirements has used the plasma amino acid response curve.[55-56] In contrast to the balance method which requires extended metabolic collections, the plasma response method requires only the measurement of free amino acids in the plasma. Plasma amino acid levels demonstrate a linear relationship with dietary amino acid levels.[55] Plasma levels fall rapidly when intake is reduced, but they finally reach a plateau level that remains constant despite further reductions in intake. The dietary intake at which this plateau occurs is considered to represent the minimum physiologic requirement for that amino acid.

Comparisons of the amino acid requirements of young and old adults based on the plasma response curve suggest that need for essential amino acids, calculated on the basis of body weight, may change with age, although the direction of change is not consistent. Minimum tryptophan requirements were 2 mg/kg body weight/day in older healthy adults, and 3 mg/kg body weight/day in younger adults.[55] Although the plasma response curve is less well defined for threonine,[56] daily requirements were estimated to be 8 mg/kg body weight/day and 7 mg/kg body weight/day in older and younger adults, respectively. Young and associates[73] em-

phasize that essential amino acid requirements when estimated per unit of body cell mass rather than per unit body weight do appear to be higher in the older adult. As noted in Chapter 3, the older adult has reduced lean body mass and proportionately more body fat than a young adult of similar body weight.

Preliminary evidence suggests that the requirement for valine may be higher in older people, if evaluated on the basis of body cell mass rather than total body weight.[73] Further work is needed to define age-related changes, if any, in essential amino acid requirements, particularly in light of changes in endocrine and adaptive responses acting upon protein and amino acid metabolism.

Practical Aspects of Protein Intake

High quality protein foods are generally among the more expensive items in the food budget. Although a portion of the protein requirement can be met with less expensive vegetable proteins such as cereals, bread, and legumes, complete proteins including meat, fish, poultry, or dairy products should be present in liberal amounts. Animal-vegetable protein combinations such as cereal and milk or macaroni and cheese, which enhance intake at reasonable cost, need to be emphasized in nutrition education for older people.

Unfortunately, convenience items, popular because they require little or no preparation, tend to be expensive sources of protein (Table 5-3). Frankfurters, less desirable choices on the basis of fat and sodium content, cost about twice as much per 20 gm portion as chicken or egg; luncheon meat costs about five times as much. Milk, one of the least expensive sources of high quality protein, also contributes calcium, riboflavin, and vitamin A to the diet. Consuming two glasses of milk each day will provide one half to one third of the daily protein needs of the older woman or man. Dairy products, eggs, ground meat, well-cooked chicken, or fish are easily handled by those with chewing problems.

Table 5-3. Comparative cost of protein (20 gm)

Food	Amount to be Consumed	Total Cost* (cents)
Beef liver	3 ounces	15
Chicken leg	3 ounces	22
Milk, dried, skim (reconstituted)	2 cups	25
Eggs	3	28
Milk, fluid	2 cups	30
Peanut butter	5 tablespoons	30
Hamburger	3 ounces	32
Bread, white, enriched	10 slices	35
Cottage cheese	¾ cup	35
American cheese	3 ounces	45
Dried beans (cooked)	1½ cups	45
Frankfurters	3	52
Haddock, fillet, frozen	3 ounces	52
Cheddar cheese	3 × 1 × 1 inch cube	63
Tuna, canned	3 ounces	66
Beef, stew meat	3 ounces	67
Luncheon meat	12 thin slices	120

*Prices in Burlington, Vt., November, 1982.

PROTEIN STATUS

Protein-Calorie Malnutrition

Incidence of Protein-Calorie Malnutrition. Protein-calorie malnutrition has been identified among hospitalized patients maintained for long periods on parenteral feeding or special diets low in nutrient content. The older person with a history of debilitating disease and/or a poor diet is likely to have poor nutrient reserves and is particularly vulnerable to overt malnutrition. The nutritional impact of chronic disease and hospitalization is suggested by the fact that institutionalized aged, in general, have poorer nutritional status than those residing nearby in the community.[21,39] The identification of protein-calorie malnutrition is difficult in this age group, as norms specific for the older population have not been developed.[35] Measurements traditionally used for evaluation such as skinfold thickness and arm circumference, creatinine index, or serum albumin and transferrin levels may change as a function of age.

Arm muscle circumference was consistently related to protein intake among nearly 800 older English subjects.[4] As arm muscle radius measurements increased from less than 30 to at least 40 mm, daily protein intakes increased as well. In general, protein intakes were higher among those below age 75 than among those age 75 and above. While only 1% of men below age 75 had muscle radius measurements below 30 mm, this was true for 7% of those age 75 or above. Daily protein intakes were 64 and 55 gm, respectively, in the younger and older groups.

The relationship between arm muscle radius and protein intake is also influenced by energy intake; as energy intake increases, protein intake is likely to increase as well. According to Anderson and coworkers,[4] however, the percentage of calories derived from protein may also increase, suggesting that the higher muscle mass is the result of increased body protein stores.

The long term consequences of low calorie and protein intakes on body build were observed in 166 English aged in an extended care hospital.[32] For emaciated or underweight people body build was related to energy intake before rather than after admission. The poorly nourished individuals frequently had problems with mobility such as rheumatoid arthritis or broken bones. It was inferred that many had some degree of disability before entering the extended care facility. The very old and those with physical disability are most vulnerable to protein-calorie problems.

Protein-Calorie Supplementation. When malnutrition is evident among older hospitalized patients, increasing their calorie and protein intakes may be difficult if usual intake is only about 1000 kcal per day and they are unable to consume more food. One hospital, evaluating 117 older patients (mean age = 73 years) over a 2-year period, found commercial liquid supplements to be of only limited value.[54] Daily energy intake increased by only 250 kcal and neither body weight nor protein status improved measurably.

As an alternative, commercial supplements found to be relatively tasteless were used in food preparation, added to soups, juices, and other beverages such as tea or eggnog. A hospital recipe for frappe made with milk, ice cream, and vanilla and containing 11.5 gm protein and 288 kcal per 12-ounce serving was increased to 42 gm protein and over 1000 kcal with added supplement powder. Items such as hot chocolate or orange juice were doubled in calories. By this method daily caloric intake increased by an average of 1200 kcal and weight loss was halted. Mean serum albumin levels increased by 0.8 gm/100 ml (range = 0.2 to 1.8 gm/100 ml), and mean serum transferrin levels by 50 mg/100 ml (range = 20 to 100 mg/100 ml), indicating an improvement in protein status.

It is evident that many malnourished older people can absorb and utilize high quality protein when caloric intake is adequate. Development of tasteless supplements that can be added to food already being served may be more productive than focusing on those offered in addition to regular meals.[54]

Protein Intake

Protein intake for most older people is generally adequate, although a recent review pointed to the problems in comparing groups because standards of evaluation are not consistent.[39] Surveys in which few or no individuals were found to have deficient intakes used 0.5 to 0.7 gm/kg body weight/day as the criterion, whereas those reporting higher numbers of people consuming less than the standard used 0.8 to 1.0 gm/kg body weight/day as the measure of adequacy. Protein status is income related; low income people are more likely to have inadequate intakes.

In a recent national survey about 10% of all men and women age 65 to 74 consumed less than two thirds the RDA, although about 18% of low income aged consumed less than that amount.[65] At greatest risk are those who may be consuming inadequate levels of both protein and calories. Over half of the low income group had less than two thirds the recommended level of calories. Although it is not possible to confirm whether those with deficient intakes of protein were also deficient in calories, it is reasonable to suggest that at least a portion of those low in one nutrient were low in the other as well. The deterioration in nutritional status resulting from such intakes can increase vulnerability to both infection and chronic disease.

Serum Protein and Albumin

Serum albumin levels tend to be lower in older versus younger adults, although total serum protein does not always change.[15,21,33-34,70] These findings are controversial, however, as the effect of age or disease cannot be separated from possible changes in protein or calorie intake. Median serum albumin decreased from 4.6 to 4.1 gm/100 ml among over 1400 clinically healthy adults between ages 20 and 60 and above evaluated by decade interval.[42] Age-related decreases were similar in over 2400 life insurance company employees ranging in age from under 35 to age 55 and over.[33] In that group albumin levels decreased from 4.4 to 4.1 gm/100 ml in men and from 4.2 to 4.0 gm/100 ml in women.

Serum albumin and protein levels continue to decline beyond age 60. In older women ages 62 to 75, 76 to 85, and 86 to 99, albumin levels were 4.0, 3.7, and 3.7 gm/100 ml, respectively.[22] Total serum protein equaled 7.0, 6.9, and 6.6 gm/100 ml, respectively. With the decrease in serum albumin, 23% had values below 3.5 gm/100 ml. Twenty-eight percent of the serum protein levels were below 6.5 gm/100 ml. Although protein intake declined with age on an absolute basis, it did not change significantly when calculated as grams per kilogram body weight (0.8 to 0.9 gm/kg). Protein-calorie ratio was positively correlated with both serum protein and albumin, although a wide range of albumin levels existed per protein-calorie ratio.

Chronic disease altering kidney or liver function can lead to changes in serum albumin levels regardless of protein status. In advanced renal disease albumin may be lost in the urine. It has been reported that albumin catabolism is accelerated in some older patients although the mechanism is unknown.[34] Others argue that catabolism of albumin is slowed in particular older individuals to compensate for reduced synthesis.[71] Such an effect has been demonstrated in younger people with low protein intakes.[26] Ricca and coworkers[43] observed that hepatocytes from aged animals synthesized less protein than those from younger animals.

It is obvious that much remains to be learned about albumin metabolism in the older individual. Reduced synthesis and/or accelerated catabolism may result in low serum albumin levels in the chronically ill, regardless of protein status. Serum albumin levels in healthy aged should be similar to young adults; low levels indicate a need for dietary and medical evaluation.

Marginal protein status and chronic disease can interact to produce clinical symptoms usually associated with protein deprivation.[4] In one report edema was present in 40% of aged with serum albumin below 3.5 gm/100 ml and in 22% with albumin levels between 3.5 and 4.5 gm/100 ml. Anderson and coworkers[4] pointed out that chronic disease exacerbates nutritional problems. For example, low serum albumin levels might not in themselves lead to edema; however, cardiac failure superimposed on marginal protein deficiency could result in fluid retention. Although fluid retention is often related to hypertension and sodium imbalance, the possible contribution of marginal or deficient protein status should not be overlooked.

The influence of nutrients other than protein or calories on albumin metabolism requires closer scrutiny. In a double blind study of 94 older patients, ascorbic acid supplementation over a 2-month period led to significant weight gain (0.4

kg) and increases in plasma albumin (0.05 gm/100 ml).[48] Over the same period patients given placebos experienced both weight loss (0.6 kg) and decreases in albumin levels (0.05 gm/100 ml). Those receiving the ascorbic acid may have had an increase in appetite and consumed more food, although the authors did not observe such a difference.

Although the effect of the ascorbic acid is unclear, these findings emphasize the importance of evaluating the entire diet when conducting a clinical trial involving a particular nutrient. Vitamin as well as protein intake appeared to influence protein metabolism and body weight.

Immunologic Function

Altered immunologic response has been associated with the aging process (see Chapter 1). Since this function involves protein synthesis, there is the possibility that poor protein status contributes to these changes. Dietary levels of calories and protein and serum levels of protein and albumin did not differ in older people having a greater or lesser immunologic response to antigen stimulation.[52] Immunoglobulin levels tended to be higher, however, in those with higher serum protein, albumin, and zinc levels. Protein supplementation had no effect on immunoglobulin levels falling within the normal range. Zinc status as well as protein status may be related to immunologic response in older individuals (see Chapter 7).

SUMMARY

Because little is known about the nutrient requirements of older people, the RDAs for this group have been extrapolated from those for younger people. Calorie requirements decrease with advancing age, and iron requirements are lower in women following menopause. Although there is no established requirement for carbohydrate, older people are encouraged to consume at least half of their calories from carbohydrate foods, with emphasis on complex carbohydrates rich in fiber. A daily source of linoleic acid providing at least 6 gm is encouraged, although a quantitative recommendation has not been developed.

Protein requirements in advanced age are influenced by changes in body compartments, previous protein intake, calorie intake, emotional stress, and chronic disease with accompanying prescription drugs. Protein metabolism tends to shift from the muscle compartment to the viscera as lean body mass is lost. Factorial evaluation of obligatory nitrogen loss indicates that older people can conserve nitrogen on low intakes, although daily nitrogen loss calculated per kilogram body cell mass is higher in older people as a result of the shift from muscle to viscera. Nitrogen loss per kilogram body weight is higher in males who have a greater proportion of lean body mass as compared to females.

Protein requirements do not differ significantly between older and younger adults when calculated using estimated obligatory nitrogen losses. Balance studies, however, indicate that many older people cannot maintain nitrogen equilibrium on intakes below 0.8 gm protein/kg body weight/day, and for some, even this level is not sufficient. Healthy older individuals with substantial calorie intakes can maintain nitrogen equilibrium on intakes within FAO/WHO guidelines. Individuals with chronic disease who are using various prescription drugs and consuming only about 1600 to 1800 kcal/day require intakes at least equal to the RDA. Protein should provide 12% to 14% of total calories.

Changes in amino acid requirements as a function of age are a matter of controversy. Although results from balance studies have pointed to both increased and reduced amino acid needs per kilogram body weight in older versus younger people, it does appear the amino acid requirements per kilogram body cell mass increase in advanced age.

Nutrition surveys suggest that some older people are at risk for protein-calorie malnutrition as intakes of both protein and calories are below 67% that recommended. The relative cost of quality protein sources may contribute to the problem. Clinical determination of protein-calorie malnutrition is complicated by the fact that albumin metabolism is altered in some older people; therefore serum albumin levels are less reliable indicators of protein status. Fortifying soups and liquids with protein supplement powders has been successful in raising the protein intake of malnourished patients.

REVIEW QUESTIONS

1. Outline the differences in the RDAs for people age 50 and below and those age 51 and above. What are the limitations of the RDAs now used for people above age 50?
2. Describe age-related changes in serum lipid levels. What factors appear to influence serum lipid levels in older people?
3. What is the basis for the shift in protein metabolism from the muscle to the viscera? How does this influence obligatory nitrogen loss calculated on the basis of (a) kilogram body weight and (b) kilogram body cell mass?
4. Discuss the relationship between protein and energy requirements. What factors other than energy intake influence protein requirements in older people?
5. Protein requirements of older people are a matter of controversy. Although some reports suggest that 0.8 gm protein/kg body weight is adequate for most older people, others indicate that many older people cannot maintain nitrogen equilibrium on that level of intake. What factors may contribute to these differences? Do you agree with the present recommendation for protein intake? Cite evidence to justify your conclusion.

REFERENCES

1. Albanese, A.A., and others: Protein requirements of old age, Geriatrics **7**:109, 1952.
2. Albanese, A.A., and others: Protein and amino acid needs of the aged in health and convalescence, Geriatrics **12**:465, 1957.
3. Albanese, A.A., and others: Steroid and dietary effects on blood lipids in elderly persons, Nut. Rep. Int. **1**:231, 1970.
4. Anderson, W.F., and others: Clinical and subclinical malnutrition in old age. In Carlson, L.A., ed.: Nutrition in old age, Symposia Swedish Nutrition Foundation X, Stockholm, 1972, Almqvist & Wiksell.
5. Beisel, W.R.: Effect of infection on human protein metabolism, Fed. Proc. **25**:1682, 1966.
6. Boberg, J., Carlson, L.A., and Froberg, S.: Serum and tissue lipids in relation to age. In Carlson, L.A., ed.: Nutrition in old age, Symposia Swedish Nutrition Foundation X, Stockholm, 1972, Almqvist and Wiksell.

7. Carlson, L.A., Froberg, S.O., and Nye, E.R.: Effect of age on blood and tissue lipid levels in the male rat, Gerontolog. **14:**65, 1968.

8. Cheng, A.H.R., and others: Comparative nitrogen balance study between young and aged adults using three levels of protein intake from a combination wheat-soy-milk mixture, Am. J. Clin. Nutr. **31:**12, 1978.

9. Crouse, S.R., Grundy, S.M., and Ahrens, E.H.: Cholesterol distribution in the bulk tissues of man: Variation with age, J. Clin. Invest. **51:**1292, 1972.

10. DaCosta, F., and Moorhouse, J.A.: Protein nutrition in aged individuals on self-selected diets, Am. J. Clin. Nutr. **22:**1618, 1969.

11. Food and Nutrition Board: Recommended dietary allowances, ed. 9, Washington, D.C., 1980, National Academy of Sciences.

12. Garza, C., Scrimshaw, N.S., and Young V.R.: Human protein requirements: The effect of variations in energy intake within the maintenance range, Am. J. Clin. Nutr. **29:**280, 1976.

13. Gersovitz, M., and others: Human protein requirements: Assessment of the adequacy of the current Recommended Dietary Allowance for dietary protein in elderly men and women, Am. J. Clin. Nutr. **35:**6, 1982.

14. Glueck, C.J., and others: Hyperalpha- and hypobeta-lipoproteinemia in octogenarian kindreds, Atherosclerosis **27:**387, 1977.

15. Greenblatt, D.J.: Reduced serum albumin concentration in the elderly: A report from the Boston collaborative drug surveillance program, J. Am. Geriatr. Soc. **27:**20, 1979.

16. Greenfield, M.S., and others: Effect of age on plasma triglyceride concentrations in man, Metabolism **29:**1095, 1980.

17. Gsell, D.: Serum cholesterol and its increase with age in a population with high fat consumption and high physical activity, Gerontol. Clin. **4:**194, 1962.

18. Harper, A.E.: Basic concepts. In Food and Nutrition Board: Improvement of protein nutriture, Washington, D.C., 1974, National Academy of Sciences.

19. Harper, A.E.: Recommended dietary allowances for the elderly, Geriatrics **33:**73, 1978.

20. Harrill, I., Jansen, C., and Barthrop, J.: Serum cholesterol and triglycerides and hyperlipoproteinemia in elderly women, J. Gerontol. **33:**347, 1978.

21. Harrill, I., and Kylen, A.: Protein intake and serum protein in elderly women, Nutr. Rep. Int. **21:**717, 1980.

22. Hegsted, D.M.: Proteins. In Beaton, G.H., and McHenry, E.W., eds.: Nutrition. A comprehensive treatise: Macronutrients and nutrient elements, vol. 1, New York, 1964, Academic Press, Inc.

23. Heiss, G., and others: Lipoprotein-cholesterol distributions in selected North American populations: The lipid research

clinics program prevalence study, Circulation **61:**302, 1980.

24. Holman, R.T., Smythe, L., and Johnson, S.: Effect of sex and age on fatty acid composition of human serum lipids, Am. J. Clin. Nutr. **32:**2390, 1979.

25. Horwitt, M.K.: Dietary requirements of the aged, J. Am. Diet. Assoc. **29:**443, 1953.

26. James, W.P.T., and Hay, A.M.: Albumin metabolism: Effect of the nutritional state and the dietary protein intake, J. Clin. Invest. **47:**1958, 1968.

27. Kountz, W.B., Ackermann, P.G., and Kheim, T.: The effect of added carbohydrate and fat on nitrogen balance in the elderly, J. Am. Geriatr. Soc. **3:**691, 1955.

28. Kountz, W.B., Hofstatter, L., and Ackermann, P.G.: Nitrogen balance studies in four elderly men, J. Gerontol. **6:**20, 1951.

29. Kritchevsky, D.: Diet, lipid metabolism, and aging, Fed. Proc. **38:**2001, 1979.

30. Kritchevsky, D.: Age-related changes in lipid metabolism, Proc. Soc. Exp. Biol. Med. **165:**193, 1980.

31. Long, C.L., and others: Metabolism of 3-methylhistidine in man, Metabolism **24:**929, 1975.

32. MacLennan, W.J., Martin, P., and Mason, B.J.: Energy intake, disability, disease and skinfold thickness in a long-stay hospital, Gerontol. Clin. **17:**173, 1975.

33. Metropolitan Life Insurance Company: More about biochemical profiles, Stat. Bull. Metropol. Life Insur. Co. **52**(1):2, 1971.

34. Misra, D.P., Laudon, J.M., and Staddon, G.E.: Albumin metabolism in elderly patients, J. Gerontol. **30:**304, 1975.

35. Mitchell, C.O., and Lipschitz, D.A.: Detection of protein-calorie malnutrition in the elderly, Am. J. Clin. Nutr. **35:**398, 1982.

36. Munro, H.N.: Major gaps in nutrient allowances: The status of the elderly, J. Am. Diet. Assoc. **76:**137, 1980.

37. Munro, H.N.: Nutrition and ageing, Br. Med. Bull. **37:**83, 1981.

38. Munro, H.N., and Young, V.R.: Protein metabolism in the elderly: Observations relating to dietary needs, Postgrad. Med. **63:**143, 1978.

39. O'Hanlon, P., and Kohrs, M.B.: Dietary studies of older Americans, Am. J. Clin. Nutr. **31:**1257, 1978.

40. Ohlson, M.A., and others: Intakes and retentions of nitrogen, calcium and phosphorus by 136 women between 30 and 85 years of age, Fed. Proc. **11:**775, 1952.

41. Ohlson, M.A., and others: Utilization of an improved diet by older women, J. Am. Diet. Assoc. **28:**1138, 1952.

42. Reed, A.H., and others: Estimation of normal ranges from a controlled sample survey. 1. Sex and age-related influence on the SMA 12/60 screening group of tests, Clin. Chem. **18:**57, 1972.

43. Ricca, G.A., and others: Rates of protein synthesis by hepatocytes isolated from rats of various ages, J. Cell. Physiol. **97**:137, 1978.

44. Roberts, P.H., Kerr, C.H., and Ohlson, M.A.: Nutritional status of older women, J. Am. Diet. Assoc. **24**:292, 1948.

45. Roe, D.: Handbook: Interactions of selected drugs and nutrients in patients, Chicago, 1982, American Dietetic Association.

46. Schlenker, E.D.: Nutritional status of older women, Ph.D. Thesis, E. Lansing, 1976, Michigan State University.

47. Schneider, J., and others: HDL cholesterol, peripheral and coronary vascular disease in high age groups, Atherosclerosis **35**:487, 1980.

48. Schorah, C.J., and others: The effect of vitamin C supplements on body weight, serum proteins, and general health of an elderly population, Am. J. Clin. Nutr. **34**:871, 1981.

49. Scrimshaw, N.S., Perera, W.D.A., and Young, V.R.: Protein requirements of man: Obligatory urinary and fecal nitrogen losses in elderly women, J. Nutr. **106**:665, 1976.

50. Shock, N.A.: Discussion. In Carlson, L.A., ed.: Nutrition in old age, Symposia Swedish Nutrition Foundation X, Stockholm, 1972, Almqvist & Wiksell, p. 68.

51. Smith, E.B.: The influence of age and atherosclerosis on the chemistry of aortic intima. 1. The lipids, J. Atheroscler. Res. **5**:224, 1965.

52. Stiedmann, M., and Harrill, I.: Relation of immunocompetence to selected nutrients in elderly women, Nut. Rep. Int. **21**:931, 1980.

53. Swanson, P.: Adequacy in old age. Part 1. Role of nutrition, J. Home Econ. **56**:651, 1964.

54. Tomaiolo, P.P., Enman, S., and Kraus, V.: Preventing and treating malnutrition in the elderly, J. Parenteral Enteral Nutr. **5**:46, 1981.

55. Tontisirin, K., and others: Plasma tryptophan response curve and tryptophan requirements of elderly people, J. Nutr. **103**:1220, 1973.

56. Tontisirin, K., and others: Plasma threonine response curve and threonine requirements of young men and elderly women, J. Nutr. **104**:495, 1974.

57. Tuttle, S.G., and others: Study of the essential amino acid requirements of men over fifty, Metabolism **6**:564, 1957.

58. Tuttle, S.G., and others: Essential amino acid requirements of older men in relation to total nitrogen intake, Metabolism **8**:61, 1959.

59. Tuttle, S.G., and others: Further observations on the amino acid requirements of older men. 1. Effects of nonessential nitrogen supplements fed with different amounts of essential amino acids, Am. J. Clin. Nutr. **16**:225, 1965.

60. Tuttle, S.G., and others: Further observations on the amino acid requirements of older men. 2. Methionine and lysine, Am. J. Clin. Nutr. **16**:229, 1965.

61. Uauy, R., Scrimshaw, N.S., and Young, V.R.: Human protein requirements: Nitrogen balance response to graded levels of egg protein in elderly men and women, Am. J. Clin. Nutr. **31**:779, 1978.

62. Uauy, R., and others: Human protein requirements: Obligatory urinary and fecal nitrogen losses and the factorial estimation of protein needs in elderly males, J. Nutr. **108**:97, 1978.

63. Uauy, R., and others: The changing pattern of whole body protein metabolism in aging humans, J. Gerontol. **33**:663, 1978.

64. United States Department of Health, Education and Welfare: Total serum cholesterol levels of adults 18-74 years. United States, 1971-74, DHEW Publication No. (PHS) 78-1652, Washington, D.C., 1978, U.S. Government Printing Office.

65. United States Department of Health, Education, and Welfare: Dietary intake source data. United States, 1971-74, DHEW Publication No. (PHS) 79-1221, Hyattsville, Md., 1979, U.S. Government Printing Office.

66. Watkin, D.M.: The assessment of protein nutrition in aged man, Ann. N.Y. Acad. Sci. **69**:902, 1958.

67. Watts, J.H., and others: Nitrogen balances of men over 65 fed the FAO and milk patterns of essential amino acids, J. Gerontol. **19**:370, 1964.

68. Winterer, J.C., and others: Whole body protein turnover in aging man, Exp. Gerontol. **11**:79, 1976.

69. Woldow, A.: Hyperlipidemia and its significance in the aged population, J. Am. Geriatr. Soc. **23**:407, 1975.

70. Woodford-Williams, E., and others: Serum protein patterns in "normal" and pathological ageing, Gerontolog. **10**:86, 1965.

71. Yan, S.H.Y., and Franks, J.J.: Albumin metabolism in elderly men and women, J. Lab. Clin. Med. **72**:449, 1968.

72. Young, V.R., and Munro, H.N.: N^ε-methylhistidine (3-methylhistidine) and muscle protein turnover: An overview, Fed. Proc. **37**:2291, 1978.

73. Young, V.R., and others: Protein and amino acid requirements of the elderly. In Winick, M., ed.: Nutrition and aging, New York, 1976, John Wiley & Sons, Inc.

74. Zanni, E., Callaway, D.H., and Zezulka, A.Y.: Protein requirements of elderly men, J. Nutr. **109**:513, 1979.

Chapter 6

Vitamins in the Aged

Changes in vitamin requirements or metabolism that may occur in the older individual are poorly understood, although biochemical changes associated with the aging process are interrelated with nutrient function. Energy storage and metabolism, dependent on the presence of vitamin cofactors, are also influenced by enzyme and hormone levels that can be altered with age. Physiologic processes such as neural function, formation of red blood cells, and visual adaptation to dim light require effective absorption and metabolism of vitamins. Common medical problems in the aged including osteoporosis and anemia are vitamin related. Unfortunately, research exploring all of these relationships has been limited and much remains to be learned.

FAT SOLUBLE VITAMINS: REQUIREMENTS AND METABOLISM

Factors Influencing Absorption

Digestive Enzymes. Absorption of the fat soluble vitamins depends on the secretion of pancreatic lipase and bile salts for the lipolysis of dietary fat and the formation of micelles. When micelle formation does not proceed normally, fat soluble vitamins cannot move into the aqueous phase and across the mucosal cell.[83] People with gallbladder disease and impaired secretion of bile salts can have impaired absorption of both fat and the fat soluble vitamins. For those unable to absorb any lipid, fat soluble vitamins can be administered in water mis-cible emulsions either orally or intramuscularly.

Dietary Constituents. Dietary fat has two important functions in the absorption of fat soluble vitamins. First, lipids serve as a transport mechanism to move the vitamin from the stomach into the intestine and eventually the micelle, and second, lipids delay gastric emptying thereby promoting micellar formation.[83] Decreased intake of fat because of health beliefs or digestive discomfort could reduce absorption of vitamins A, E, K, and D, although this has not been studied in older people. Polyunsaturated fatty acids, recommended in favor of saturated fats, lower absorption of the fat soluble vitamins, although the mechanism by which this occurs is unknown.[83] Vitamin A appears to compete with vitamins E and K for binding sites and at high levels of supplementation has been shown to depress absorption of those two vitamins in rats.[83] Highly concentrated vitamin A supplements therefore have potential for creating imbalance as well as general toxicity.

Vitamin A

Dietary Intake and Serum Levels. Increasing age does not appear to either increase the requirement for vitamin A or hinder vitamin A absorption in normal individuals. Serum vitamin A levels are not lower in older than in younger adults.[35,40,69,75,77] In fact, in recent national surveys serum vitamin A levels actually rose with increasing age; incidence of deficiency declined.[75,77] In the HANES report,[77] less than 1% of those above age 60 had serum levels below 20 μg/100 ml (considered to be indicative of deficiency). In the Ten-State Nutrition Survey,[75] 12% of older low income Spanish-Americans had deficient serum vitamin A levels; however, this most likely related to intake as nearly half were consuming less than 50% of the recommended level of vitamin A.[76] Mean serum levels did not differ between independent-living and institutionalized women[40] of similar age (55 versus 50 μg/100 ml) or between those 60 to 84 years of age (42 μg/100 ml) and 85 to 98 years of age (39 μg/100 ml).[69] Twelve percent of the younger and 14% of the older subjects had serum levels classed as deficient.[69] Low serum vitamin A levels in older people usually respond to vitamin supplementation, suggesting poor prior intake.[18] Although statistical correlations are low, older individuals with higher intakes tend to have higher serum vitamin A levels.[35,75] Serum carotene levels, suggestive of recent intake, are of no value in predicting vitamin A status.

Metabolism of Vitamin A. Animal studies have established that serum vitamin A levels may not fall below normal until liver vitamin stores are practically exhausted (<10 μg/gm).[52,73] This suggests that serum level is not a sensitive measure to identify people at risk of vitamin A deficiency. Evaluation of liver vitamin A stores in 102 persons dying of unnatural causes revealed that 60% had less than 100 μg/gm tissue (100-300 μg/gm is considered normal), although adults above age 50 had higher mean vitamin levels (147 μg/gm) than young adults (96 μg/gm).[73] Liver vitamin A was lower in individuals representing (in the judgment of Underwood and coworkers) deprived populations.

Animal work suggests that plasma response to vitamin A administration is significantly greater in those with low as compared to adequate liver stores.[52] Apparently, recently ingested vitamin A is efficiently mobilized to meet immediate tissue needs. The increase in human plasma levels observed on supplementation may be reflecting this pattern. The level and period of supplementation

required to replete low liver stores are not known.

Data from HANES[78] indicate that 39% of those age 65 and above consume less than 2500 IU vitamin A per day (RDA = 5000 IU for men; 4000 IU for women). An intake less than 67% the RDA suggests that normal serum levels are being maintained at the expense of liver stores. Clinical abnormalities can exist when serum levels range from 20 to 40 μg/100 ml.[15] One third of 18 adults with serum levels between 30 and 39 μg/100 ml had impaired dark adaptation, which became normal on vitamin A supplementation and an increase in serum levels to 40 μg/100 ml or above. This raises questions concerning the use of 20 μg/100 ml as the cut-off point for evaluating vitamin A status.

In view of the inadequate vitamin intake, problems in absorption of dietary fat, and unknown changes in the efficiency of liver storage or mobilization of vitamin A in some aged individuals, a method to more precisely define vitamin A status should be a research priority.

Vitamin E

Health Claims. Distorted claims suggesting that vitamin E delays the onset or severity of age changes or prevents cardiovascular and other chronic problems often appear in the popular press.[58,60] Although vitamin E does function as a biologic antioxidant preventing lipid peroxidation damage to enzymes and membranes, no benefit has been observed in animal species from supplementation with high levels of either this vitamin or similar compounds.[70] Although vitamin E deficiency leads to cardiac damage in some (but not all) experimental animals, this has not been observed in humans.[60] In fact, vitamin E deficiency is rare in adults and when it does occur is usually the result of a malabsorption syndrome.

Serum Levels. Surveys of both aged and general populations have not revealed significant numbers of people with vitamin E deficiency (serum level below 0.5 mg/100 ml).[10,37,79] Among 47 men (age 21 to 76) in a Veterans Administration facility there was no relationship between serum vitamin E and age; only one had a value below standard (mean = 1.15 mg/100 ml).[79] Barnes and Chen[10] evaluated 84 independent-living and 22 institutionalized aged between 60 and 90 years of age and found no significant serum differences on the basis of age by decade, sex, or institutionalization. Vitamin E levels ranged from 0.85 to 3.84 mg/100 ml although both serum vitamin E and cholesterol levels were lower in the oldest subjects.

The vitamin E requirement is influenced by the level of intake of polyunsaturated fatty acids (PUFAs).[28] This is usually not a problem, however, as the primary sources of PUFAs, vegetable oils or margarine, are also good sources of vitamin E. Evaluation of liver tocopherol in persons dying of unnatural causes revealed the highest concentration (14.8 μg/gm) in those above age 50.[72] When expressed on the basis of liver lipid, tocopherol values were still higher in older as compared to younger adults. Serum tocopherol was positively related to liver tocopherol when expressed on the basis of liver tissue rather than liver lipid content. Liver vitamin E was not influenced by ethnic or economic group, leading Underwood and coworkers to conclude that vegetable oils rather than green vegetables are the primary source of this vitamin.

Vitamin D

Sources. Although vitamin D can be obtained from food or exposure to sunlight, the vitamin D status of many aged evaluated on the basis of either dietary intake[26,51] or serum vitamin D metabolite levels[9] is less than optimum. The problem is complicated by the series of biochemical steps required to convert either ingested vitamin D_2 or the vitamin D_3 produced in the skin from ultraviolet light to the active metabolite. Most reported levels of serum 25 (OH)D and 1, 25 (OH)$_2$ D include both the D_2 and D_3 forms.[30-31]

Dietary sources appear to make only a limited contribution to the vitamin D requirement. Among older Britons living at home average daily intake was 135 IU;[26] one fourth of independent-living New Mexico aged consumed less than 50% of the recommended level.[33]

The seasonal variation in serum vitamin D metabolite levels emphasizes the importance of sunlight in meeting the vitamin D requirement.[21,27,51] Serum 25-hydroxy vitamin D (25[OH]D) levels were three times higher in summer than winter in 23 people tested (age 72 to 86 years).[51] Winter serum levels were in the range associated with development of osteomalacia.

Serum vitamin D metabolites are lower in older than younger people and are lowest in those confined indoors (Table 6-1).[85] Although exposure to sunlight increases serum 25(OH)D, older farm workers spending several hours each day in the fields still had lower levels than young controls. Institutionalized aged who sat outdoors occasionally did have improved serum levels over those totally confined indoors. Weisman and associates[85] concluded that age-related changes in the skin, as well as decreased ability to convert vitamin D to the 25-hydroxy form, contributed to the lower levels observed among those with high exposure to sunlight.

Indoor lighting providing ultraviolet exposure has been tried in institutions as an alternative to sunlight. Calcium absorption was improved in older men exposed to high levels of fluorescent light-

Table 6-1. Vitamin D serum levels and exposure to sunlight

	Serum 25(OH)D Levels (ng/ml)
Aged confined indoors	8.0
Aged spending some time outdoors	11.4
Aged farm workers	14.6
Young controls	21.5

Data from Weisman, Y., and others: Inadequate status and impaired metabolism of vitamin D in the elderly, Isr. J. Med. Sci. **17**:19, 1981.

ing (in the ultraviolet range) for several hours each day, although the long term use of high light levels has been questioned on the basis of possible eye damage.[20,59] Lower levels of ultraviolet light, on a daily basis, may be an adequate supplement for those who cannot go outdoors.

Conversion to Active Form. Metabolic alterations in both the intestinal absorption of vitamin D and the conversion of 25(OH)D to 1,25(OH)$_2$D in the kidney, occur with age. Serum vitamin levels in aged subjects following an oral dose of radioactive cholecalciferol were only 60% those of young controls.[11] This difference was not related to transit time or gastric emptying, as a triglyceride peak representing the lipid given with the test vitamin appeared at the same time in both age groups.

Gallagher and coworkers[30-31] reported that older subjects with normal serum levels of 25(OH)D have depressed levels of 1,25(OH)$_2$D suggesting either lack of kidney hydroxylase enzyme or decreased secretion of parathyroid hormone, which normally stimulates production of kidney hydroxylase and 1,25(OH)$_2$D. In some individuals with normal or elevated parathyroid hormone, 1,25(OH)$_2$D levels are still depressed pointing to a metabolic problem in the conversion step requiring kidney hydroxylase. This raises questions concerning the efficacy of vitamin D supplementation or increased exposure to ultraviolet light for older people, as the vitamin either supplied or synthesized is of no value if not converted to the active 1,25-dihydroxy form.

MacLennan and Hamilton[53] observed that 500 IU of vitamin D per day given to long term geriatric patients led to an increase in serum 25(OH)D levels, although rate of calcium absorption or serum 1,25(OH)$_2$D levels were not measured. When initial serum 25(OH)D levels were low (<8 ng/ml), supplementation resulted in a twofold increase in serum levels. When initial levels were high (≥8 ng/ml) the supplement had little effect. According to those authors, this suggests a feedback inhibition after physiologic levels have been achieved.[53] Sup-

plements of 2000 IU/day as compared with 500 IU/day had the same results. Pharmacologic doses (20 μg/day) of the metabolite 25(OH)D given to older women with poor calcium absorption led to significant increases in both calcium absorption (from 38% to 49% of a test dose) and serum 1,25(OH)$_2$D levels.[50]

Both the form of the vitamin fed and the vitamin D status of the individual influence the results obtained with supplementation. Administration of either 500 or 10,000 IU/day of vitamin D had no effect on calcium absorption in older individuals (mean age = 83 years) or young controls (mean age = 35 years), although serum 25(OH)D levels increased in both groups.[68] Those older individuals, however, had normal calcium absorption and serum 25(OH)D levels prior to supplementation, suggesting adequate absorption and metabolic conversion of vitamin D. Supplementation appears to have no particular benefit for people with adequate vitamin D status.

Age-related problems with vitamin D focus on two events: (1) absorption of vitamin D, which may be less efficient in some older people, and (2) conversion of 25(OH)D to 1,25(OH)$_2$D in the kidney. Low 25(OH)D serum levels may result from poor vitamin intake and often increase on supplementation with dietary levels of vitamin D (500 IU). In those individuals vitamin absorption and formation of the monohydroxy metabolite in the liver appear to proceed normally.[53] The defect exists in the enzymatic conversion to the dihydroxy form, although it can be overcome with pharmacologic doses of 25(OH)D.[50] The active form of vitamin D (1,25(OH)$_2$D) is being evaluated in the clinical treatment of bone disorders (see Chapter 8).

Recommended Intake. For healthy aged a daily intake of 400 IU (10 μg) appears adequate to maintain normal serum D levels, even if exposure to sunlight is minimal.[20,53] The Food and Nutrition Board recommends an intake of 200 IU or 5 μg cholecalciferol for all adults.[28] Encouraging clients to use vitamin D–fortified dairy products and spend time outdoors, even if physical activity is limited, is appropriate advice. Many multivitamin supplements now on the market contain the recommended level of vitamin D. In light of the danger of vitamin D toxicity and subsequent hypercalcemia, supplements containing more than 400 IU are hazardous unless the individual is being treated for a bone disorder and under constant medical supervision.[62]

WATER SOLUBLE VITAMINS: REQUIREMENTS AND METABOLISM

Thiamin, Riboflavin, and Niacin

Thiamin Requirements. Little is known about age-related changes, if any, in the requirements and metabolism of thiamin. Animal studies have suggested that thiamin absorption is less efficient in advanced age although absorption does not appear to be impaired in older humans unless associated with use of alcohol.[44] Horwitt,[42] comparing thiamin and riboflavin metabolism in younger (mean age = 34) and older (mean age = 70) men found no differences in (1) rate of decrease in vitamin excretion when placed on a deficient diet, (2) appearance of clinical signs during 3 months of depletion, and (3) rate of increase in urinary excretion following vitamin supplementation. Horwitt concluded that older men were able to absorb and retain thiamin and riboflavin to the same extent as younger men.

The minimum requirement for thiamin established by Sauberlich and coworkers[67] is 0.3 mg/1000 kcal with the recommended level 0.5 mg/1000 kcal. It is best, however, that daily intake not fall below 1.0 mg despite an energy intake under 2000 kcal.[28] Thiamin appears to be involved in fatty acid metabolism and therefore is required regardless of calorie intake.[82] Obligatory thiamin loss further emphasizes the need for adequate dietary levels. Finally, it has been suggested that older people use thiamin less efficiently than younger people.[67] An intake of 1 mg daily therefore provides a margin of safety. Thiamin requirements and utilization in alcoholism will be discussed in Chapter 9.

Thiamin Intake and Biochemical Status. Both thiamin intake[78] and excretion decrease with age,[49] although incidence of deficiency is related to institutionalization[13] and the biochemical method of evaluation.[13,44] In the Ten-State Nutrition Survey over half of the men and nearly three fourths of the women age 60 and above had thiamin intakes below 1.0 mg, although less than 2% had deficient urinary excretion levels.[75-76] Less than 10% had urinary excretion levels classified as low. A recent review of available literature estimated that 10% of older people are thiamin deficient.[44] Urinary thiamin is poorly correlated with dietary intake.[75] To some extent people with higher intakes have higher levels of excretion; however, in the Ten-State Survey the quarter of older people with the highest excretion (>489 μg/gm creatinine) had a mean intake of only 1.01 mg.[75]

Thiamin excretion declines throughout adulthood, although values are similar in both sexes.[40,49,69] In a Mississippi survey people above age 60 excreted less thiamin than those age 18 to 34 or 35 to 60.[49] Among 70 women not receiving supplements (Table 6-2) thiamin excretion continued to decline between ages 62 and 99, and the proportion with inadequate excretion levels increased threefold between the age ranges of 76 to 85 and 86 to 99.[40] None in the youngest group (age 62 to 75) had excretion levels rated as deficient or low. Poor thiamin status related to dietary intake, although the oldest group appeared to either absorb or utilize thiamin less efficiently than the younger

Table 6-2. Thiamin levels in older women

Age (yr)	Mean Thiamin Intake (mg)	Percent with Low Excretion
62-75	0.83	0
76-85	0.70	20
86-99	0.64	69

Modified from Harrill, I., and Cervone, N.: Vitamin status of older women, Am. J. Clin. Nutr. **30:**431, 1977.

women with similar intakes. Nursing home residents, more likely to have low excretion levels than the noninstitutionalized women (36% versus 15% were low), also had lower intakes (0.69 versus 0.80 mg)[40] from food.

The apparent incidence of thiamin deficiency differs according to the biochemical method used (red blood cell transketolase activity or urinary thiamin excretion per gram creatinine).[13] In an evaluation of 234 New York aged including both institutionalized and noninstitutionalized individuals, 18% were deficient based on urinary thiamin compared to only 1% based on transketolase activity.[13] The transketolase test is highly sensitive; enzyme activity will remain normal on an intake of 0.5 mg thiamin daily. In contrast urinary thiamin levels will fall to near deficiency levels on a similar intake. Another problem in evaluating urinary thiamin levels is the age-related decrease in creatinine excretion used as a standard. Although urinary thiamin levels are useful as a screening tool, the enzyme assay provides a more precise indication of thiamin status.

Although thiamin excretion increases with supplementation, the functional significance of high intakes has not been demonstrated. Vir and Love[81] reported that daily intakes of 2.5 mg did not restore erythrocyte transketolase activity to normal in an older person who was consuming alcohol regularly and deficient in folic acid. Good sources of dietary thiamin should be emphasized to older clients in view of the apparent numbers consuming less than the recommended level of 1 mg.

Riboflavin Requirements and Metabolism. Riboflavin metabolism as evaluated by erythrocyte glutathione reductase activity (FAD effect) does not necessarily deteriorate with age. Screening of 667 people ranging from 20 to 87 years of age at a state fair revealed that 6% of those above 50 years of age who were not taking supplements had less than acceptable levels as compared to 11% of those age 20 to 49.[32] Riboflavin status improved with advancing age in both supplemented and unsupplemented individuals, with the most striking change

occurring beyond age 50.[32] The relationship between total riboflavin intake and enzyme activity is more closely defined at lower levels of intake; little change occurs when intake reaches 3 to 4 mg daily and the enzyme system is saturated with riboflavin cofactor.

Dietary intake and enzyme activity levels appear to be remarkably constant. In 23 aged adults evaluated over 18 months, a single week's dietary record provided a reasonable estimate of riboflavin intake with a variation of less than 20%.[66] Over a month's period intake and enzyme activity were highly related within individuals; however, correlations of intake and enzyme activity between individuals are less obvious unless the range of intakes is very broad.

Riboflavin Intake and Excretion. Evaluation of urinary excretion levels per gram creatinine reveals lower riboflavin excretion levels in aged men than women.[49] In a national survey 15% to 30% of persons age 60 and above consumed less than 67% of the RDA for riboflavin.[76] Blacks were more likely to have both low intakes and excretion levels, possibly reflecting lower use of dairy products.[75-76] Biochemical evidence of deficiency usually relates to poor intake and can be reversed when dietary riboflavin is increased.[81] The potential benefit of supplementation when enzyme and excretion values are in the normal range is not known.

Niacin Intake and Excretion. Biochemical evaluation of niacin status in older people based on urinary excretion of N-methylnicotinamide per gm creatinine reveals little evidence of deficiency. (N-Methylnicotinamide is a major product of niacin metabolism.) Among 116 institutionalized and independent-living subjects, only 3 had niacin metabolite excretions below the acceptable level.[40,69] However, in a national survey over one third of low income aged consumed less than 67% the RDA for niacin.[78] Since tryptophan was found to be one of the three limiting amino acids in the diets of older individuals, it may not be available for niacin synthesis.[57] Therefore good dietary sources of preformed niacin are indicated.

Ascorbic Acid

Dietary Intake and Biochemical Levels. Ascorbic acid status defined on the basis of either plasma or leukocyte vitamin levels has been related to age,[3,14] sex,[34,56] income,[56] smoking,[46-47] season of the year,[2,23] and dietary intake.[12,34] The relationship between diet and plasma levels is more apparent for ascorbic acid than most other vitamins. Bates and associates[12] evaluated ascorbic acid metabolism in 23 older people over 18 months and reported high correlations between dietary and plasma vitamin levels both within and between individuals.

Ascorbic acid is stored in the leukocytes and to some extent in the platelets. Andrews and coworkers[2] found no significant relationship between dietary ascorbic acid and storage levels in the leukocytes of older people. This inconsistency could relate to the measurement itself if the platelets are not included. For individuals with daily or seasonal variations in dietary ascorbic acid, plasma levels will reflect immediate intake. Leukocyte stores are a better indicator of long term status.

Requirements. Older men and women appear to differ in metabolism of ascorbic acid as men have lower plasma levels despite intakes equal to or higher than those of women.[34,56] Morgan and

coworkers[56] suggested the increased requirement related to the higher proportion of lean body mass in males. Data from 270 healthy, independent-living aged confirm that plasma ascorbic acid levels are influenced by both level of intake and sex.[34] Although dietary intakes (from food only) were similar in men and women (over two times the RDA) plasma levels were significantly higher in women as compared to men (1.14 versus 0.91 mg/100 ml) (see Table 6-3). Differences in plasma level were less apparent at higher levels of intake.

The total body pool of ascorbic acid is estimated to reach a maximum at 20 mg/kg with a plasma concentration of about 1.0 mg/100 ml.[46] Calculation of plasma vitamin concentration per unit of ascorbic acid intake suggests that older women require 75 mg and older men 150 mg daily to maintain a body pool of 20 mg/kg.[34] Garry and coworkers[34] concluded that the different requirements of older men and women for ascorbic acid should be considered when establishing the RDA. The effect of smoking, known to increase ascorbic acid requirements, did not influence these recommendations, as less than 10% of that population smoked regularly. In men between ages 21 and 69 smoking increased the ascorbic acid intake required for maintenance of the body metabolic pool from 100 to 140 mg;[47] therefore older people who smoke would appear to have a requirement about 40% above nonsmokers.

Factors Influencing Status. Ascorbic acid intake, smoking habits, and biochemical levels are related in older people. Burr and associates[14] found that men above age 75 who smoked more than 15 cigarettes per day had lower leukocyte ascorbic acid levels than nonsmokers (13.8 versus 17.5 $\mu g/10^8$ cells). Those smoking less than 15 cigarettes daily had vitamin levels intermediate between the heavy smokers and nonsmokers. Those authors maintain that older men with equal ascorbic acid intakes have similar plasma levels regardless of smoking habits.[14] Older men who smoked consumed fewer vitamin C–rich fruits and vegetables than non-

Table 6-3. Ascorbic acid intake and plasma levels

	Men	Women
Ascorbic Acid Intake		
Food only	142 mg	137 mg
Food and supplements	738 mg	734 mg
Plasma Ascorbic Acid		
Food only	0.91 mg/100 ml	1.14 mg/100 ml
Food and supplements	1.31 mg/100 ml	1.41 mg/100 ml

Modified from Garry, P.J., and others: Nutritional status in a healthy elderly population: Vitamin C, Am. J. Clin. Nutr. **36:**332, 1982.

smokers; in general intakes of both groups of older men were lower than older women. Although those authors concluded that level of fruit consumed did not totally explain the sex- and smoking-related differences in plasma ascorbic acid, food selection should be evaluated carefully in relation to biochemical values observed.[14] Season influences plasma ascorbic acid in older individuals possibly because of the availability of fresh produce.[2]

In older people socioeconomic status and ascorbic acid status are related.[56] Among 270 healthy aged in New Mexico, above average in education, less than 2% had serum ascorbic acid levels below 0.2 mg/100 ml (high risk) and 2% had values between 0.2 and 0.39 mg/100 ml (moderate risk).[34] In contrast, 7% and 14% of white low income women and men, respectively, had serum ascorbic acid levels below 0.2 mg/100 ml.[75] Over half of low income black men were below 0.4 mg/100 ml.[75] Although several British papers have reported

ascorbic acid deficiency in institutionalized aged,[2-3] evaluation of 46 nursing home residents in the United States found no individuals with serum levels below 0.2 mg/100 ml.[69] Ascorbic acid is lost if cooked vegetables are held at serving temperature for several hours, as sometimes happens in institutional settings or home-delivered meals programs (see Chapter 12). Citrus fruits are a better choice under such circumstances.

Vitamin B₆

Dietary Intake and Plasma Levels. Vitamin B₆ status evaluated on the basis of plasma pyridoxal phosphate,[1,64] serum or erythrocyte glutamic oxaloacetic transaminase (SGOT or EGOT),[38,63-64] or the tryptophan load test[38,63] declines with advancing age. The decrease in plasma pyridoxal phosphate (PLP) among 617 independent-living men is described in Fig. 6-1.[64] In those not taking supplements, plasma levels decreased by 0.9 ng/ml per

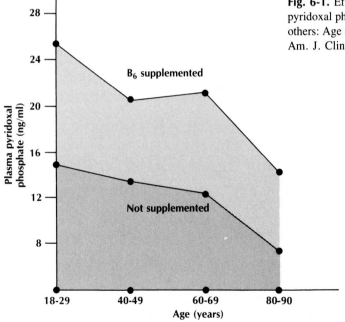

Fig. 6-1. Effect of age and supplementation on plasma pyridoxal phosphate levels. (Data from Rose, C.S., and others: Age differences in vitamin B₆ status of 617 men, Am. J. Clin. Nutr. **29**:847, 1976.)

decade. Plasma levels were higher in supplemented individuals at all ages and did not decrease significantly in older versus younger subjects. In the unsupplemented group, values below 5 ng/ml (considered less than optimum) increased from 3% to 12% between ages 40 and 80. In a recent evaluation of 119 persons in Central Kentucky (age 60 to 95), 57% of the institutionalized and 44% of the independent-living were judged vitamin B_6 deficient on the basis of red blood cell glutamic-pyruvic transaminase (EGPT) activity.[16] Dietary levels of vitamin B_6 were not reported.

Basis of Age-Related Change. Reasons proposed for the age-related change in vitamin B_6 parameters include decreased intake, impaired absorption, or impaired pyridoxine phosphorylation (conversion of the vitamin to the active form).[38] Although data are limited, many older people do consume less than the recommended level of vitamin B_6. In a Virginia survey one half of older women and one fifth of older men had less than 50% of the RDA. In a recent USDA survey of 394 low income persons age 75 and over, mean intake was about half that recommended.[74]

Biochemical abnormalities are reversed with vitamin B_6 supplementation. Administration of 15 mg[63] to 100 mg[38] of pyridoxine restored low SGOT and PLP levels to those of young controls and decreased the excretion of xanthurenic acid following a tryptophan load. According to Ranke and coworkers[63] restoration of normal SGOT function following addition of pyridoxine suggests that the apoenzyme was available; what was missing was the pyridoxal coenzyme. Hamfelt[38] pointed out that absorption may be a problem since high levels of supplementation are successful in reversing deficiency symptoms; however, daily supplements of 2.5 mg (about the RDA) have been shown to significantly influence SGOT levels.[80] Prescription drugs influence vitamin B_6 absorption and metabolism (see Chapter 9).

Although all factors described above may be involved in the age-related changes in vitamin B_6

metabolism, decreased use of meat, poultry, and fish because of problems with chewing or reduced income could result in low intakes. Because vitamin B_6 can be destroyed by heat processing, convenience foods can be poor sources.[28] Further study of the metabolic role of this vitamin in advancing age is urgently needed.

Folic Acid

Absorption. Presently, there are differing opinions regarding impaired folate absorption in healthy older people. A recent review concluded that low serum folate results from inadequate intake or use of alcohol or other drugs rather than impaired absorption.[65] Baker and coworkers[7] suggest that older people have decreased ability to absorb naturally occurring forms of folate. Absorption of folate (measured by circulating serum folate levels following ingestion) appeared to be significantly less when older people were fed yeast as compared to a synthetic vitamin (see Table 6-4).[7] Younger people absorbed the natural (yeast) and synthetic forms equally well. Naturally occurring folate in the form of folylpolyglutamate must be hydrolyzed to a monoglutamate to be absorbed.

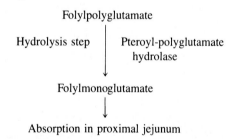

Baker and associates[7] concluded that older people lack sufficient enzyme to adequately hydrolyze naturally occurring folate forms. Folate fed in the monoglutamate form, requiring no prior hydrolysis, was readily absorbed. Recent work has suggested that hydrolase levels are 4 to 5 times higher in the intestinal lumen of young (2 to 3 months) versus aged (28 to 30 months) rats.[48]

Poor folate status itself impairs folate absorp-

Table 6-4. Serum levels following ingestion of naturally occurring and synthetic folate

	Serum Folate Levels	
	Following Yeast (ng/ml)	Following Synthetic Folate (ng/ml)
Young subjects (age 24-42 yr)	34.0	32.8
Older subjects (age 73-101 yr)	4.6	46.5

Modified from Baker, H., Jaslow, S.P., and Frank, O.: Severe impairment of dietary folate utilization in the elderly, J. Am. Geriatr. Soc. **26**:218, 1978.

tion.[24] Folate deficiency leads to both structural and functional changes in the upper jejunum, primary site of folate absorption. Atrophy of the mucosa and impaired enzyme secretion put in motion a vicious cycle in which declining folate status results in lowered folate absorption and eventual folate depletion. If mucosal damage is severe, even folylmonoglutamate absorption is limited. Intestinal changes are reversed with folate supplementation.

Liver folate stores, determined at autopsy of people who died of unnatural causes, declined with advancing age.[41] Although only 12% of those above age 60 were below the normal range, 2% were severely deficient in liver folate. Institutionalized or hospitalized aged consuming high levels of prescription drugs known to interfere with folate absorption (see Chapter 9) are at higher risk of folate deficiency.[65]

Dietary Intake and Serum Levels. Although information defining dietary folate levels in independent-living older people is limited (recent national surveys have not reported folate intake), available evidence suggests that a large proportion are consuming less than the recommended level of 400 μg.[65] Among 270 healthy aged in New Mexico,

over three fourths had less than 300 μg of folate daily and about 40% had less than 200 μg.[65] Folic acid intake also relates to income. In a Florida survey 65% of low income aged had less than half the RDA as compared to only 37% of those with higher incomes.[65] Moreover, over one third of low income groups had intakes that fell below 25% the RDA; this was true for only 3% of the upper income groups. Good sources of folic acid such as fruits, leafy vegetables, and whole grains are more likely to be selected by those with more money to spend for food.

Regardless of low intake, deficient plasma folate levels are not always observed. Less than 10% of the healthy aged in New Mexico had deficient plasma folate despite intakes below the recommended level (quoted by Rosenberg and coworkers).[65] This suggests either that the RDA is unrealistic in terms of actual requirements or that plasma levels are being maintained at the expense of body stores. Jagerstad and Westesson[45] reported that mean daily intakes of 145 to 175 μg folate prevented a decline in whole blood folate in 35 healthy Swedish pensioners observed over a period of six years.

Low serum folate levels in older people seem to be a nutritional rather than a physiologic response associated with aging. Incidence of folate deficiency is highest among institutionalized aged.[8,36,54,84] Older people living at home have folic acid levels more like those of young controls.[8,54] Hospitalized aged are more than twice as likely to be deficient.[36] This difference has been attributed to higher food intake among those in the community. Folic acid intake of institutionalized aged has been estimated to be less than half that of those at home.[54] Although nutritious meals are planned and served, the confined individual because of illness or food preferences may not consume what is provided. Use of prescription drugs is also greater among the chronically ill.

Red cell folate, representing tissue stores, provides an index of body folate as compared to serum values, which reflect recent intake. A majority of

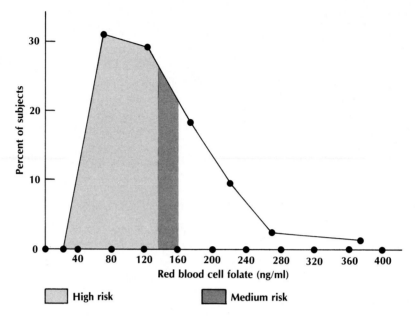

Fig. 6-2. Red blood cell folate levels in urban aged. (From Bailey, L.B., and others: Folacin and iron status and hematological findings in predominately black elderly persons from urban low-income households, Am. J. Clin. Nutr. **32:**2346, 1979.)

urban low income aged were at risk of folate deficiency (Fig. 6-2) according to red cell folate concentrations.[5] Food records revealed that intakes of folate-rich foods were low; only 17% regularly used fresh vegetables and only 30% regularly used citrus fruits. It was customary to boil vegetables for long periods of time, resulting in destruction of folate. Irregular shopping habits can limit use of fresh fruits and vegetables. Low cost sources of folic acid with emphasis on nutrient retention should be stressed in nutrition education programs.

Vitamin B$_{12}$

Absorption. Intrinsic factor found in the gastric juice of normal individuals is required for the absorption of vitamin B$_{12}$. Lack of intrinsic factor leads to pernicious anemia (see Chapter 8). Vita-

min B$_{12}$ deficiency results in degenerative changes in the myelin sheath and irreversible neurologic damage, in addition to hematologic changes.

Older individuals who do not have pernicious anemia may poorly absorb vitamin B$_{12}$. Gastrectomy, achlorhydria, chronic gastritis, or decreased secretion of gastric juices reduces intrinsic factor and subsequent vitamin B$_{12}$ absorption.[61,71] The problem is sometimes associated with general malabsorption, steatorrhea, and iron and folate deficiency.[25,55] Absorption is sometimes but not always improved by administration of intrinsic factor.[17] In some cases there is atrophy of the intestinal mucosa although physical findings may be similar in older people with normal absorption. Use of laxatives that reduce transit time can interfere with vitamin B$_{12}$ absorption.[71]

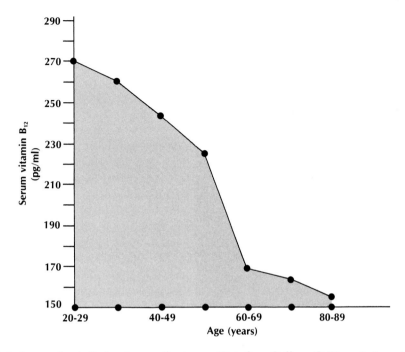

Fig. 6-3. Serum vitamin B_{12} levels according to age. (Data from Gaffney, G.W., and others: Vitamin B_{12} serum concentrations in 528 apparently healthy human subjects of ages 12-94, J. Gerontol. **12:**32, 1957.)

Impaired absorption exists in some but not all older people. Hyams[43] evaluated labeled vitamin B_{12} absorption in 13 aged men (73 to 90 years) and 10 young controls (28 to 50 years) and found no differences. Older men absorbed 62% of the test dose as compared with 57% for the control group. Only one older man absorbed less than half of the test dose (26%); this was true for 4 of the 10 younger men. That author suggests that percentage of absorption relates to need and the younger individuals may have had a more adequate diet, thus accounting for the lower percentage of absorption. At the level of vitamin administered (0.6 μg) normal absorption is estimated to be 63% (range 20% to 92%).[28] Therefore all of the older individuals were within the normal range.

Serum Vitamin B_{12} Levels. The nutritional significance of the age-related decline in serum vitamin B_{12} levels observed in both independent-living[8,29] and institutionalized[8,17,19,25] aged has not been resolved (Fig. 6-3). This could reflect (1) a decrease in vitamin intake, (2) malabsorption of the vitamin, or (3) a physiologic change in vitamin metabolism. Although this age-related decrease was observed in prisoners who had all been exposed to the same diet for a period of at least 5 years, it cannot be assumed that all consumed equal amounts of the food served.[29] The decline in calorie intake and problems with mastication observed in older people at home can also occur in older prisoners, resulting in lower consumption of animal products.

Low income aged consume less meat and may

not compensate by increasing their intakes of milk or cheese; therefore in one report consumption of animal products decreased by 20%.[26] Low serum vitamin B_{12} levels are more likely to be found in those over age 75 and living alone.[22,26] In one evaluation 2.5% of young controls as compared to 24% of the aged examined had inadequate vitamin B_{12} status.[8] Elsborg and coworkers[25] reported an improvement in previously deficient serum vitamin B_{12} levels when older individuals were placed on a normal hospital diet and concluded that their prior intake had not been adequate.

In a recent USDA survey of low income aged, however, dietary vitamin B_{12} was not a problem; mean intake for both sexes including those age 75 and over equaled the RDA.[74] Among aged in New Mexico over 85% consumed at least half the RDA.[33] A problem contributing to the conflicting evidence regarding vitamin B_{12} intakes is the limited information available regarding the vitamin B_{12} content of both fresh and processed foods.

The question of vitamin B_{12} intake versus aging or chronic disease in determining serum levels is far from being resolved. Among 473 institutionalized and independent-living aged vitamin B_{12} deficiency (based on serum vitamin levels) was more frequent in those at home (20% versus 32%), suggesting that problems with food preparation may limit vitamin B_{12} intake.[8] Some of those individuals residing in the community were participating in congregate or home-delivered meals programs, which do not serve meals everyday or provide for all meals of the day (see Chapter 12). If other food resources are very limited, dietary intake could be inadequate. Among those at home, vitamin B_{12} deficiency was reduced by half when vitamin supplements were reported, although 19% of those taking supplements still had inadequate serum levels suggesting problems in absorption.

The sex of the individual could be a factor in vitamin B_{12} status because older men appear to be more likely to become vitamin B_{12} deficient than older women.[4] Race and ethnic group should also be explored in relation to vitamin B_{12} intake and metabolism, as an evaluation of high risk, low income aged blacks and Spanish-Americans found no one with serum vitamin B_{12} levels below normal.[6]

SUMMARY

Metabolic studies evaluating vitamin requirements in older people have been few in number. For the most part requirements have been inferred from the blood or excretion levels of metabolites as related to general intake. Inability to ascertain liver stores, problems in fat digestion and absorption, and heavy use of laxatives complicate evaluation of the fat soluble vitamins. Vitamin A appears to be consumed in less than optimal amounts, although deficient serum levels are infrequent. Although vitamin E deficiency is not a problem, supply of vitamin D obtained through food or exposure to ultraviolet light is frequently less than desirable.

Requirements of the B complex vitamins and ascorbic acid are influenced by sex, smoking, and use of drugs. Thiamin and riboflavin excretion decrease with age and institutionalization, although intake decreases similarly. Red cell enzyme assays as compared to urinary excretion provide a more accurate indication of true status. Ascorbic acid requirements appear to be somewhat elevated in males, regardless of smoking, and it is suggested that RDAs be adjusted to reflect sex differences.

Folic acid and vitamin B_{12} absorption are impaired in some aged. Levels of the hydrolase required to convert folylpolyglutamates to folylmonoglutamates for absorption appear to be reduced. Use of prescription drugs and low folate intake further contribute to reduced serum folate. Serum vitamin B_{12} levels decrease with age; however, the cause of the change—reduced intake, impaired absorption, or the aging process per se—has not been resolved. Failure to secrete intrinsic factor does increase in frequency with advancing age.

Low serum pyridoxine levels in older individuals respond to supplementation, suggesting a problem with intake rather than absorption, although this vitamin is poorly absorbed in the presence of certain prescription drugs. Further studies of the vitamin requirements of older individuals as influenced by both the aging process and other dietary factors are desperately needed.

REVIEW QUESTIONS

1. How is fat soluble vitamin absorption influenced by (a) dietary fat (both level and type), (b) exaggerated intake of one fat soluble vitamin, and (c) use of mineral oil cathartics?
2. What is the relative contribution of dietary vitamin D and sunlight in meeting the vitamin requirement in older people? How is vitamin D metabolism related to calcium absorption?
3. It has been proposed that the RDA for ascorbic acid be specific according to sex and age in older adults. What evidence exists to support this idea? How is smoking related to the ascorbic acid requirement?
4. How does (a) caloric intake, (b) institutionalization, and (3) method of evaluation influence thiamin status and/or requirements of older people? Which groups appear most vulnerable to poor riboflavin status? Explain.
5. Serum pyridoxine, folic acid, and vitamin B_{12} levels tend to be lower in older than in younger adults. This has been related to (a) inadequate intake, (b) impaired absorption, and (c) normal aging. Which of these explanations do you support? (Be specific for each vitamin.) Cite evidence to justify your conclusion.

REFERENCES

1. Anderson, B.B., Peart, M.B., and Fulford-Jones, C.E.: The measurement of serum pyridoxal by a microbiological assay using *Lactobacillus casei*, J. Clin. Pathol. **23**:232, 1970.
2. Andrews, J., Brook, M., and Allen, M.A.: Influence of abode and season on the vitamin C status of the elderly, Gerontol. Clin. **8**:257, 1966.
3. Andrews, J., Letcher, M., and Brook, M.: Vitamin C supplementation in the elderly: A 17-month trial in an old persons' home, Br. Med. J. **2**:416, 1969.
4. Armstrong, B.K., and others: Hematological, vitamin B_{12}, and folate studies on Seventh-day Adventist vegetarians, Am. J. Clin. Nutr. **27**:712, 1974.
5. Bailey, L.B., and others: Folacin and iron status and hematological findings in predominately black elderly persons from urban low-income households, Am. J. Clin. Nutr. **32**:2346, 1979.
6. Bailey, L.B., and others: Vitamin B_{12} status of elderly persons from urban low-income households, J. Am. Geriatr. Soc. **28**:276, 1980.
7. Baker, H., Jaslow, S.P., and Frank, O.: Severe impairment of dietary folate utilization in the elderly, J. Am. Geriatr. Soc. **26**:218, 1978.
8. Baker, H., and others: Vitamin profiles in elderly persons living at home or in nursing homes, versus profile in healthy young subjects, J. Am. Geriatr. Soc. **27**:444, 1979.
9. Baker, M.R., Peacock, M., and Nordin, B.E.: The decline in vitamin D status with age, Age Ageing **9**:249, 1980.
10. Barnes, K.J., and Chen, L.H.: Vitamin E status of the elderly in central Kentucky, J. Nutr. Elderly **1**(3-4):41, 1981.
11. Barragry, J.M., and others: Intestinal cholecalciferol absorption in the elderly and in younger adults, Clin. Sci. Mol. Med. **55**:213, 1978.
12. Bates, C.J., and others: Long-term vitamin status and dietary intake of healthy elderly subjects. 2. Vitamin C, Br. J. Nutr. **42**:43, 1977.
13. Brin, M., and others: Some preliminary findings on the nutritional status of the aged in Onondaga County, New York, Am. J. Clin. Nutr. **17**:240, 1965.
14. Burr, M.L., and others: Plasma and leukocyte ascorbic acid levels in the elderly, Am. J. Clin. Nutr. **27**:144, 1974.
15. Carney, E.A., and Russell, R.M.: Correlation of dark adaptation test results with serum vitamin A levels in diseased adults, J. Nutr. **110**:552, 1980.
16. Chen, L.H., and Fan-Chiang, W.L.: Biochemical evaluation of riboflavin and vitamin B_6 status of institutionalized and non-institutionalized elderly in Central Kentucky, Int. J. Vitam. Nutr. Res. **51**:232, 1981.
17. Chernish, S.M., and others: The effect of intrinsic factor on the absorption of vitamin B_{12} in older people, Am. J. Clin. Nutr. **5**:651, 1957.
18. Chieffi, M., and Kirk, E.: Vitamin studies in middle-aged and old individuals. 2. Correlation between vitamin A plasma content and certain clinical and laboratory findings, J. Nutr. **37**:67, 1949.
19. Chow, B.F., and others: Agewise variation of vitamin B_{12} serum levels, J. Gerontol. **11**:142, 1956.
20. Conely, J., and Summer, D.: Prevention of vitamin D deficiency in the elderly (letter), Br. Med. J. **2**:1668, 1977.
21. Corless, D., and others: Vitamin D status in long-stay geriatric patients, Lancet **1**:1404, 1975.
22. Dawson, A.A., and Donald, D.: The serum vitamin B_{12} in the elderly, Gerontol. Clin. **8**:220, 1966.
23. Dibble, M.V., and others: Evaluation of the nutritional status of elderly subjects, with a comparison between fall and spring, J. Am. Geriatr. Soc. **15**:1031, 1967.
24. Elsborg, L.: Reversible malabsorption of folic acid in the

elderly with nutritional folate deficiency, Acta Haematol. **55:**140, 1976.

25. Elsborg, L., Lund, V., and Bastrup-Madsen, P.: Serum vitamin B_{12} levels in the aged, Acta Med. Scand. **200:**309, 1976.

26. Exton-Smith, A.N.: A nutrition survey of the elderly, Reports on Health and Social Subjects No. 3, London, 1972, Her Majesty's Stationery Office.

27. Fairney, A., Fry, J., and Lipscomb, A.: The effect of darkness on vitamin D in adults, Postgrad. Med. J. **55:**248, 1979.

28. Food and Nutrition Board: Recommended dietary allowances, ed. 9, Washington, D.C., 1980, National Academy of Sciences.

29. Gaffney, G.W., and others: Vitamin B_{12} serum concentrations in 528 apparently healthy human subjects of ages 12-94, J. Gerontol. **12:**32, 1957.

30. Gallagher, J.C., Riggs, B.L, and Deluca, H.F.: Effect of estrogen on calcium absorption and serum vitamin D metabolites in post-menopausal osteoporosis, J. Clin. Endocrinol. Metab. **51:**1359, 1980.

31. Gallagher, J.C., and others: Intestinal calcium absorption and serum vitamin D metabolites in normal subjects and osteoporotic patients: Effect of age and dietary calcium, J. Clin. Invest. **64:**729, 1979.

32. Garry, P.J., Goodwin, J.S., and Hunt, W.C.: Nutritional status in a healthy elderly population: Riboflavin, Am. J. Clin. Nutr. **36:**902, 1982.

33. Garry, P.J., and others: Nutritional status in a healthy elderly population: Dietary and supplemental intakes, Am. J. Clin. Nutr. **36:**319, 1982.

34. Garry, P.J., and others: Nutritional status in a healthy elderly population: Vitamin C, Am. J. Clin. Nutr. **36:**332, 1982.

35. Gillum, H.L., Morgan, A.F., and Sailer, F.: Nutritional status of the aging. 5. Vitamin A and carotene, J. Nutr. **55:**655, 1955.

36. Girdwood, R.H., Thompson, A.D., and Williamson, J.: Folate status in the elderly, Br. Med. J. **2:**670, 1967.

37. Gontzea, I., and Nicolau, N.: Relationship between serum tocopherol level and dyslipidemia, Nut. Rep. Int. **5:**225, 1975.

38. Hamfelt, A.: Age variation of vitamin B_6 metabolism in man, Clin. Chim. Acta **10:**48, 1964.

39. Hampton, D.J., Chrisley, B.M., and Driskell, J.A.: Vitamin B_6 status of the elderly in Montgomery County, Va., Nut. Rep. Int. **16:**743, 1977.

40. Harrill, I., and Cervone, N.: Vitamin status of older women, Am. J. Clin. Nutr. **30:**431, 1977.

41. Hoppner, K., and Lampi, B.: Folate levels in human liver from autopsies in Canada, Am. J. Clin. Nutr. **33:**862, 1980.

42. Horwitt, M.K.: Dietary requirements of the aged, J. Am. Diet. Assoc. **29:**443, 1953.

43. Hyams, D.E.: The absorption of vitamin B_{12} in the elderly, Gerontol. Clin. **6:**193, 1964.

44. Iber, F.L., and others: Thiamin in the elderly: Relation to alcoholism and neurological degenerative disease, Am. J. Clin. Nutr. **36**(suppl.):1067, 1982.

45. Jagerstad, M., and Westesson, A.K.: Folate, Scand. J. Gastroenterol. **14**(suppl. 52):196, 1979.

46. Kallner, A.B., Hartmann, D., and Hornig, D.H.: Steady-state turnover and body pool of ascorbic acid in man, Am. J. Clin. Nutr. **32:**530, 1979.

47. Kallner, A.B., Hartmann, D., and Hornig, D.H.: On the requirements of ascorbic acid in man: Steady-state turnover and body pool in smokers, Am. J. Clin. Nutr. **34:**1347, 1981.

48. Kesavan, V., and Noronha, J.M.: Folate malabsorption in aged rats related to low levels of pancreatic folyl conjugase, Am. J. Clin. Nutr. **37:**262, 1983.

49. Koh, E.T.: Selected blood components and urinary B vitamins as related to age and sex of black population in Southwest Mississippi, Am. J. Clin. Nutr. **33:**670, 1980.

50. Lawoyin, S., and others: Ability of 25-hydroxyvitamin D_3 therapy to augment serum 1,25- and 24,25-dihydroxyvitamin D in postmenopausal osteoporosis, J. Clin. Endocrinol. Metab. **50:**593, 1980.

51. Lawson, D.E., and others: Relative contributions of diet and sunlight to vitamin D state in the elderly, Br. Med. J. **4:**303, 1979.

52. Loerch, J.D., Underwood, B.A., and Lewis, K.C.: Response of plasma levels of vitamin A to a dose of vitamin A as an indicator of hepatic vitamin A reserves in rats, J. Nutr. **109:**778, 1979.

53. MacLennan, W.J., and Hamilton, J.C.: Vitamin D supplements and 25-hydroxy vitamin D concentrations in the elderly, Br. Med. J. **2:**859, 1977.

54. Meindok, H., and Dvorsky, R.: Serum folate and vitamin B_{12} levels in the elderly, J. Am. Geriatr. Soc. **18:**317, 1970.

55. Montgomery, R.D., and others: The ageing gut: A study of intestinal absorption in relation to nutrition in the elderly, Q.J. Med. (New Series) **47**(186):197, 1978.

56. Morgan, A.F., Gillum, H.L., and Williams, R.I.: Nutritional status of the aging. 3. Serum ascorbic acid and intake, J. Nutr. **55:**431, 1955.

57. Nair, B.M., and Andersson, I.: Quantitative and qualitative evaluations of protein intake in a geriatric subpopulation from a southern Swedish community, Am. J. Clin. Nutr. **31:**1280, 1978.

58. National Dairy Council: Fat-soluble vitamins, Dairy Council Digest **53:**1, May/June 1982.

59. Neer, R.M., and others: Stimulation by artificial lighting of calcium absorption in elderly human subjects, Nature **229:**255, 1971.

60. Olson, R.E.: Vitamin E and heart disease, Food Nutr. News **5-6:**1, Feb./March 1973.

61. Pathy, M.S., Kirkman, S., and Molloy, M.J.: An evaluation of simultaneously administered free and intrinsic factor bound radioactive cyanocobalamin in the diagnosis of pernicious anaemia in the elderly, J. Clin. Pathol. **32**:244, 1979.
62. Patterson, C.R.: Vitamin-D poisoning: Survey of causes in 21 patients with hypercalcaemia, Lancet **1**:1164, 1980.
63. Ranke, E., and others: Vitamin B_6 deficiency in the aged, J. Gerontol. **15**:41, 1960.
64. Rose, C.S., and others: Age differences in vitamin B_6 status of 617 men, Am. J. Clin. Nutr. **29**:847, 1976.
65. Rosenberg, I.H., and others: Folate nutrition in the elderly, Am. J. Clin. Nutr. **36**(suppl.):1060, 1982.
66. Rutishauser, I.H., and others: Long-term vitamin status and dietary intake of healthy elderly subjects. 1. Riboflavin, Br. J. Nutr. **42**:33, 1979.
67. Sauberlich, H.E., and others: Thiamin requirement of the adult human, Am. J. Clin. Nutr. **32**:2237, 1979.
68. Somerville, P.J., Lien, J.W., and Kaye, M.: The calcium and vitamin D status in an elderly female population and their response to administered supplemental vitamin D_3, J. Gerontol. **32**:659, 1977.
69. Stiedemann, M., Jansen, C., and Harrill, I.: Nutritional status of elderly men and women, J. Am. Diet. Assoc. **73**:132, 1978.
70. Tappel, A.L.: Reactions of vitamin E, ubiquinol, and seleno-amino acids, and protection of oxidant-labile enzymes. In DeLuca, H.F., and Suttie, J.W., eds.: The fat-soluble vitamins, Madison, 1970, University of Wisconsin Press.
71. Thomas, J.H., and Powell, D.E.: Blood disorders in the elderly, Bristol, 1971, John Wright & Sons, Ltd.
72. Underwood, B.A., and others: Liver stores of α-tocopherol in a normal population dying suddenly and rapidly from unnatural causes in New York City, Am. J. Clin. Nutr. **23**:1314, 1970.
73. Underwood, B.A., and others: Liver stores of vitamin A in a normal population dying suddenly or rapidly from unnatural causes in New York City, Am. J. Clin. Nutr. **23**:1037, 1970.
74. United States Department of Agriculture: Food and nutrient intakes of individuals in 1 day, low-income households, November 1979-March 1980, National Food Consumption Survey 1977-78, Preliminary Report No. 13, Washington, D.C., 1982, U.S. Government Printing Office.
75. United States Department of Health, Education and Welfare: Ten-State Nutrition Survey 1968-1970. 4. Biochemical, DHEW Publication No. (HSM) 72-8132, Atlanta, 1972, Centers for Disease Control.
76. United States Department of Health, Education and Welfare: Ten-State Nutrition Survey 1968-70, 5. Dietary, DHEW Publication No. (HSM) 72-8133, Atlanta, 1972, Centers for Disease Control.
77. United States Department of Health, Education and Welfare: Preliminary findings of the first Health and Nutrition Examination Survey, United States, 1971-1972: Dietary intake and biochemical findings, DHEW Publication No. (HRA) 74-1219-1, Washington, D.C., 1974, U.S. Government Printing Office.
78. United States Department of Health, Education and Welfare: Dietary intake source data, United States, 1971-74, DHEW Publication No. (PHS) 79-1221, Hyattsville, Md., 1979, U.S. Government Printing Office.
79. Vatassery, G.T., Alter, M., and Stadlan, E.M.: Serum tocopherol levels and vibratory threshold changes with age, J. Gerontol. **26**:481, 1971.
80. Vir, S.C., and Love, A.H.: Vitamin B_6 status of the hospitalized aged, Am. J. Clin. Nutr. **31**:1383, 1978.
81. Vir, S.C., and Love, A.H.: Nutritional status of institutionalized and noninstitutionalized aged in Belfast, Northern Ireland, Am. J. Clin. Nutr. **32**:1934, 1979.
82. Volpe, J.J., and Marasa, J.C.: A role for thiamin in the regulation of fatty acid and cholesterol biosynthesis in cultured cells of neural origin, J. Neurochem. **30**:975, 1978.
83. Weber, F.: Absorption mechanisms for fat-soluble vitamins and the effect of other food constituents. In Nutrition in health and disease and international development, Symposia from the XII International Congress of Nutrition, New York, 1981, Alan R Liss, Inc.
84. Webster, S.G., and Leeming, J.T.: Erythrocyte folate levels in young and old, J. Am. Geriatr. Soc. **27**:451, 1979.
85. Weisman, Y., and others: Inadequate status and impaired metabolism of vitamin D in the elderly, Isr. J. Med. Sci. **17**:19, 1981.

Chapter 7

Minerals in the Aged

In past years limited attention was directed toward the mineral requirements of older individuals. Balance techniques traditionally used to ascertain mineral requirements are both costly and tedious and demand extraordinary cooperation on the part of the subject. Recent advances in methodology including use of radioactive isotopes and quantitative measurement of minute levels of the trace minerals have brought renewed interest in both the structural and the metabolic role of minerals. This is especially true in relation to older people because age-related degenerative problems including bone disease, and alterations in glucose tolerance and immune function are associated with mineral requirements and metabolism. Unfortunately, it is difficult to differentiate between changes related to normal aging and those resulting from chronic disease.

This chapter will focus on current knowledge relating to changes in mineral requirements in the later years. For various minerals including magnesium, manganese, selenium, and molybdenum there has been no work addressing the particular needs of the aged. For general information relating to those minerals see reference 18.

MINERAL REQUIREMENTS AND METABOLISM

Iron

Iron Absorption. Absorption of dietary iron is a complicated and inefficient process in people of all ages. Because there is no established route for the excretion of iron, control is exerted at the point of entry.[18] In young adults average iron absorption was estimated by the Food and Nutrition Board to be about 10%,[18] although Kuhn and associates[42] have reported absorption levels of 6.5% in men and 16% in women. Iron absorption is influenced by body need, body stores, stomach pH, and other foods in the meal.[11,68] Although evaluation of absorption in older people has been limited, heme iron was reported to be absorbed equally well by people of all ages (11% of labeled dose).[37] Absorption of inorganic iron, however, was significantly lower in older (>age 50) versus younger (<age 30) subjects. Greater absorption by the younger group could reflect the elevated iron needs of menstruating women. (The number of women in each group was not indicated.)

Animal studies suggest an age-related decrease in iron absorption.[71] Absorption of ^{59}Fe decreased from 46% to 20% of a given dose in rats between the ages of 6 and 20 months. Although older animals retained the ability to increase the percentage absorbed in response to increased need (in this case reduced atmospheric pressure) total absorption was still less than in young controls.

Achlorhydria and reduced secretion of gastric juice decrease absorption, as components within the gastric juice bind to iron and enhance absorption and the hydrochloric acid maintains an acid environment that promotes the reduction of inorganic iron from the ferric to the ferrous form.[11,38,68]

The incidence of achlorhydria increases with age[62] and partial or complete gastrectomy is more common in older people. The intestinal brush border, prominently involved in the absorption process,[8] undergoes age-related morphologic changes that could modify rate of absorption.[52] Antacids raising pH levels[16] and certain drugs (e.g., cholestyramine) binding both inorganic and organic iron complexes decrease iron uptake.[25]

Highly processed bread and cereal items are attractive to older people because they have a long shelf life, are easily chewed, and require little preparation. Naturally occurring iron, however, is lost in the milling process and replaced with inorganic iron compounds, which are less easily absorbed.[9] A liberal intake of fiber, to promote normal bowel function, may bind trace minerals and decrease iron absorption.[12]

Iron Metabolism. After being absorbed iron has several possible destinations: (1) to replace cells lost through the skin, gastrointestinal tract, or urine; (2) to replace or produce red blood cells (average life span 120 days); or (3) to be stored in the liver. Normal iron losses in the young adult have been estimated to be 1.0 and 1.5 mg daily in men and women, respectively.[18] Finch,[17] using labeled iron, estimated daily iron loss to be 0.61 mg in older men (mean age = 70) and 0.64 mg in nonmenstruating women (mean age = 66).

Iron is less rapidly assimilated into red blood cells in older individuals and high levels of iron in the bone marrow suggest that slowed production of red blood cells is not always the result of iron deficiency;[47] active hemopoietic tissue may decrease as a consequence of age. Liver iron stores in a Spanish population dying of unnatural causes were similar in young and aged men[10] and in aged of both sexes. Only 3% of older men and 8% of older women had liver stores indicative of deficiency. Depletion of iron stores is usually the result of pathologic conditions or practices that cause continual blood loss such as gastrointestinal ulcers or excessive use of aspirin (see Chapter 9).

Practical Aspects of Iron Intake. Iron is found in the average American diet at a level of 6 mg/1000 kcal.[47] Unless iron-rich foods are deliberately selected, an energy intake of nearly 2000 kcal is required to obtain the recommended level. Men who consume more calories are less vulnerable to poor iron intake than women who often consume only 1200 to 1600 kcal (see Chapter 3). In a recent survey 94% of older men as compared to 67% of older women consumed at least 100% the RDA for iron.[23] Income level and iron intake levels are correlated in older women. In the HANES study both white and black older men regardless of income had median intakes of at least 9 mg.[66] For white and black older women of low income, median intakes were 7.2 and 6.7 mg, respectively. For higher income women these values were 8.6 and 7.4 mg, respectively. Half of all low income black women age 65 and over had less than two thirds the RDA.

For low income people a greater proportion of dietary iron may come from fortified cereal products rather than heme-containing animal foods. Over one fourth of low income Food Stamp recipients age 75 or above reported consuming a ready-to-eat cereal on the day of record in a recent USDA food survey.[65]

Both ascorbic acid and heme iron facilitate absorption of nonheme iron.[50-51] One gram of cooked meat, fish, or poultry is equivalent to 1 mg of ascorbic acid in promoting absorption of nonheme iron; maximum absorption is achieved with more than 75 units of enhancing factors: 75 gm cooked meat, fish, or poultry; 75 mg ascorbic acid; or an equivalent combination of the two. The percentage of iron absorbed from a low, medium, and high availability meal is illustrated in Table 7-1. In a low availability meal (containing less than 1 ounce of meat, poultry, or fish or less than 25 mg of ascorbic acid) only 3% of the nonheme iron present will be absorbed. Percentage of absorption is proportionally increased as these items are added. The addition of more than 3 ounces of meat, poultry,

Table 7-1. Improving absorption of nonheme iron

Meal Type	Food Content	Nonheme Iron Absorbed*
Low availability meal	Less than 1 ounce cooked meat, poultry, or fish or less than 25 mg ascorbic acid	3%
Medium availability meal	1-3 ounces meat, poultry, or fish or 25-75 mg ascorbic acid	5%
High availability meal	More than 3 ounces meat, poultry, or fish or more than 75 mg ascorbic acid or 1-3 ounces cooked meat, poultry, or fish plus 25-75 mg ascorbic acid	8%

*In persons with adequate iron stores.

Modified from Monsen, E.R., and others: Estimation of available dietary iron, Am. J. Clin. Nutr. **31**:134, 1978.

or fish or more than 75 mg of ascorbic acid or a combination can increase the level of absorption of nonheme iron to 8%. Heme iron is usually absorbed at a level of 23%. Absorption is enhanced even more in individuals with poor iron stores.

Older clients should be taught to combine their foods to best advantage for maximum iron absorption. Having orange juice along with a fortified breakfast cereal will effectively promote the absorption of the inorganic iron in the grain product. Identification of low and moderate cost iron-rich foods should be a priority with all clients.

Calcium and Phosphorus

Calcium metabolism has important implications for both nutritional and physical health. Aging is accompanied by a gradual loss of calcium from the bones, which if accelerated leads to the clinically defined bone disease osteoporosis (see Chapter 8). For those with less degree of loss bone strength is still diminished, increasing the risk of fracture.

Control of Calcium Metabolism. Serum calcium must be maintained within very narrow limits (9 to 11 mg/100 ml) to ensure normal function of the heart and nervous system. This is regulated by parathyroid hormone (PTH), which controls calcium absorption, excretion, and metabolism in bone. A decrease in serum calcium or increase in serum phosphate leads to secretion of PTH and subsequent (1) release of calcium from bone (bone resorption), (2) increase in calcium absorption in the intestine, and (3) increase in calcium reabsorption in the kidney tubule with a concomitant increase in phosphate excretion, thereby restoring serum calcium to normal levels.[4] The action of PTH in resorbing calcium from the bone is balanced by the protective effect of estrogen suppressing bone resorption. Following menopause and estrogen withdrawal, bone becomes increasingly sensitive to PTH, and calcium mobilization is accelerated.[21,32,34] As bone resorption continues, bringing about high serum calcium levels, secretion of PTH is reduced, resulting in lowered absorption of dietary calcium and reabsorption of calcium in the kidney. Loss of skeletal calcium was estimated to be 21 mg/day in premenopausal as compared to 38 mg/day in postmenopausal women.[32-33] Estrogen therapy reduced calcium losses to premenopausal levels.

Effect of Estrogen. Gallagher and coworkers[20-22] propose that estrogen improves calcium balance by decreasing bone resorption. This effectively decreases serum calcium and promotes PTH secretion. The final step in this sequence is increased production of the active metabolite of vitamin D, required for active calcium transport across the mucosa.[21]

Estrogen replacement

↓

Decreased calcium mobilization from bone

↓

Increased release of parathyroid hormone

↓

Activation of renal 1α-hydroxylase

↓

Stimulated conversion of 25(OH)D to 1,25(OH)$_2$D

↓

Increased calcium absorption

Calcium absorption can be increased by administration of either estrogen or 1,25(OH)$_2$D. It has been shown that estrogen leads to increased levels of the active vitamin D metabolite. Whether estrogen acts by slowing bone resorption or directly increasing the activity of the renal hydroxylase required for the conversion of 25(OH)D to 1,25(OH)$_2$D is not known. Another possible action is slowing the rate at which 1,25(OH)$_2$D is degraded. According to Gallagher and coworkers,[21] all actions are possible, based on current data.

Calcium Intake and Absorption. It has been recognized for many years that calcium absorption decreases with age, although to a greater extent in women.[5,53] Younger women may absorb as much as 67% of a given dose; those age 80 and above may absorb 26% or less.[53] The problem is complicated further by the fact that calcium intakes also decrease (658 to 568 mg/day) in women between ages 25 and 65.[66] Therefore considerably less calcium becomes available for bone maintenance.

Younger individuals have the ability to adapt the rate of calcium absorption to level of intake.[2] Among younger people with calcium intakes ranging from 200 to 1800 mg/day serum 1,25(OH)$_2$D levels and the percentage of calcium absorbed increased as intake decreased.[54] Older individuals, especially those with osteoporotic bone disease, are less able to respond to changes in dietary calcium,

particularly low levels of intake.[59] Among women consuming 400 mg calcium daily, serum 1,25(OH)$_2$D levels were 20 and 34 pg/ml in older versus younger groups.[22] Regulation of absorption rate appears to be mediated through changes in parathyroid secretion and eventual production of 1,25(OH)$_2$D. The ileum appears to be the site of regulation protecting against variations in calcium intake.[54]

Calcium balance can be improved in older women by increasing dietary intake. Although the rate of absorption may be low, the net amount absorbed from a larger as compared to a smaller intake will be greater. Heaney and coworkers,[32] after studying calcium balance in 168 healthy women, concluded that postmenopausal women could achieve calcium balance on a daily intake of 1.5 gm. For premenopausal or estrogen-treated postmenopausal women the requirement was 0.99 gm/day. These levels are substantially above those currently recommended (0.8 gm daily) for, or consumed by, women of all ages.[18] HANES[66] found median calcium intakes of white and black older women to be 504 and 373 mg/day, respectively. Older men have higher intakes (median levels = 620 mg in whites and 476 mg in blacks). Based on the recommendations of Heaney and coworkers, postmenopausal women are consuming only 25% to 34% of the calcium needed.

Protein-Calcium Interaction. The calciuric effect of high protein diets has been observed in adults of all ages.[45] Catabolism and excretion of sulfate, arising from the sulfur-containing amino acids, interfere with renal tubular reabsorption of calcium resulting in elevated urinary calcium. Urinary calcium nearly doubled in older men and women when dietary protein increased from 47 to 112 gm daily.[45] The calciuric effect of a high protein diet is less dramatic if phosphorus also increases, as when meat is the protein source, because a greater proportion of calcium is reabsorbed in the renal tubule. However, protein intakes above recommended levels are not generally appropriate (see Chapter 5).

Controversy Regarding Requirements. Epidemiologic studies suggest that daily intakes of 400 to 500 mg calcium are sufficient to maintain calcium balance on a vegetable-grain diet low in protein and phosphorus.[14] This level may not be adequate, however, for an individual consuming a typical acid-producing Western diet.[14] The common use of phosphate-containing food additives and increasing consumption of meat and soft drinks have led to a calcium/phosphorus ratio estimated to be 1:1.5.[18] Ratios of 1:2 fed to experimental animals were detrimental to bone health although this has not been demonstrated in humans.[14]

The more important question relating to the current recommended intake of calcium is whether bone loss can be either prevented or reduced in severity by increasing dietary calcium. Heaney and coworkers[32] propose, on the basis of their experimental evidence, that older women require more than 800 mg calcium daily to maintain calcium balance and prevent calcium depletion. In their opinion, if the RDA is expected to provide a margin of safety for all healthy people, it should be increased.

A further argument for increasing the calcium recommendation is based on comparative requirements for animal species. Animals similar in body weight to humans have calcium requirements of 52 to 62 mg/kg/day; the present recommendation for humans is 11 mg/kg/day, only 20% that predicted.[34] Up to this time the Food and Nutrition Board has taken the position that (1) people have been shown to maintain calcium balance on intakes less than the recommended level and (2) high intakes of calcium have not been shown to prevent or reverse osteoporosis.[18]

Recent studies (see Chapter 8) do suggest that calcium intakes of 1.0 and 1.5 gm can prevent calcium loss and may lead to calcium deposition, although long term studies are required to confirm the latter. Although higher intakes of calcium may be beneficial at younger ages and increase bone mineralization, they appear to be especially pertinent for the postmenopausal woman to prevent bone loss. Calcium is a nutrient for which an age- and sex-specific requirement might be considered.

Chromium

Body Functions. Chromium is essential for maintaining normal glucose tolerance, interacting with insulin at the receptor site on the cell membrane.[30,48] Impaired glucose tolerance occurs in chromium deficiency and is reversed upon supplementation. With this in mind chromium supplementation has been tried both with older individuals exhibiting abnormal glucose tolerance and with diagnosed diabetics; however, success has been limited.[24]

Double-blind studies evaluating use of inorganic chromium[43,56] or chromium-rich brewer's yeast[55] indicate that abnormal glucose tolerance can be marginally improved in some older people. Levine and coworkers[43] reported improved glucose tolerance in 4 of 10 institutionalized aged (age range = 74 to 96 years). Offenbacher and Pi-Sunyer[55] in a double-blind evaluation of 24 older persons from a retirement home (mean age = 78 years) observed an improvement in both mildly diabetic and nondiabetic groups. In nondiabetics supplementation led to a slower increase and more rapid decline in serum glucose following a 100 gm dose; however, serum glucose at 120 minutes was about 120 mg/100 ml prior to supplementation and decreased only slightly following treatment. Although serum glucose at 120 minutes was lower in diabetics following supplementation, values still approached 200 mg/100 ml. Those responding to chromium have reduced blood glucose levels after 2 hours; serum insulin levels are either reduced or unchanged. Therefore the improvement in removal of glucose is brought about not by increased secretion of insulin but rather by increased effectiveness of available insulin.

Although chromium deficiency may in some instances contribute, abnormal glucose tolerance in older people is usually age- or disease-related.

(Age-related changes in glucose tolerance will be discussed in Chapter 8.) Chromium supplementation does not appear to be clinically useful in treating older individuals with impaired glucose tolerance.

Chromium Intake. The suggested daily intake of chromium is 50 to 200 μg.[18] Mean daily intake reported for institutionalized aged was 52 μg.[43] Data are lacking for healthy aged living in the community; however, people treated for abnormal glucose tolerance sometimes required supplementation for periods of 2 months or more, suggesting poor previous intake and low body stores.[24] At present there is no simple procedure for assessing chromium status, although hair chromium concentration appears to decrease as a function of age.[30] Although hair analysis is still being evaluated as an indicator of body chromium, this suggestion of reduced chromium levels in older individuals warrants further attention. Chromium tends to be lost in food processing and will likely be present at low levels in diets comprised mainly of highly processed items. Older people should be encouraged to consume whole grains whenever possible. Brewer's yeast, meat products, and cheese are other good sources.[48]

Fluoride

Fluoride is required for optimum mineral crystallization in bones and teeth.[49] Epidemiologic comparisons of people residing in areas with high or low levels of naturally occurring fluoride point to a positive effect of fluoride in maintaining bone density throughout life.[6] Large bone crystals as developed in the presence of fluoride are less susceptible to resorption than smaller crystals. The potential toxicity of fluoride, however, has limited its use in treating bone disorders (see Chapter 8).

Zinc

Zinc Intake. The RDA for zinc is 15 mg.[18] Daily zinc intake of older people estimated from dietary records obtained in recent national surveys ranged from 7 to 13 mg.[58] Forty-four participants in a congregate meals program (mean age = 69 years) had an average intake of 10.1 mg.[28] In that study neither sex nor race was a factor, although 59% consumed less than two thirds the RDA. Institutionalized aged (mean age = 75 years) from the same geographical region consumed about 8 mg daily, although the meals provided contained nearly 19 mg.[26] Snacks including fruit, breadstuffs, and milk contributed to total dietary zinc.

Dietary zinc is influenced by total calorie intake and money spent for food, as well as food selection.[58] Zinc intake increases proportionately with energy intake. It was estimated[58] that older men with an energy intake of 1800 kcal consume about 10.6 mg of zinc. Older women consuming about 1300 kcal take in only 7.2 mg zinc (less than 50% the RDA). People with low calorie intake can compensate by selecting foods rich in zinc (Table 7-2), such as whole grains, dark poultry meat, and liver. In the average American diet about 40% of the zinc is provided by meat, fish, and poultry, relatively expensive items in the food budget.[58] The

Table 7-2. Zinc content of selected foods

Food Item (edible portion)	Zinc (mg)
Grain products	
Oatmeal, cooked (1 cup)	1.2
Bran flakes, 40% (1 oz.)	1.0
Corn flakes (1 oz.)	0.1
Whole wheat bread (1 slice)	0.5
White bread (1 slice)	0.2
Dairy foods	
Cheese, cheddar (1 ½ oz.)	1.6
Milk, whole (1 cup)	0.9
Meat or meat alternatives	
Liver, beef (3 oz.)	4.4
Beef, ground (3 oz.)	3.8
Chicken, dark meat (3 oz.)	2.4
Fish, white (3 oz.)	0.9
Peanut butter (2 T)	0.9
Frankfurter (1)	0.7

most common food source is beef. A diet based on dairy products and highly processed breads and cereals will be limited in zinc. Older people with low intakes of meat or poultry, as a result of limited income or chewing difficulties, are at risk of deficient intake.

Zinc Status. Hair and plasma zinc concentrations are used to evaluate zinc status, although both have limitations. Plasma zinc levels do not always relate to body stores and may not provide an accurate assessment of zinc status.[60] Sampling technique is critical when obtaining hair for zinc analysis.[70] Gregor[26] found that hair zinc concentrations in older persons related to dietary protein levels rather than dietary zinc. Among 135 aged low income blacks, 8% had hair zinc concentrations below 71 μg/gm (indicative of deficiency) and 29% had concentrations below 101 μg/gm (considered to be low).[70]

The influence of age per se on serum zinc levels is currently unclear. Sandstead and coworkers,[58] comparing plasma zinc levels in 61 healthy aged (mean age = 72 years) and 71 controls (mean age = 31 years), found significantly higher values in the younger (86 μg/100 ml) versus the older (80 μg/100 ml) group. In a recent HANES report serum zinc levels decreased in men between ages 18 and 64.[67] Women at younger ages have lower serum zinc levels than men, but values in women do not change appreciably with increasing age. Thirty-two percent of men and 39% of women age 65 and above had serum zinc levels below 80 μg/100 ml (considered to be less than adequate). Levels were consistently lower in poverty versus nonpoverty groups. Whether the serum zinc levels observed reflect reduced intake or a metabolic response of the aging process requires continued study. A recent report indicated that healthy older men were able to maintain zinc balance on the recommended intake of 15 mg.[64]

These data support the earlier suggestion that those on a reduced income are at particular risk of zinc deficiency. Decreasing calorie intake further jeopardizes zinc intake unless there is special attention given to zinc-rich foods. When assisting older clients with meal planning, good sources of this nutrient should be included.

Zinc and Physiologic Function. Zinc plays a role in the taste mechanism and immunologic response.[58] Because these functions are sometimes altered in older people, the question is raised whether such changes result from the aging process or zinc deficiency.

Taste Acuity. Dietary and hair zinc levels have not been related to taste acuity in either institutionalized or independent-living aged.[26,28] Zinc supplementation (15 mg daily) of 49 institutionalized aged in a double-blind pattern over a 3-month period did not significantly improve taste acuity, although taste thresholds for both salt and sucrose decreased slightly.[27] Hair zinc concentration did increase, confirming that dietary zinc was being absorbed. Hair zinc concentration, smoking, or use of dentures did not influence taste threshold.[27] Changes in the taste buds as a consequence of age or drugs used in treatment of chronic disease could contribute to the reduced taste acuity observed in many older people.[27]

Immune Function. Zinc supplementation did influence immune function in one group of older individuals. Immune response can be tested on the basis of skin reactions (diameter of skin responses) to common antigens and on the basis of the level of antibodies produced following injection of a standard vaccine. Supplementation of 30 institutionalized persons over 70 years of age with 440 mg zinc sulfate daily (approximately 175 mg zinc) significantly improved both antibody and skin responses to standard immunologic tests.[15] This improvement could reflect correction of a zinc deficiency or a short-term direct stimulation of the immunologic system; zinc status was not evaluated prior to supplementation. Zinc deficiency in animals is accompanied by a loss of immune function that can be restored with administration of dietary levels of zinc.

Age-related changes in zinc metabolism may be

mediated at the cellular level, as adipocytes from aged rats (24 months of age) transported and retained 40% less zinc from an incubation medium than adipocytes from younger animals (12 months of age); serum zinc was decreased by 15% in the older group.[61] Changes in the cellular metabolism of zinc may lead to physiologic alterations despite adequate intake. Long-term evaluation of healthy older people given zinc supplements falling within dietary rather than pharmacologic ranges would provide valuable information relating to the possible influence of zinc status on observed changes in immune function.

Wound Healing. Zinc supplementation has been evaluated in relation to wound healing in older patients. When zinc status was adequate (based on serum zinc levels), supplementation had no effect on rate of healing. When zinc status was less than adequate, healing was significantly improved in those given zinc supplements as compared to those given a placebo.[58] Zinc nutriture is therefore particularly important in older persons who have decubitus ulcers or are recovering from surgery.

Copper

The role of copper in formation of red blood cells makes this a nutrient of importance among older individuals at risk for iron-deficiency anemia (see Chapter 8). Plasma copper in 53 Belfast aged ranged from 75 to 166 μg/100 ml and was not related to either hair copper concentrations or hemoglobin levels, although the number of people low in hemoglobin was not indicated.[69] Balance studies in six older men suggest that copper requirements do not differ (RDA = 2 to 3 mg) in older versus younger individuals.[64] Those authors expressed the concern, however, that errors in measurement may obscure gain or loss of body copper. Balance varied from −0.27 to +0.22 mg among the individuals studied.

In the general population, copper intake of 22 adults (determined by biochemical diet analysis) was about 1 mg daily, and 81% of this urban group consumed less than 1.3 mg or 67% the RDA.[36] This would suggest inadequate copper intake among all age groups if current recommended levels are reasonable estimates of need.

WATER AND ELECTROLYTE BALANCE

Fluid Balance

Fluid Intake. Water is supplied to the body by food, liquids consumed, and water of oxidation.[18] In younger people the thirst mechanism ensures adequate fluid intake. Diminished sensitivity to dehydration can reduce fluid intake in the older client. The individual with physical problems who cannot drink without help is particularly vulnerable to low fluid intake. Those subject to incontinence may consciously restrict fluid intake to avoid embarrassment.[3] Patients with high protein intakes are subject to dehydration if fluids are limited.[44] Because older people are less able to concentrate urine (see Chapter 1) fluid intake becomes more critical.

Physical signs of dehydration include dry tongue, flushing, and fever leading to personality changes or delirium as the condition increases in severity.[44] Unless advised otherwise because of cardiac or renal complications, older people should be encouraged to drink six to eight glasses of water each day (water intake as related to constipation is discussed in Chapter 4).

Sodium Intake and Fluid Retention. Age-related changes alter cardiac function (see Chapter 1) and reduce the blood volume delivered to major arteries. Reduced perfusion of the renal arteries and a subsequent decline in glomerular filtrate can stimulate the renin-angiotensin system to secrete aldosterone, and sodium and water reabsorption is increased in the distal tubule. At the same time decreased pressure in the baroreceptors can stimulate release of antidiuretic hormone (ADH) by the posterior pituitary, increasing water reabsorption in the distal tubule.[7] Continued sodium and fluid reabsorption and retention can result in edema and a rise in blood pressure.

Older individuals with cardiac problems are usually treated with (1) drugs to increase the strength of the heart as a pump, (2) diuretics, and/or (3) sodium restriction.[7,31] Diuretics preventing sodium reabsorption in the kidney increase excretion of both sodium and water. Restricting salt intake to 3 to 4 gm (50 to 70 mEq sodium) per day,[31,57] reduces the osmolarity of extracellular fluids, further contributing to loss of water.

Bine[7] has pointed to the danger of sodium depletion (hyponatremia) in older people on severe sodium restriction (500 mg sodium; 1.3 gm salt/day). Symptoms may include weakness and aches in the muscles, anorexia, abdominal cramps, and disorientation.

Sodium Intake and Hypertension. Although evidence is conflicting, excessive intakes of sodium lead to elevated blood pressure in susceptible individuals. The Food and Nutrition Board recommends that sodium intake not exceed 1 to 3 gm/day (2.5 to 7.5 gm NaCl).[18] Fregley[19] estimated that intakes of sodium chloride among the general population can go as high as 10 to 14.5 gm/day. Data from HANES suggest that sodium intake from food decreases with age.[1] Among men 18 to 74 years of age, sodium intake from food decreased from 3032 to 2229 mg. Women consume less sodium at all ages; intakes within adult age cohorts ranged from 1863 to 1526 mg. For both sexes grain products provided about one fourth of sodium intake from food. Soups, a common convenience item, contributed 11% to 13% of food sodium consumed by older men and women. No estimates of sodium intake from table salt were included. These older women, if limiting their discretionary use of table salt to about 4 gm, would fall within the recommended guidelines for sodium intake.

Recent evidence suggests the renin-angiotensin system, controlling sodium reabsorption in the kidney, is disturbed in some older individuals.[29] Among 401 persons (age 13 to 60) with mild hypertension, plasma renin activity decreased by about half over adulthood, whereas aldosterone levels did not change.[29] Because the renin-angiotensin system controls the secretion of aldosterone, both renin and aldosterone would be expected to decline simultaneously in the normal individual. Continued aldosterone secretion and sodium reabsorption in the presence of high sodium intake would contribute to increased blood pressure.[35,46] An age-related change in control of aldosterone could contribute to the incidence of hypertension in older age cohorts (changes in the cardiovascular system and hypertension are discussed in Chapter 1).

Potassium Balance

The average American diet is estimated to contain 50 to 150 mEq of potassium;[19] however, intakes of older individuals have not been evaluated. For older English subjects in long term care facilities mean potassium intake was less than 50 mEq per day and was attributed to low consumption of meat, milk, and fruits.[13] Among Glasgow aged living at home daily potassium intakes were 58 mEq in men and 48 mEq in women.[41] Low potassium intake coupled with long term use of potassium-losing diuretics can result in decreased serum potassium levels and hypokalemia.

Serum potassium levels below 3.5 mEq/L are often associated with impairment of several organ systems.[44] Changes in the resting membrane potential and excitability of both nerves and muscles can lead to (1) disorientation and confusion, (2) decreased motility of the gastrointestinal tract, (3) inability of the kidney to concentrate urine, (4) cardiac arrhythmias, and (5) deterioration in glucose tolerance. Susceptibility to digitalis intoxication increases in potassium deficiency. Potassium has been suggested to have a protective effect in reducing the hypertensive action of sodium.[7] Unfortunately, hypokalemia can go unnoticed as many of the clinical signs are associated with aging and older patients in general.

The relative incidence of hypokalemia is still debated.[41] Judge,[39-40] in a double-blind study of older patients, reported that potassium chloride supplementation improved both grip strength (muscle strength) and mental function. Cardiac patients receiving long term diuretic therapy were reported to have 20% to 30% less body potassium (determined by whole body counting) than controls;[63] however, patients and controls were not matched for age and body build; therefore potassium loss could have reflected normal aging rather than drug-induced depletion. In a further evaluation with age-matched controls, cardiac patients were found to have only about 5% less body potassium.[63] Encouraging frequent use of foods rich in potassium, such as bananas or orange juice, is appropriate for all older clients. The relative advantages and disadvantages of potassium supplements for those on diuretics will be discussed in Chapter 9.

SUMMARY

Decreased calcium absorption in older women following menopause results from an alteration in vitamin D metabolism. Estrogen withdrawal leads to a decrease in conversion of 25(OH)D to 1,25(OH)$_2$D, the active vitamin form stimulating calcium absorption. Increasing calcium intake does increase net calcium absorption regardless of estrogen levels. On this basis it is argued that calcium recommendations are too low and should be raised to 1.0 to 1.5 gm/day.

Intakes of iron, chromium, and zinc are less than desirable in many older people. Although daily iron losses do not increase in healthy aged, iron intake declines with the age-related decrement in calorie intake, and absorption of ingested iron can be compromised by an increase in stomach pH or use of drugs. Increased use of highly processed foods, easy to prepare and easy to chew, contributes to reduced intakes of zinc. A reduction in total calories and lesser intakes of red meat further limit dietary zinc. Although poor zinc status does not appear to be the cause of reduced taste acuity in older people, it may be related to altered immune response. Poor chromium status may contribute to

impaired glucose tolerance in some older people; however, chromium supplementation does not correct the problem.

Fluid balance can be precarious in the older individual as a result of altered control systems. Decreased sensitivity of the thirst mechanism increases risk of dehydration, particularly in those with limited access to water. Cardiac problems and altered control of aldosterone can lead to sodium and water retention. Potassium depletion resulting from low intake or diuretic-induced loss has serious consequences for cardiac, kidney, gastrointestinal, and neural function.

REVIEW QUESTIONS

1. What factors may interfere with iron absorption in the older adult? What advice would you give an older client toward improving iron absorption?
2. Calcium requirements of older women are a source of controversy. Would you support an increase in the RDA for calcium? Cite evidence to justify your conclusion. What is the relationship between calcium intake and calcium loss following menopause?
3. What is the relationship between chromium status and glucose tolerance in older people?
4. What socioeconomic and nutritional factors have been related to zinc intake and status in older adults? What is the influence of zinc status on (a) taste acuity and (b) immune function in older people?
5. What factors influence potassium balance in older adults? What problems are associated with hypokalemia? Discuss the relationship between sodium intake, sodium retention, and fluid balance in older adults.

REFERENCES

1. Abraham, S., and Carroll, M.D.: Fats, cholesterol, and sodium intake in the diet of persons 1-74 years: United States, National Center for Health Statistics Advanced Data, DHHS Publication No. (PHS) 81-1250, Washington, D.C., 1981, U.S. Government Printing Office.
2. Adams, N.D., Gray, R.W., and Lemann, J.: The effects of oral CaCO$_3$ loading and dietary calcium deprivation on plasma 1,25-dihydroxy-vitamin D concentration in healthy adults, J. Clin. Endocrinol. Metab. **48**:1008, 1979.
3. Agate, J.: Special hazards of illness in later life. In Rossman, I., ed: Clinical geriatrics, ed. 2, Philadelphia, 1979, J.B. Lippincott Co.
4. Albanese, A.A., and others: Calcium throughout the life cycle, Rosemont, Ill., 1978, National Dairy Council.

5. Avioli, L.V., McDonald, J.E., and Lee, S.W.: The influence of age on the intestinal absorption of ^{47}Ca in women and its relation to ^{47}Ca absorption in post-menopausal osteoporosis, J. Clin. Invest. **44**:1960, 1965.

6. Bernstein, D.S., and others: Prevalence of osteoporosis in high- and low-fluoride areas in North Dakota, JAMA **198**:499, 1966.

7. Bine, R.: Cardiology. In Schneider, H.A., Anderson, C.E., and Coursin, D.B., eds: Nutritional support of medical practice, Hagerstown, 1977, Harper & Row, Publishers, Inc.

8. Callender, S.: The intestinal mucosa and iron absorption, Br. Med. J. **23**:263, 1967.

9. Callender, S.T., and Warner, G.T.: Iron absorption from bread, Haematologia **5**:369, 1971.

10. Celada, A., Herreros, V., and DeCastro, S.: Liver iron storage in Spanish aging population, Am. J. Clin. Nutr. **33**:2662, 1980.

11. Crosby, W.H.: Control of iron absorption by intestinal luminal factors, Am. J. Clin. Nutr. **21**:1189, 1968.

12. Cummings, J.H.: Nutritional implications of dietary fiber, Am. J. Clin. Nutr. **31**:S21, 1978.

13. Dall, J.L., Paulose, S., and Fergusson, J.A.: Potassium intake of elderly patients in hospital, Gerontol. Clin. **13**:114, 1971.

14. Draper, H.H., and Scythes, C.A.: Calcium, phosphorus and osteoporosis, Fed. Proc. **40**:2434, 1981.

15. Duchateau, J., and others: Beneficial effects of oral zinc supplementation on the immune response of old people, Am. J. Med. **70**:1001, 1981.

16. Ekenved, G., Halvorsen, L., and Solvell, L.: Influence of a liquid antacid on the absorption of different iron salts, Scand. J. Haematol. **28**(suppl.):65, 1976.

17. Finch, C.A.: Body iron exchange in man, J. Clin. Invest. **38**:392, 1959.

18. Food and Nutrition Board: Recommended dietary allowances, ed. 9, Washington, D.C., 1980, National Academy of Sciences.

19. Fregley, M.J.: Sodium and potassium, Ann. Rev. Nutr. **1**:69, 1981.

20. Gallagher, J.C., and Riggs, B.L.: Nutrition and bone disease, N. Engl. J. Med. **298**:193, 1978.

21. Gallagher, J.C., Riggs, B.L., and Deluca, H.F.: Effect of estrogen on calcium absorption and serum vitamin D metabolites in post-menopausal osteoporosis, J. Clin. Endocrinol. Metab. **51**:1359, 1980.

22. Gallagher, J.C., and others: Intestinal calcium absorption and serum vitamin D metabolites in normal subjects and osteoporotic patients: Effect of age and dietary calcium, J. Clin. Invest. **64**:729, 1979.

23. Garry, P.J., and others: Nutritional status in a healthy elderly population: Dietary and supplemental intakes, Am. J. Clin. Nutr. **36**:319, 1982.

24. Glinsmann, W.H., and Mertz, W.: Effect of trivalent chromium on glucose tolerance, Metabolism **15**:510, 1966.

25. Greenberger, N.J.: Effects of antibiotics and other agents on the intestinal transport of iron, Am. J. Clin. Nutr. **26**:104, 1973.

26. Greger, J.L.: Dietary intake and nutritional status in regard to zinc of institutionalized aged, J. Gerontol. **32**:549, 1977.

27. Greger, J.L., and Geissler, A.H.: Effect of zinc supplementation on taste acuity of the aged, Am. J. Clin. Nutr. **31**:633, 1978.

28. Greger, J.L., and Sciscoe, B.S.: Zinc nutriture of elderly participants in an urban feeding program, J. Am. Diet. Assoc. **70**:37, 1977.

29. Guthrie, G.P., and others: Dissociation of plasma renin activity and aldosterone in essential hypertension, J. Clin. Endocrinol. Metab. **3**:446, 1976.

30. Hambidge, K.M.: Chromium nutrition in man, Am. J. Clin. Nutr. **27**:505, 1974.

31. Harris, R.: Special problems of geriatric patients with heart disease. In Reichel, W., ed.: Clinical aspects of aging, Baltimore, 1978, Williams & Wilkins.

32. Heaney, R.P., Recker, R.R., and Saville, P.D.: Menopausal changes in calcium balance performance, J. Lab. Clin. Med. **92**:953, 1978.

33. Heaney, R.P., Recker, R.R., and Saville, P.D.: Menopausal changes in bone remodeling, J. Lab. Clin. Med. **92**:964, 1978.

34. Heaney, R.P., and others: Calcium nutrition and bone health in the elderly, Am. J. Clin. Nutr. **36**(suppl.):986, 1982.

35. Hiramatsu, K., and others: Changes in endocrine activities relative to obesity in patients with essential hypertension, J. Am. Geriatr. Soc. **29**:25, 1981.

36. Holden, J.M., Wolf, W.R., and Mertz, W.: Zinc and copper in self-selected diets, J. Am. Diet. Assoc. **75**:23, 1979.

37. Jacobs, A.M., and Owen, G.M.: The effect of age on iron absorption, J. Gerontol. **24**:95, 1969.

38. Jacobs, A., and others: Gastric acidity and iron absorption, Br. J. Haematol. **12**:728, 1966.

39. Judge, T.G.: Hypokalaemia in the elderly, Gerontol. Clin. **10**:102, 1968.

40. Judge, T.G.: Potassium metabolism in the elderly. In Carlson, L.A., ed.: Nutrition in old age, Symposia of the Swedish Nutrition Foundation X, Stockholm, 1972, Almqvist & Wiksell.

41. Judge, T.G., and Cowan, N.R.: Dietary potassium intake and grip strength in older people, Gerontol. Clin. **13**:221, 1971.

42. Kuhn, I.N., and others: Iron absorption in man, J. Lab. Clin. Med. **71**:715, 1968.

43. Levine, R.A., Streeten, D.H., and Doisy, R.J.: Effects of oral chromium supplementation on the glucose tolerance of elderly human subjects, Metabolism **17**:114, 1968.

44. Lindeman, R.D.: Application of fluid and electrolyte balance principles to the older patient. In Reichel, W., ed.: Clinical aspects of aging, Baltimore, 1978, Williams & Wilkins.

45. Linkswiler, H.M., and others: Protein-induced hypercalciuria, Fed. Proc. **40**:2429, 1981.

46. Luft, F.C., and others: Cardiovascular and humoral responses to extremes of sodium intake in normal black and white men, Circulation **60**:697, 1979.

47. Lynch, S.R., and others: Iron status of elderly Americans, Am. J. Clin. Nutr. **36**(suppl.):1032, 1982.

48. Mertz, W.: Chromium and its relation to carbohydrate metabolism, Med. Clin. North Am. **60**:739, 1976.

49. Messer, H.H., and Singer, L.: Fluoride. In Present knowledge in nutrition, ed. 2, New York, 1976, The Nutrition Foundation, Inc.

50. Monsen, E.R., and Balintfy, J.L.: Calculating dietary iron bio-availability: Refinement and computerization, J. Am. Diet. Assoc. **80**:307, 1982.

51. Monsen, E.R., and others: Estimation of available dietary iron, Am. J. Clin. Nutr. **31**:134, 1978.

52. Mukherjee, T.: Factors affecting iron attachment to microvilli, Med. J. Aust. **2**:378, 1972.

53. Nordin, B.E., and others: Calcium and bone metabolism in old age. In Carlson, L.A., ed.: Nutrition in old age, Symposia Swedish Nutrition Foundation X, Stockholm, 1972, Almqvist & Wiksell.

54. Norman, D.A., and others: Jejunal and ileal adaptation to alterations in dietary calcium: Changes in calcium and magnesium absorption and pathogenic role of parathyroid hormone and 1,25-dihydroxyvitamin D, J. Clin. Invest. **67**:1599, 1981.

55. Offenbacher, E.G., and Pi-Sunyer, F.X.: Beneficial effect of chromium-rich yeast on glucose tolerance and blood lipids in elderly subjects, Diabetes **29**:919, 1980.

56. Riales, R., and Albrink, M.J.: Effect of chromium chloride supplement on glucose tolerance and serum lipids including high-density lipoprotein of adult men, Am. J. Clin. Nutr. **34**:2670, 1981.

57. Rodstein, M.: Heart disease in the aged. In Rossman, I., ed.: Clinical geriatrics, ed. 2, Philadelphia, 1979, J.B. Lippincott Co.

58. Sandstead, H., and others: Zinc nutriture in the elderly in relation to taste acuity, immune response, and wound healing, Am. J. Clin. Nutr. **36**:1046, 1982.

59. Slovik, D.M., and others: Deficient production of 1,25-dihydroxyvitamin D in elderly osteoporotic patients, N. Engl. J. Med. **305**:372, 1981.

60. Solomons, N.W.: On the assessment of zinc and copper nutriture in man, Am. J. Clin. Nutr. **32**:856, 1979.

61. Sugarman, B., and Munro, H.M.: Altered ^{65}Zn chloride accumulation by aged rats' adipocytes in vitro, J. Nutr. **110**:2317, 1980.

62. Thomas, J.H., and Powell, D.E.: Blood disorders in the elderly, Bristol, 1971, John Wright & Sons, Ltd.

63. Thomas, R.D., and others: Potassium depletion and tissue loss in chronic heart-disease, Lancet **2**:9, 1979.

64. Turnlund, J., Costa, F., and Margen, S.: Zinc, copper, and iron balance in elderly men, Am. J. Clin. Nutr. **34**:2641, 1981.

65. United States Department of Agriculture: Food and nutrient intakes of individuals in 1 day, low-income households, November 1979-March 1980. National Food Consumption Survey 1977-78, Preliminary Report No. 13, Washington, D.C., 1982, U.S. Government Printing Office.

66. United States Department of Health, Education and Welfare: Dietary intake source data, United States, 1971-74, DHEW Publication No. (PHS) 79-1221, Hyattsville, Md., 1979, U.S. Government Printing Office.

67. United States Department of Health and Human Services: Hematological and nutritional biochemistry reference data for persons 6 months - 74 years of age: United States, 1976-80, DHHS Publication No. (PHS) 83-1682, Hyattsville, Md., 1982, U.S. Government Printing Office.

68. VanCampen, D.: Regulation of iron absorption, Fed. Proc. **33**:100, 1974.

69. Vir, S.C., and Love, A.H.: Zinc and copper status of the elderly, Am. J. Clin. Nutr. **32**:1472, 1979.

70. Wagner, P.A., and others: Zinc status of elderly black Americans from urban low-income households, Am. J. Clin. Nutr. **33**:1771, 1980.

71. Yeh, S.D., Soltz, W., and Chow, B.F.: The effect of age on iron absorption in rats, J. Gerontol. **20**:177, 1965.

Chapter 8

Nutritional Disorders in the Aged

Although nutrition-related diseases exist in all age groups, they are particularly difficult to both diagnose and treat in the aged. The vulnerability of the older individual to nutritional disorders is influenced by a variety of factors. If vitamin B_{12} absorption is impaired, anemia will result despite an adequate vitamin intake. Disorders in bone metabolism such as osteoporosis, thought to be inevitable consequences of the aging process, are now being evaluated in terms of both nutrition intervention and prevention. The fundamental problem is the inability to separate physiologic changes reflecting normal aging from functional disease processes. Altered glucose tolerance, considered pathologic in younger individuals, may be "normal" for the older adult. Age-related standards for clinical evaluation based on observations of healthy, independent-living aged are essential for effective diagnosis and treatment of nutritional disorders in older people. Unfortunately, such standards are seldom available.

CARBOHYDRATE METABOLISM AND GLUCOSE TOLERANCE

Glucose tolerance, or the ability to metabolize a glucose load, deteriorates with age. Using general standards it has been estimated that 50%[8,88] to 80%[26] of people above age 60 have abnormal glucose tolerance. In younger individuals abnormal glucose tolerance is associated with development of overt diabetes. In the older individual the differentiation between pathologic consequences of disease and normal aspects of aging is less clear, as is the decision regarding appropriate treatment.

Glucose Tolerance Test

Standards for Test. The oral glucose tolerance test consists of oral administration of a standard dose of glucose (75 gm is currently recommended[65]) with blood samples taken every half hour for 2 to 3 hours thereafter. Defined conditions include (1) minimum daily carbohydrate intake of 150 gm for 3 days preceding the test, (2) 8- to 16-hour fast before the test, and (3) avoidance of exercise, coffee, or smoking prior to and during the test.[22] Caffeine, nicotine, and physical activity raise blood glucose levels, as do some drugs commonly used by older people such as aspirin and diuretics. Lack of adequate dietary preparation contributes to the incidence of abnormal glucose tolerance in older individuals. Among institutionalized aged about one half had abnormal glucose tolerance when tested without dietary preparation; this decreased to one third when a high carbohydrate diet was fed for several days prior to the test.[42]

Blood Glucose Levels in the Aged. Fasting blood glucose levels do not significantly differ between old and young; when differences do exist they range from 1 to 2 mg/100 ml/decade.[26] In contrast, blood levels 2 hours following administration of

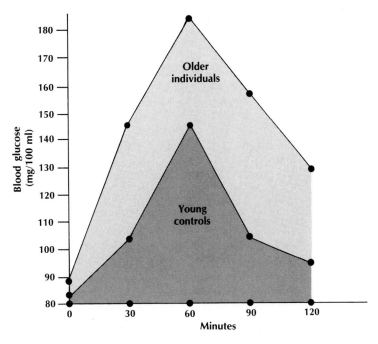

Fig. 8-1. Age-related changes in oral glucose tolerance. (Data from Pagano, G., and others: Insulin resistance in the aged: The role of the peripheral insulin receptors, Metabolism **30**:46, 1981.)

glucose increase as much as 11 mg/100 ml/decade with a mean of 5 mg/100 ml/decade.[9,26] Two hours following a 100 gm glucose load, blood glucose levels were significantly higher in those age 70 as compared to those age 32; fasting blood glucose levels were similar (Fig. 8-1).[67] Values do not differ according to sex, although there is a disproportionate increase in postprandial levels after age 50.[26]

Basis for Change in Glucose Tolerance. General health patterns as well as molecular abnormalities contribute to the age-related change in glucose tolerance. Low carbohydrate intake has been linked to the problem, although in one report, prior diets containing only 50 gm carbohydrate had only limited influence on test results.[22] Obesity and the age-related decrease in lean body mass have been im-

plicated in glucose removal. Excessive body fat in younger people leads to impaired glucose tolerance and weight loss brings about improvement.[47] Lean body mass itself influences the glucose pattern, as overweight individuals with large muscle mass did not differ from lean controls in fasting and postprandial glucose and insulin levels.[46] Swedish researchers suggest that physical training, regardless of change in body weight or body fat, improves glucose tolerance.[52,78] Increased physical activity is believed to enhance metabolic activity and glucose uptake in the skeletal muscle thereby lowering blood glucose levels. It has been shown that bed rest decreases glucose tolerance.[22]

Because the older person has less lean body mass, glucose movement into cells may be slowed simply because there is less muscle for it to enter.

Silverstone and coworkers,[82] estimating lean body mass on the basis of intracellular water, concluded that glucose tolerance declined by 42% whereas lean body mass declined by only 18%. This suggests that alterations apart from changes in body composition contribute to impaired glucose tolerance. Potassium depletion resulting from inadequate intake or prolonged use of diuretics influences glucose tolerance, because movement of glucose into the cell requires potassium ions. Within any individual several factors are likely to be involved.

Insulin Levels and Glucose Tolerance

Secretion of Insulin. Insulin facilitates both the entry and the metabolism of glucose within the cell. Abnormal glucose tolerance in the aged, however, is generally not the result of low insulin secretion; insulin levels are not decreased in older versus younger people following oral glucose.[9,23,26,45] In fact, after 60 minutes serum insulin levels are often higher in the older group. Others have noted a delayed response in insulin secretion during the first few minutes following glucose ingestion.[23,62] However, this does not completely explain the change in glucose tolerance, for although the pancreas may be initially less sensitive to glucose, the total amount of insulin produced is similar in all age groups.

Effectiveness of Secreted Insulin. The resistance or reduced sensitivity of peripheral tissues (fat and muscle) to the action of insulin has been studied by administering known levels of insulin and observing over a period of time the amount of glucose required to maintain a specific blood glucose level.[9,27] This "hyperglycemic clamp" technique provides a means of calculating the amount of glucose metabolized and measures the effectiveness of insulin secreted. Rate of glucose metabolism is inversely related to age. Glucose entry in peripheral tissues was significantly reduced in groups with mean ages of 43 and 60 as compared to the group aged 25.[27] According to DeFronzo,[27] insulin resistance occurs primarily in fat and muscle rather than in the liver.

Insulin resistance relates in part to the enhanced obesity and larger fat cells of the older individual. Enlarged fat cells are less sensitive to insulin than smaller fat cells. When younger and older people are matched on the basis of fat cell diameter, age differences in glucose and insulin levels are only minor.[20] Fat cells of even normal weight aged do have fewer insulin receptors than cells from younger people,[67] suggesting that age-related biochemical changes may also contribute to the differences observed.

The form of insulin secreted also differs in younger and older people.[26,42] Proinsulin, a precursor of insulin that has only limited effectiveness on fat and muscle cells, is present in greater proportions in older people following a glucose challenge. In vitro animal studies of pancreatic cells indicate that particular cell groups differ in secretory response to glucose. The form of insulin produced depends on the age of the donor; forms differ in their degree of stimulation of fat, muscle, or liver cells.[79]

The islets of Langerhans are variable in size with large islets secreting more insulin in response to glucose than small islets, regardless of age. Aging promotes the accumulation of large islets with increased numbers of beta cells. Although the insulin secretion of large islets is somewhat reduced in advanced age, secretion from small islets is decreased by half.[48]

Accumulation of large islets may be a physiologic compensation for the age-related impairment of small islets. However, somatostatin, a known inhibitor of glucose-stimulated insulin release,[79] is secreted at an enhanced rate by the pancreas of older animals. These findings, however, have not been confirmed in human subjects.

In general there appear to be age-related differences in the forms of insulin secreted, although the total amount remains relatively stable throughout the aging process. The effect of the various forms on particular cell types is poorly understood but could result in a shift in carbohydrate metabolism from one tissue to another or a preference for one energy source over another. These relationships require further study.

Diagnosis of Diabetes

The practitioner working with older people is presented with a dilemma regarding treatment of those with abnormal glucose tolerance. Being designated a diabetic carries with it both social and employment consequences, as well as complications with insurance.[26] On the other hand, untreated diabetes leads to both visual and renal vascular complications.[65] One approach has been age-corrected standards, by which an individual's performance on the oral glucose tolerance test is judged according to that of his peers.[9] This assumes that age-related changes in glucose tolerance are a normal consequence of the aging process. If impairment in glucose tolerance is considered pathologic and predictive of true diabetes, then any adjustment for age is inappropriate.

Recent recommendations of the National Diabetes Data Group limit diagnosis of diabetes to those with one of the following:

1. Classical symptoms of diabetes (i.e., polyuria, polydipsia, ketonuria, extreme hyperglycemia)
2. Fasting plasma glucose levels greater than or equal to 140 mg/100 ml on at least two tests
3. Glucose levels greater than or equal to 200 mg/100 ml at some point within 2 hours and 2 hours following ingestion of 75 gm glucose under standard conditions[65]

Using these criteria there are no adjustments for age. Individuals with plasma glucose levels between 140 and 200 mg/100 ml 2 hours following a 75 gm glucose challenge and an intermediate level greater than or equal to 200 mg/100 ml are considered to have impaired glucose tolerance but not diabetes. Normal levels are less than 140 mg/100 ml after 2 hours with no intermediate level equal to or greater than 200 mg/100 ml.

Longitudinal studies suggest that only 1% to 5% of people with impaired glucose tolerance develop overt diabetes per year.[65] Some revert to normal levels if tested at a later time and others remain the same. The higher the glucose levels observed, however, the more likely the individual is to develop overt diabetes.[26] It should be recognized that people with impaired glucose tolerance, while not diabetic, are at greater risk of atherosclerotic disease, usually related to hypertension, hyperlipidemia, and obesity.[65] Therefore dietary intervention focusing on weight control, and moderate intakes of sodium and fat, would be appropriate.

Dietary Considerations

General dietary treatment for both the insulin-dependent and noninsulin-dependent diabetic are described in detail elsewhere.[5]

Diets containing 50 gm plant fiber and 55% to 60% carbohydrate have improved glucose tolerance and reduced the insulin required by older diabetics.[7] Fiber was provided by a variety of foods including whole wheat bread, breakfast cereals high in bran, rice, beans, other vegetables and fruits. Fiber slows the rate at which glucose is released into the blood from the small intestine, thereby lowering postprandial glucose levels.[6] A further result of the high fiber diet was the lowering of plasma cholesterol (206 versus 148 mg/100 ml).

High carbohydrate high fiber regimens are also effective in improving glucose tolerance in nondiabetics. Other benefits of such a diet are increased satiety, helpful in weight control, and decreased incidence of constipation (see Chapter 4). Because of the abdominal distress caused by excessive levels of bran, Anderson and Sieling[7] recommend that fiber be derived from a variety of sources. Long term follow-up (2 to 4 years) has not revealed detrimental changes in vitamin or mineral status in those on a high fiber maintenance diet. Those authors,[7] however, do recommend daily use of a vitamin and mineral supplement containing vitamin B_{12}.

DISORDERS IN BONE METABOLISM

Changes in Bone Structure

General Considerations. Loss of bone mineral and matrix, a physiologic accompaniment of aging, has been identified in prehistoric skeletons from the year 2000 B.C.[70] Osteoporosis (porous bone) is the clinical syndrome resulting when over one third of the bone is lost.[11] Beginning at age 30 to 40, women lose about 10% of their bone mass per decade; men lose about 3%.[11] Although all people lose bone as a consequence of aging, not all develop osteoporosis. What biochemical or physiologic factors differ between ''slow losers'' and ''rapid losers'' is not understood.[12] Metabolic etiology also differs in loss of bone in the spine as compared to loss in the hip or femur.[57,76]

Public Health Aspects. Loss of bone matrix and mineral increases susceptibility to bone fracture and disability. Spontaneous fractures (resulting from little or no trauma) occur at the rate of over 6 million per year among people above age 45.[1] Fractures of the pelvis increase in incidence among white women from 2/1000 between ages 50 and 64, to 5/1000 between ages 65 and 74, to 10/1000 among those age 75 and above.[12] Mortality from medical complications of bone fractures is 15% to 30%. The medical cost is over 1 billion dollars per year.[12] The personal cost of resulting immobility and inactivity can be a change in life-style, as in the case of the older woman who is forced to enter a nursing home after breaking her hip.

Osteoporosis with compression of the vertebrae causes chronic back pain and difficulty in locomotion. It is estimated that 25% of older women have orthopedic problems.[12] Weakened vertebrae can result in deformity of the spine or kyphosis, sometimes referred to as dowager's hump.[1] Spinal changes are involved in the decrease in standing height observed in many aged.[84] Loss of bone mass and deterioration of the jaw contribute to periodontal disease and subsequent loss of teeth.

Physical Characteristics. Osteoporosis, the most common bone disorder among older people, is characterized by decreased bone mass with no change in the chemical ratio of mineral to protein matrix. Existing bone is normal, there is just less of it.[1,11] In osteomalacia (adult rickets) bone density is decreased because of poor mineralization of available matrix. Although the etiology of osteomalacia is well known, the combination of factors implicated in the development of osteoporosis is not understood.

Relative bone mass at older ages is influenced by the total bone laid down during periods of growth.[33] Men at all ages have greater bone mass than women and lose bone less rapidly. Blacks have more bone than whites and are less likely to develop osteoporosis. The reduced bone found in low-income as compared to high income people has been attributed to a diet less adequate in nutrients.[33]

Bone as a Tissue

Bone Dynamics. Bone disorders are better understood in relation to the normal physiology of bone. There are two types of bone in the mature skeleton.[91]

1. Spongy (cancellous) bone is characterized by numerous interwoven partitions called trabeculae, each containing red or fatty marrow. It includes the vertebrae, flat bones of the ribs and pelvis, and ends of the long bones such as the femur.
2. Hard, compact (cortical) bone is a circular, layered structure with a blood vessel through the center. It appears as a solid mineralized area on a normal x-ray film with a structural pattern visible only at higher magnification. The skull, the jaw, and the shafts of the long bones are compact bone.

Once thought to be relatively inert, bone is now recognized as a dynamic active tissue undergoing constant remodeling throughout life.[68] Active removal of both mineral and matrix (resorption) is occurring at one location while deposition of matrix material and subsequent mineralization (apposition) is occurring in another.[59,91] What mechanism triggers resorption and apposition at a particular surface is not known, as some areas remain unchanged for long periods of time. Remodeling is more active in trabecular than compact bone and the relative rates of resorption and replacement figure prominently in age-related bone loss.[39]

Garn[33] developed a model for the gain and loss of cortical bone, suggesting that increases in bone thickness occur through lifelong apposition on the outer (subperiosteal) bone surface. Although gain is most rapid during the growth period, it continues at a slower rate throughout adulthood. While bone apposition is constant at the outer surface, the inner (endosteal) surface undergoes a rapid phase of resorption beginning about age 30 and continuing throughout life. The aged woman may be left with less bone than she had in early adolescence. The rate or degree of change within an individual, however, cannot be predicted.[59]

Mechanism of Bone Loss. Bone mass depends on a balance in the rate of formation and resorption. Osteoblasts, active cells which lay down bone, (1) synthesize the protein matrix and (2) promote calcification by storing calcium to be passed into the bone matrix.[91] Osteoclasts are instrumental in bone resorption; exactly how they work is not well understood. It appears that these cells secrete acids that dissolve the bone mineral; the remaining collagen is digested by lysosomes.[91]

Bone turnover occurs in loci called bone remodeling units covering less than 1 cu mm. Each includes an advancing series of osteoclasts, an inactive segment, and a closing series of osteoblasts. The entire process requires 4 to 6 months.[68] Radiocalcium experiments showed bone resorption in postmenopausal women to equal 425 mg/day of calcium, whereas bone formation equaled only 387 mg/day, for a net daily loss of 38 mg.[39] At this rate the individual loses 1.5% of her bone per year.

Osteoblasts may be less efficient in replacing bone in some remodeling units, or completion of the resorption phase may not be followed by the usual apposition phase, leaving a surface unrepaired.[68]

Factors Influencing Bone Loss

General Theories. Since clinical bone loss was first described in 1941,[4] a variety of factors have been identified that contribute to bone resorption:

Dietary
  Calcium
  Protein
  Calcium-phosphorus ratio
  Fluoride
  Vitamin D
  Vitamin C
Hormonal
  Estrogen
  Parathyroid hormone
  Calcitonin
Other
  Age
  Race
  Sex
  Economic status
  Physical exercise

The most obvious predisposing condition is being female. Albanese and coworkers[3] suggest that the abnormally low bone density of some women may be a consequence of (1) weight reduction diets inadequate in nutrients, (2) calcium costs of pregnancy, and (3) calcium costs of breast feeding, if calcium is not replaced. In population studies, however, bone density has not been related to number of children or breast feeding.[33]

Heaney and coworkers[38] summarized two general theories describing age-related bone loss, both focusing on the known decrease in calcium absorption (see Chapter 7). The first considers the problem to be a deficiency of $1,25(OH)_2D$, the vitamin metabolite required for active transport of calcium in the upper small intestine. The primary defect is reduced production of this metabolite by the kidney, as a result of decreased synthesis of the required enzyme, estrogen withdrawal, or unknown factors. Reduced supply of calcium to the blood, resulting in lowered serum calcium stimulates the secretion of parathyroid hormone (PTH) leading to continued bone resorption and development of osteoporosis.

The second theory proposes an imbalance favoring bone resorption over bone formation as the primary cause of loss. Age, estrogen withdrawal, reduced physical activity, or unknown factors contribute to this pattern. Constant flux of calcium from the bone suppresses secretion of PTH and subsequent production of $1,25(OH)_2D$. Calcium absorption decreases as a homeostatic response to the increased availability of calcium being released from the bone.

Both theories agree on the concept of reduced calcium absorption and reduced serum levels of active vitamin D metabolites, with excessive resorption of bone. The first theory presumes elevated PTH levels whereas the second sees PTH levels as suppressed. Both situations have been observed in specific groups of osteoporotics. In one report about 15% had elevated PTH levels.[38] Analysis of available evidence led Heaney and coworkers[38] to conclude that both theories may be correct depending on the individual. Differing etiologies may also explain why a method of treatment is successful with some osteoporotics and not others or why bone loss differs in severity among people of similar age.

Physical Exercise. Absence of physical stress or muscle pull on the bone causes rapid mineral loss, with increased urinary and fecal calcium.[93-94] Whether this results from altered neurologic or circulatory stimuli is not known. Physical exercise alone will not prevent mineral loss; body weight must be exerted on the bone tissue.[93] Weightlessness, as shown by space flights, results in mineral loss similar to bed rest despite normal calcium intakes and efforts at exercise. During full bed rest, losses can equal 200 to 300 mg calcium daily.[38]

Even general inactivity can contribute to calcium loss, as older people who participated only infrequently in physical exercise (less than twice per week) had, over 1 year, significant bone loss in contrast to those with greater levels of activity (exercising at least twice per week).[80] In older individuals exercise appears to be more effective in retarding bone loss than in promoting net gain, although in one report even mild exercise (30 minutes per day, 3 days per week) over a 3-year period led to a 2% increase in bone mineral content in women ranging from 69 to 95 years of age.[83] Control subjects of similar age lost 3% of their bone mineral over the same period.

Dietary Calcium. The influence of calcium or other nutrients in reducing or accelerating bone loss has been debated extensively. Limitations of existing studies include (1) focusing on calcium only, with less consideration of dietary protein and phosphorus or environmental factors such as sunlight or level of physical activity; (2) relatively short periods of observation; and (3) using dairy foods only, as indicators of calcium intake, neglecting the possible contribution of other foods, beer, drinking water, or medications.[33,38] (One popular antacid contains 200 mg of calcium per tablet.)

Moreover, bone density in one area of the skeleton may not be representative of losses in other sites. Bone mass in the metacarpal bones (bones of the hand), often measured in large scale surveys because of the ease of measurement, may not reflect bone density in the vertebrae or elsewhere.[38,57] As a result population studies have found limited, if any, correlation between calcium intake and bone loss.[33,84] Clinical evaluations, however, agree that osteoporotic women are more likely to have calcium intakes below 400 mg daily[74] or lactase deficiency.[19]

An evaluation of two communities in Yugoslavia, having similar exposure to sunlight, exercise patterns, and life-style and differing only in food

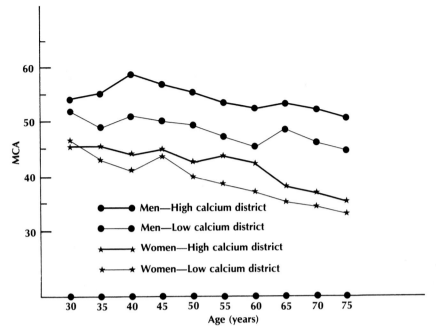

Fig. 8-2. Calcium intake and metacarpal cortical area (MCA) of bone by age and sex. (From Matkovic, V., and others: Bone status and fracture rates in two regions of Yugoslavia, Am. J. Clin. Nutr. **32:**540, 1979.)

pattern (either high or low calcium), does suggest that a generous intake of calcium throughout life offers some protection against developing osteoporosis in later life.[57] Calcium intakes equaled about 450 and 1000 mg in men from the low and high calcium regions, respectively, and about 400 and 875 mg in women.

The differences in bone mass between women with high or low calcium intakes continued throughout life (Fig. 8-2). Those with greater bone mass at younger ages had more bone remaining in later life, despite age-related bone loss. The rate of femur fracture in those communities was inversely proportional to bone mass, emphasizing the value of increased bone, although no differences in wrist fracture rates existed between high and low calcium groups. The latter reflects loss of trabec-

ular rather than cortical bone, not generally apparent by methods used in epidemiologic surveys.

In general, bone mass remaining in old age is influenced by the amount of bone deposited in young adulthood and the rate of loss. Although bone deposition is controlled to some extent by genetic factors, generous intakes of calcium (see Chapter 7) and continued physical activity appear to retard bone loss in older age groups.

Management of Osteoporosis

No ideal pattern of treatment now exists for those with clinical osteoporosis and fragile bones. Although estrogen reduces bone resorption, it does not enhance bone formation; therefore the net effect is a slowing of bone loss.[73,93] Because of the influence of estrogen on blood coagulation and possibly the development of uterine cancer, its long term use, even at low levels, is still under evaluation. Fluoride coupled with calcium and vitamin D was considered to have promise for increasing bone formation and replacing lost bone. Unfortunately, the new bone formed can have less strength than normal bone and further fractures can occur.[93] Fluoride therapy has produced undesirable side effects including gastritis and anemia.[15,75]

Dietary Calcium and Vitamin D. Calcium supplementation has been shown to slow bone resorption and promote positive calcium balance. Among 12 older women (mean age = 80) on intakes of 1.0 to 1.5 gm calcium, not only did calcium loss decrease but also bone density actually increased over a 3-year period.[2-3] Nonsupplemented women of similar age (mean age = 82) lost bone during the same period. Dietary calcium from food equaled 450 mg/day, and in the supplemented group 750 mg/day was provided in the form of calcium carbonate. Vitamin D intake from the supplement was 375 IU per day; the vitamin D intake from food was not specified. The bone density coefficient of the supplemented group increased from 91 to 96 mils; the unsupplemented group decreased from 90 to 84 mils.

A regimen adding 710 mg calcium and 405 IU vitamin D to the diet, in the form of 2.2 ounces processed cheese (360 mg calcium and 6 IU vitamin D) and calcium phosphate capsules (350 mg calcium and 399 IU vitamin D) was tested with older women (mean age = 70 years) living at home.[51] These women consumed an additional 452 mg calcium and 127 IU vitamin D daily in their self-selected diets, making their total intake similar to that reported above. Over a 6-month period, bone density improved significantly in about half of the participants and decreased in about one third. It has been suggested, however, that calcium supplementation programs should be evaluated over a period of at least 2 to 3 years to differentiate between short term and long term responses.[38] Initiated changes in bone remodeling may require 6 to 18 months for completion.

In individuals with no previous history of kidney problems, calcium intakes of 1.0 to 2.5 gm daily appear to have no adverse effects.[3,38,92] Whedon[93] sees little risk of urinary stone formation, as urinary calcium increases only slightly (69 mg) per gram of calcium supplement. Although hypercalcemia has been reported in people consuming large amounts of both calcium and alkali (sodium bicarbonate), this is not likely to occur at levels up to 2.5 gm calcium daily administered in divided doses.[38] However, individuals should check with their physicians before using calcium supplements as to the presence of any condition contraindicating their use.

Administration of 1,25(OH)$_2$D. Experimental work indicates that supplementation with the active form of vitamin D may have potential for treatment of osteoporosis.[32] In a double-blind study of 12 osteoporotic women given physiologic doses of 1,25(OH)$_2$D$_3$, the percentage of calcium absorbed returned to normal (increased from 7% to 27%) within 6 to 8 months and continued at this level over a period of 2 years. On a short term basis calcium balance improved (-59 to $+2$ mg/day); however, on a long term basis calcium balance declined to a level about midway between initial values and short term levels (-27 mg/day). Initially bone resorption was significantly reduced but returned to base line levels. Trabecular bone volume did increase over the 2-year period and incidence of new fractures among these patients was about one third that expected in untreated patients. Because calcium balance was not positive throughout the treatment period, Gallagher and coworkers[32] suggest that bone may have been reallocated between cortical and trabecular compartments. No unfavorable effects on kidney function were observed.

According to those workers, long term studies with larger numbers of patients are required before any conclusions can be drawn regarding the general feasibility and effectiveness of this treatment.[32]

Osteomalacia

Osteomalacia, characterized by demineralization of the bone matrix, is usually nutritional in origin resulting from vitamin D deficiency. Among older people this can relate to (1) low vitamin D intake coupled with nonexposure to ultraviolet light, (2) malabsorption of ingested vitamin D, or (3) liver or renal disease, which interferes with conversion of the vitamin to its active form.[29] In the young individual, newly formed bone matrix is not mineralized as a result of inadequate calcium absorption and subsequent lowered serum calcium and phosphate levels.[66] In the older individual the situation is compounded by the fact that reduced serum calcium and phosphate levels not only result in failure to calcify matrix formed in bone remodeling but also stimulate secretion of PTH which causes resorption of previously formed bone.[66] Nordin[66] suggests that the extensive bone loss observed in osteomalacia relates to secondary hyperparathyroidism. Although bone loss often begins in the vertebrae or trunk region in osteoporosis, losses in osteomalacia are most apparent in the peripheral skeleton.

British workers have described older subjects with osteomalacia resulting from lack of vitamin D.[28,30] Reduced incidence of vitamin D deficiency in the United States has been attributed to the vitamin fortification of both fluid and dried milk.[18] In the United States osteomalacia is more likely the result of malabsorption, related disease, or drug-related problems.[69] Excessive use of aluminum hydroxide antacids that bind dietary phosphate has been implicated in the etiology of this condition.[43]

The active form of vitamin D (1,25[OH]$_2$D) or an analogue is being used in treatment of osteomalacia. Alleviation of the secondary hyperparathyroidism associated with the problem in older adults may require daily calcium supplementation (1.5 gm) in addition to vitamin D therapy.[24]

NUTRITIONAL ANEMIA

Causes of Anemia

Anemia results from changes in either the number or characteristics of the erythrocyte.[95] A decrease in the oxygen-carrying capacity of the blood and the consequent oxygen deficit in the tissues leads to increased heart rate, shortness of breath, and weakness. Nutritional anemia in the aged usually relates to (1) lack of iron or a vitamin cofactor required for production and maturation of the erythrocyte or (2) occult blood loss.[85] In advanced iron-deficiency anemia cells are hypochromic and microcytic. In the early stages the bone marrow continues to produce cells normal in size and hemoglobin concentration but compensates by producing fewer cells.

Lack of vitamins B$_6$ or B$_{12}$ or folic acid interrupts the DNA synthesis required for the maturation of the erythroblast precursor to the erythrocyte with normal oxygen-carrying capacity. Megaloblastic cells are easily recognized on a blood smear by their large size and discrete particles, as compared with the smaller size and dense chromic material of the mature erythrocyte.[95]

Iron-Deficiency Anemia

Basis of Problem. The most common nutritional cause of anemia in older people is iron deficiency, although vitamin deficiencies may complicate the problem. In 100 consecutive older persons admitted to a hospital with deficient hemoglobin levels

45 were deficient in iron

18 were deficient in vitamin B$_{12}$

7 were deficient in folic acid

27 were deficient in iron and/or vitamin B$_{12}$ and folate

3 had anemias nonnutritional in origin[85]

Iron deficiency can result from (1) poor dietary

intake, (2) poor iron absorption, or (3) increased erythropoiesis resulting from blood loss or correction of folic acid or vitamin B_{12} deficiency. Blood loss through the gastrointestinal tract is a frequent and critical cause of iron deficiency in older people. Excessive blood in the stool may go unnoticed, discovered only on examination for anemia or other problems.[41] Normal daily blood loss in the stool is less than 3.0 ml; values above this level are pathologic.[25] Blood losses of 50 to 75 ml impart a dark red or black color to the stool; however, abnormal losses below this level are frequently not visible,[25] and require chemical analysis of the stool for detection.

Patients with hiatus hernia may lose up to 15 ml of blood daily.[41] Many of these individuals are free of gastric symptoms and do not seek medical attention until the anemia is severe. As 1 ml of blood (hemoglobin = 15 gm/100 ml) contains about 0.5 mg iron, such losses could over a 6-month period equal 20% of body iron stores (total body iron is about 6000 mg). Conditions associated with gastrointestinal bleeding include stomach or duodenal ulcers, diverticulitis, hiatus hernia, hemorrhoids, and undiagnosed cancer.[85] Long term use of aspirin with irritation of the stomach lining can lead to significant blood loss.[77]

Identifying Anemia. Hemoglobin levels, serum iron, transferrin levels and percent saturation, and red blood cell indices are used in diagnosis of iron-deficiency anemia; however, there is disagreement regarding normal values in older people. Although Wintrobe and coworkers[95] consider hemoglobin levels below 12 gm/100 ml to be deficient, some authors[87] regard levels between 10 and 11.9 gm/100 ml in women as marginal rather than deficient. Hemoglobin levels between 11.5 and 12.9 gm/100 ml were proposed to be normal for some older individuals who did not respond to iron supplementation.[35] Another approach to this dilemma involves establishing percentiles based on observations of large numbers of individuals.[34] People between the 5th and 15th percentile would be classified as low and those below the 5th percentile as deficient. Race also influences biochemical levels as blacks of all ages have lower hemoglobin levels than whites independent of socioeconomic status.

Freedman and Marcus[31] maintain that anemia is frequently one of the first signs of illness in the older person; therefore lowering the range of normal values could delay recognition and treatment. Among 292 aged ambulatory hospital patients, 80% had hemoglobin and red cell indices within normal ranges.[31] The cause of the apparent anemia in those with below normal values was not reported. Among 73 relatively fit independent-living aged (63 to 94 years of age), only 1 had a hemoglobin level below 12 gm/100 ml, although 12 (16%) had serum iron levels below 75μg/100 ml, and 10 (14%) had transferrin levels above 350 μg/100 ml.[44] For six (8%) the percentage of saturation fell below 20%.

These evaluations of both hospitalized and relatively healthy older people suggest that the majority fall within the normal standards established for younger individuals. Therefore an older individual with below normal hematologic values should be evaluated further as to dietary intake, presence of disease or infection, or occult blood loss. If no apparent reason can be found for the anemia, the individual should be reexamined periodically to reaffirm the absence of problems. Although hematologic values outside the normal range may be related to age and not nutritional or health problems, this should never be assumed without further examination.

Incidence of Iron-Deficiency Anemia. In healthy older people, including those above age 90, hemoglobin levels remain similar to those found in younger individuals; nevertheless, several trends are apparent.[29,30,44,60] In men, hemoglobin levels decrease with age and the incidence of anemia is higher after age 65. Women have lower hemoglobin levels throughout the child-bearing years but improve in iron status when menstruation ceases. In the Ten State Nutrition Survey, older black men had a higher incidence of deficient hemoglobin than older white men (15% versus 4%) although both were low income.[87] Fewer older women were deficient in hemoglobin (5% of blacks versus 1% of whites). This relates in part to the standards used, as the level of adequacy was 12 gm/100 ml for men and 10 gm/100 ml for women.

Recent data from HANES indicate a higher incidence of iron problems among aged blacks than whites, with black women at particular risk.[89] Although blacks are more likely to have lower hemoglobin levels (considered to reflect genetic differences), proportionately more black women have hemoglobin levels below 12 gm/100 ml compared to black men (22% versus 7%). Two percent of white men and 4% of white women, age 65 to 74, had hemoglobin levels below 12 gm/100 ml.

Number of red blood cells (RBCs) and mean cell hemoglobin concentration (MCHC) provide an index of both erythropoiesis and iron status. (RBC count is expressed as the number $\times 10^{12}$ per liter of blood; MCHC is expressed as grams of hemoglobin per 100 ml RBCs.) Older people regardless of sex or ethnic group have reduced numbers of RBCs according to established standards.[89] Twenty-one and 36% of white and black women, respectively, had less than 4.2×10^{12} RBCs/L, considered the lower limit of normal for women. About one fourth of older black men and 15% of older white men had values below 4.4×10^{12} RBCs/L (4.5×10^{12} RBCs/L is the lower limit for men). Mean cell hemoglobin concentration decreased less, as only 2% of whites and 6% of blacks had MCHC values below 31.0 gm/100 ml RBCs (31.5 gm/100 ml RBCs is the lower limit of normal). This suggests that the erythrocytes present have normal hemoglobin concentration.

As noted in Chapter 7, erythropoiesis is less efficient in advanced age. Harrison[37] suggests this reflects a lack of available nutrients or changes in the internal environment of the bone marrow, because stem cells from young animals had depressed erythropoietic response when transplanted to older animals. Timaffy[86] reported fatty infiltration of the bone marrow in older people examined at autopsy. Such a change could interfere with the flow of nutrients or of control proteins to active erythropoietic sites.

Decreased erythrocyte production can also result from unavailability of body iron. Beisel[16] pointed out that body iron stores become unavailable for hemoglobin synthesis during infection, and erythropoiesis is halted. Several authors consider this a body defense mechanism making iron less available to the disease organism.[58,64] This response is usually accompanied by a decrease in serum iron and a significant increase in serum transferrin to achieve binding of all available iron. Although in the HANES report serum iron below 60 μg/100 ml was observed in less than 10% of those age 65 to 74, nearly half had transferrin levels above 350 μg/100 ml.[89] Increase in transferrin also occurs in simple iron-deficiency anemia and can be a consequence of poor iron intake. As noted earlier, a significant number of aged are consuming less than 67% the recommended level of iron.

Benzie,[17] observing a progressive increase in the iron content of bone marrow between ages 31 to 50, 51 to 70, and 71 and over, suggested that stored iron is less available for hemoglobin synthesis in the older individual, as marrow iron stores were high in some individuals with low hemoglobin levels. The defect in utilization could be a failure in ferritin or transferrin release.

Chronic low-grade infection produces a type of anemia characterized by normochromic, normocytic cells; low serum iron; and reduced erythropoiesis.[49] Anemia of chronic disorders is associated with fever, inflammation, and other conditions found in the aged such as renal disease and rheumatoid arthritis.[85] Differentiating between this anemia and uncomplicated iron-deficiency anemia may be difficult since serum iron levels and total iron-binding capacity (TIBC) vary greatly in older people. In general TIBC is elevated in iron-deficiency anemia and reduced in chronic-disorder anemia. Uncomplicated iron-deficiency anemia will respond to iron therapy; anemia of chronic disorders is highly resistant to treatment.[21,95]

A recent report suggests that depressed erythropoiesis in older people can be the result of protein-calorie malnutrition.[53] Animal studies have shown that erythrocyte production decreases in protein deficiency as a result of reduced erythropoietin; administration of erythropoietin or refeeding protein returns red blood cell production to normal.[72] The number of cells in the bone marrow capable of producing red blood cells is reduced in experimental protein-calorie malnutrition and appears to be reduced in malnourished aged.[53] Another contributing factor may be reduced survival time of existing red blood cells.[50] In protein deficient young adults the half life of chromium labeled red blood cells was 12 days and increased to 24 days on protein repletion.[50] In healthy older people above 80 years of age, red blood cell survival time is unchanged as compared to survival time in people age 18 to 25.[96]

Differences in hemoglobin levels might be used to distinguish between well nourished and protein-calorie deficient older people.[53] Among healthy, community-living men, only 5% had hemoglobin levels below 12 gm/100 ml as compared to 90% of a hospitalized malnourished group. For older women the criterion of 10 gm/100 ml was used. Chronic disease, however, could also have influenced hemoglobin levels in the malnourished group.

In general the causes of anemia in older people are poorly understood. Although iron deficiency may be an obvious cause in some individuals, in others the problem is unexplained. Chronic disease, the aging process, and protein-calorie malnutrition can all interact, precluding a simple interpretation. Lipschitz and coworkers[54] propose that older people with apparently unexplained anemia resulting from reduced capability of the bone marrow are also at risk of infection, as leukocyte response is also impaired.

Prevention and Treatment of Iron-Deficiency Anemia

Iron Supplementation. Treatment of iron-deficiency anemia should be preceded by careful evaluation and supervised by a physician. Administering supplemental iron to people who in fact have megaloblastic anemia precipitated by lack of folic acid or vitamin B_{12} has serious consequences, as the vitamin B_{12} deficiency eventually leads to neural damage. Equally unwise is the shotgun approach including iron and all necessary vitamin cofactors. A healthy, nonanemic individual who is not consuming adequate iron should be encouraged to select iron-rich foods. If the diet cannot be improved, the individual with the advice of his physician could select a supplement containing the daily recommended allowance for iron (10 mg). Self-medication with iron supplements above the recommended intake is extremely dangerous and can lead to hemochromatosis and liver damage[56] or mask a pathologic condition causing gastrointestinal blood loss.

Intervention Programs. Intervention programs with older people having hemoglobin levels below optimum have had only limited success. In a Boston study of over 200 older persons (hemoglobin levels between 9 and 12.9 gm/100 ml), iron was provided in fortified cereal, crackers, and cookies containing 15 to 22 mg per serving.[35] One third of the participants received items containing only 1 to 2.5 mg iron per serving. Participants were encouraged to eat one serving daily from the foods provided.

At the end of 6 months both groups had an average increase in hemoglobin of 1.4 gm/100 ml. This was interpreted to be a general effect of the intervention program and not attributed to the iron provided. People could have become more conscious of their food habits and improved their general food selection as a result of participation. The personal attention, in the form of a weekly visit and counseling about health problems in general, could have improved well-being in these individuals. Over half of the participants reported feeling better after 6 months; none felt worse.

Despite the general increase in hemoglobin levels, over 25% still had values below 13 gm/100 ml after 6 months and at that time were treated with ferrous sulfate. There was no measurable change in hemoglobin level after 3 months of supplementation. Serum iron and TIBC levels were normal. Gershoff and coworkers[35] concluded that such individuals are not iron deficient despite low hemoglobin and suggested that current standards when applied to the aged may be too high.

Exton-Smith[29] observed that hemoglobin levels of 11.7 mg/100 ml appeared to be normal for some healthy older women. individuals with low hemoglobin levels resistant to change may have low grade infections or inflammation associated with chronic disease or decreased erythropoietic capacity.

Megaloblastic Anemia

Although pernicious anemia occurs in less than 1% of the population, incidence increases with age.[95] It is seldom found in those below 30 years of age; the average age of onset is 60 years. The pathologic aspects of this condition relate to both the anemia and the role of vitamin B_{12} in maintenance of neural tissue. The severely reduced oxygen-carrying capacity of the blood results in tissue anoxia. Lack of the vitamin leads to myelin degeneration, which can be halted but not reversed when vitamin is restored.[40] Vitamin B_{12} deficiency eventually results in behavior changes and mental deterioration.

Serum vitamin B_{12} levels below 100 pg/ml are indicative of pernicious anemia, while borderline levels (100 to 200 pg/ml) are not always accompanied by anemia.[14,29,36,60-61] Because serum vitamin B_{12} measurements are costly and not always available on a routine basis, mean corpuscular volume (MCV), readily obtained by automated procedures, has been considered as a means of evaluating vitamin B_{12} status.[63] Although older men with borderline serum vitamin B_{12} levels had an MCV significantly greater than men with higher serum vitamin B_{12}, mean values were still within normal range.[10,63]

The value of borderline serum vitamin B_{12} levels as predictors of risk of pernicious anemia is still unclear. If vitamin B_{12} is poorly absorbed and body stores are systematically being depleted, overt deficiency is imminent. One clinician described this condition as latent pernicious anemia.[85] On the other hand, many people with vitamin B_{12} levels below normal, observed over periods of time, have not developed overt anemia.[10] Whether depressed serum vitamin B_{12} is an individual characteristic or representative of the aging process is not known. Increasing numbers of aged are being treated with intramuscular injections of vitamin B_{12} as a preventive measure, although serum vitamin levels do not always increase. Pernicious anemia will de-

Table 8-1. Relationships among hematologic measurements

	Persons with Normal Hemoglobin (No. = 606)	Persons with Deficient Hemoglobin (No. = 46)
Deficient serum iron	95	32
Deficient serum folate	83	11
Deficient serum vitamin B_{12}	6	1

Modified from Exton-Smith, A.N.: A nutrition survey of the elderly, Reports on Health and Social Subjects No. 3, London, 1972, Her Majesty's Stationery Office.

velop following a gastrectomy (18 to 24 months) if vitamin B_{12} is not administered. Subclinical vitamin deficiencies can contribute to both physical and mental dysfunction.[13]

Because of cost, screening procedures are often restricted to simple automated analyses such as hemoglobin. As suggested in Table 8-1, older people with normal hemoglobin levels can be deficient in serum iron, vitamin B_{12}, or folate.[29] Even mild iron deficiency significantly reduces the activity level of enzyme systems such as cytochrome c.[81] Experimental folate deficiency in humans indicates that low serum levels are followed by clinical deficiency and anemia.[40] A screening tool with specificity and sensitivity for identification of anemia is a current need.

Serum ferritin is now recognized as a valuable index of iron stores.[90] Qvist and associates[71] observed a significant relationship between serum ferritin and dietary iron among 54 older subjects (mean age = 73); ferritin levels did not differ between older men and young controls, although older women, as might be expected, had higher serum ferritin than younger women. Conversely, a recent report on 82 aged indicated that ferritin levels increased with age, particularly after age 70, regardless of iron deficiency and suggested that factors other than iron status influenced values.[55] The influence of chronic disease or age-related changes in erythropoiesis on serum ferritin levels must be clarified. Nevertheless, this method holds promise as a means of differentiating between simple iron-deficiency anemia and anemias resulting from other age-related or dietary causes.

SUMMARY

Age-related decreases in nutrient intake combined with degenerative changes relating to chronic disease make the older individual increasingly vulnerable to nutritional disorders. Decreased sensitivity of the beta cells of the pancreas to serum glucose levels, insulin resistance resulting from enlarged adipocytes, and decreased lean body mass have been implicated in the alterations in glucose tolerance in older individuals. Weight loss, physical activity, and high fiber diets have been successful in clinical management.

Changes in calcium or vitamin D intake and metabolism lead to bone disorders. Osteoporosis is characterized by a loss of both bone mineral and matrix. Although all older people lose bone, losses are greater in women. Estrogen withdrawal, immobility, calcium/phosphorus ratio and dietary protein have all been implicated in the problem. Daily intakes of 1.0 to 1.5 gm calcium appear to reverse bone loss; supplementation with $1,25(OH)_2D_3$ is being explored. Osteomalacia occurs less commonly and usually relates either to deficient vitamin D intake or absorption or to excessive use of antacids.

The etiology of nutritional anemia in the aged person is often obscure. Although iron-deficiency anemia is often the result of occult blood loss, chronic infection, protein deficiency, or impaired erythropoiesis can lead to decreased hemoglobin or unacceptable levels of red blood cells. Hemoglobin levels below 12 gm/100 ml may be normal for certain older people as iron supplementation does not always lead to increases in blood levels. Although many older people have less than acceptable numbers of red blood cells, hemoglobin concentration per cell appears to be within normal limits. Further work is needed to define the nutritional and metabolic processes contributing to these observations.

Incidence of pernicious anemia increases with age. Borderline serum vitamin B_{12} levels, however, are not always indicative of risk; some individuals remain healthy despite below average serum vitamin B_{12}. Hemoglobin levels, commonly used in screening, are not sensitive to developing anemia as indicated by deficient serum iron, folic acid, and vitamin B_{12} levels.

REVIEW QUESTIONS

1. How does glucose tolerance change over adulthood? Briefly describe current theories relating to this change. Give suggestions for dietary management of the older individual with impaired glucose tolerance.
2. Differentiate between osteoporosis and osteomalacia. What is the etiology of each?
3. Describe current treatment strategies for osteoporosis. Give suggestions for possible prevention of osteoporosis.
4. What is the most common form of anemia in older people? What factors contribute to the development of this anemia? Discuss problems in diagnosis of anemia in old people.
5. It has been suggested that reduced hemoglobin and red blood cell levels are natural consequences of the aging process and are not nutrition related. Do you agree? Cite experimental evidence to justify your conclusion.

REFERENCES

1. Albanese, A.A.: Calcium nutrition in the elderly, Postgrad. Med. **63:**167,1978.
2. Albanese, A.A., and others: Effect of a calcium supplement on serum cholesterol, calcium and phosphorus and bone density of "normal healthy" elderly women, Nut. Rep. Int. **8:**119, 1973.
3. Albanese, A.A., and others: Problems of bone health in elderly, N.Y. State J. Med. **75:**326, 1975.
4. Albright, F., Smith, P.M., and Richardson, A.M.: Postmenopausal osteoporosis, its clinical features, JAMA **116:**2465, 1941.
5. American Diabetes Association: Principles of nutrition and dietary recommendations for individuals with diabetes mellitus: 1979, Diabetes **28:**1027, 1979.
6. Anderson, J.W., and Chen, W.J.: Plant fiber: Carbohydrate and lipid metabolism, Am. J. Clin. Nutr. **32:**346, 1979.
7. Anderson, J.W., and Sieling, B.: High-fiber diets for diabetics: Unconventional but effective, Geriatrics **36**(5):64, 1981.
8. Andres, R.: Aging and diabetes, Med. Clin. North Am. **55:**835, 1971.
9. Andres, R.: Aging and carbohydrate metabolism. In Carlson, L.A., ed.: Nutrition in old age, Symposia Swedish Nutrition Foundation X, Stockholm, 1972, Almqvist & Wiksell.
10. Armstrong, B.K., and others: Hematological vitamin B_{12} and folate studies on Seventh-day Adventist vegetarians, Am. J. Clin. Nutr. **27:**712, 1974.
11. Avioli, L.V.: Aging, bone and osteoporosis. In Steinberg, F.U., ed.: Cowdry's care of the geriatric patient, ed. 6, St. Louis, 1982, The C.V. Mosby Co.
12. Avioli, L.V.: Postmenopausal osteoporosis: Prevention versus cure, Fed. Proc. **40:**2418, 1981.
13. Baker, H., and others: Vitamin profiles in elderly persons living at home or in nursing homes, versus profile in healthy young subjects, J. Am. Geriatr. Soc. **27:**444, 1979.
14. Batata, M., and others: Blood and bone marrow changes in elderly patients with special reference to folic acid, vitamin B_{12}, iron, and ascorbic acid, Br. Med. J. **2:**667, 1967.
15. Baylink, D.J., and Ivey, J.L.: Sodium fluoride for osteoporosis: Some unanswered questions (editorial), JAMA **243:**463, 1980.
16. Beisel, W.R.: Trace elements in infectious processes, Med. Clin. North Am. **60:**831, 1976.
17. Benzie, R.M.: The influence of age upon the iron content of bone marrow, Lancet **1:**1074, 1963.
18. Berry, W.T.: General discussion, part I. In Exton-Smith, A.N., and Scott, D.L., eds.: Vitamins in the elderly, Bristol, 1968, John Wright & Sons, Ltd.
19. Birge, S.J., and others: Osteoporosis, intestinal lactase deficiency and low dietary calcium intake, N. Engl. J. Med. **276:**445, 1967.
20. Björntorp, P., Berchtold, P., and Tibblin, G.: Insulin secretion in relation to adipose tissue in men, Diabetes **20:**65, 1971.
21. Cartwright, G.E., and Lee, G.R.: The anemia of chronic disorders, Br. J. Haematol. **21:**147, 1971.
22. Committee on Statistics of the American Diabetes Association: Standardization of the oral glucose tolerance test, Diabetes **18:**299, 1969.
23. Crockford, P.M., Harbeck, R.J., and Williams, R.H.: Influence of age on intravenous glucose tolerance and serum immunoreactive insulin, Lancet **1:**465, 1965.
24. Cundy, T., and others: Failure to heal vitamin D-deficiency rickets and suppress secondary hyperparathyroidism with conventional doses of 1,25-dihydroxy vitamin D_3, Br. Med. J. **284:**883, 1982.
25. Davidsohn, I., and Henry, J.B.: Todd-Sanford clinical diagnosis by laboratory methods, ed. 14, Philadelphia, W.B. Saunders Co.
26. Davidson, M.B.: The effect of aging on carbohydrate metabolism: A review of the English literature and a practical approach to the diagnosis of diabetes mellitus in the elderly, Metabolism **28:**688, 1979.
27. DeFronzo, R.A.: Glucose intolerance and aging. Evidence for tissue insensitivity to insulin, Diabetes **28:**1095, 1979.
28. Exton-Smith, A.N.: The problem of subclinical malnutrition in the elderly. In Exton-Smith, A.N., and Scott, D.L., eds.: Vitamins in the elderly, Bristol, 1968, John Wright & Sons, Ltd.
29. Exton-Smith, A.N., Chrm., Panel on Nutrition of the Elderly: A nutrition survey of the elderly, Reports on Health and Social Subjects No. 3, London, 1972, Her Majesty's Stationery Office.

30. Exton-Smith, A.N., and Stanton, B.R.: Report of an investigation into the dietary of elderly women living alone, London, 1965, King Edward's Hospital Fund for London.

31. Freedman, M.L., and Marcus, D.L.: Anemia and the elderly: Is it physiology or pathology? Am. J. Med. Sci. **280**:81, 1980.

32. Gallagher, J.C., and others: 1,25-dihydroxy vitamin D_3: Short- and long-term effects on bone and calcium metabolism in patients with postmenopausal osteoporosis, Proc. Natl. Acad. Sci. USA **79**:3325, 1982.

33. Garn, S.M.: The earlier gain and the later loss of cortical bone in nutritional perspective, Springfield, Ill., 1970, Charles C Thomas, Publisher.

34. Garn, S.M., and others: Suggested sex and age appropriate values for low and deficient hemoglobin levels, Am. J. Clin. Nutr. **34**:1648, 1981.

35. Gershoff, S.N., and others: Studies of the elderly in Boston. 1. The effects of iron fortification on moderately anemic people, Am. J. Clin. Nutr. **30**:226, 1977.

36. Girdwood, R.H., Thomson, A.D., and Williamson, J.: Folate status in the elderly, Br. Med. J. **2**:670, 1967.

37. Harrison, D.E.: Defective erythropoietic responses of aged mice not improved by young marrow, J. Gerontol. **30**:286, 1975.

38. Heaney, R.P., and others: Calcium nutrition and bone health in the elderly, Am. J. Clin. Nutr. **36**:986, 1982.

39. Heaney, R.P., Recker, R.R., and Saville, P.D.: Menopausal changes in bone remodeling, J. Lab. Clin. Med. **92**:964, 1978.

40. Herbert, V.: The nutritional anemias, Hosp. Pract. **15**:65, 1980.

41. Holt, J.M., and others: Iron absorption and blood loss in patients with hiatus hernia, Br. Med. J. **3**:22, 1968.

42. Horwitt, D.L.: Diabetes and aging, Am. J. Clin. Nutr. **36**:803, 1982.

43. Insogna, K.L., and others: Osteomalacia and weakness from excessive antacid ingestion, JAMA **244**:2544, 1980.

44. Jernigan, J.A., and others: Reference values for blood findings in relatively fit elderly persons, J. Am. Geriatr. Soc. **28**:308, 1980.

45. Joffe, B.I., Vinik, A.I., and Jackson, W.P.: Insulin reserve in elderly subjects, Lancet **1**:1292, 1969.

46. Kalkhoff, R., and Ferrou, C.: Metabolic differences between obese overweight and muscular overweight men, N. Engl. J. Med. **284**:1236, 1971.

47. Kalkhoff, R.K., and others: Metabolic effects of weight loss in obese subjects. Changes in plasma substrate levels, insulin and growth hormone responses, Diabetes **20**:83, 1971.

48. Kitahara, A., and Adelman, R.C.: Altered regulation of insulin secretion in isolated islets of different sizes in aging rats, Biochem. Biophys. Res. Commun. **87**:1207, 1979.

49. Kumar, R.: Mechanism of the anaemia of chronic infection: A reexamination of the role of functional iron deficiency in its causation, Indian J. Med. Res. **64**:1046, 1976.

50. Lanzkowsky, P., and others: Erythrocyte abnormality induced by protein malnutrition. II. 51-chromium labelled erythrocyte studies, Br. J. Haematol. **13**:639, 1967.

51. Lee, C.J., Lawler, G.S., and Johnson, G.H.: Effects of supplementation of the diets with calcium and calcium-rich foods on bone density of elderly females with osteoporosis, Am. J. Clin. Nutr. **34**:819, 1981.

52. Lindgarde, F., and Saltin, B.: Daily physical activity, work capacity and glucose tolerance in lean and obese normoglycaemic middle-aged men, Diabetologia **20**:134, 1981.

53. Lipschitz, D.A., and Mitchell, C.O.: Hematologic measurements in nutritional assessment of the elderly. In Assessing the nutritional status of the elderly: State of the art, Report of the Third Ross Roundtable on Medical Issues, Columbus, Oh., 1982, Ross Laboratories.

54. Lipschitz, D.A., Mitchell, C.O., and Thompson, C.: The anemia of senescence, Am. J. Hematol. **11**:47, 1981.

55. Loria, A., Hershko, C., and Konijn, A.M.: Serum ferritin in an elderly population, J. Gerontol. **34**:521, 1979.

56. Lynch, S.R., and others: Iron status of elderly Americans, Am. J. Clin. Nutr. **36**:1032, 1982.

57. Matkovic, V., and others: Bone status and fracture rates in two regions of Yugoslavia, Am. J. Clin. Nutr. **32**:540, 1979.

58. McFarlane, H., and others: Immunity, transferrin, and survival in kwashiorkor, Br. Med. J. **4**:268, 1970.

59. McLean, F.C., and Urist, M.R.: Bone: Fundamentals of the physiology of skeletal tissue, ed. 3, Chicago, 1968, University of Chicago Press.

60. McLennan, W.J., and others: Anaemia in the elderly, Q.J. Med. (New Series) **42**(165):1, 1973.

61. Meindok, H., and Dvorsky, R.: Serum folate and vitamin B_{12} levels in the elderly, J. Am. Geriatr. Soc. **18**:317, 1970.

62. Metz, R., and others: Glucose tolerance, plasma insulin, and free fatty acids in elderly subjects, Ann. Intern. Med. **64**:1042, 1966.

63. Munasinghe, D.R., and Pritchard, J.G.: The relationship between mean corpuscular volume, serum B_{12} and serum folate status in aged persons admitted to a geriatric unit, Br. J. Clin. Prac. **32**:16, 1978.

64. Murray, M.J., and others: The adverse effect of iron repletion on the course of certain infections, Br. Med. J. **2**:1113, 1978.

65. National Diabetes Data Group: Classification and diagnosis of diabetes mellitus and other categories of glucose intolerance, Diabetes **28**:1039, 1979.

66. Nordin, B.E.: Metabolic bone and stone disease, Baltimore, Md., 1973, The Williams & Wilkins Co.

67. Pagano, G., and others: Insulin resistance in the aged: The role of the peripheral insulin receptors, Metabolism **30:**46, 1981.

68. Parfitt, A.M.: Quantum concept of bone remodeling and turnover: Implications for the pathogenesis of osteoporosis, Calcif. Tissue Int. **28:**1, 1979.

69. Parfitt, A.M., and others: Vitamin D and bone health in the elderly, Am. J. Clin. Nutr. **36:**1014, 1982.

70. Perzigian, A.J.: The antiquity of age-associated bone demineralization in man, J. Am. Geriatr. Soc. **21:**100, 1973.

71. Qvist, I., Norden, A., and Olofsson, T.: Serum ferritin in the elderly, Scand. J. Clin. Lab. Invest. **40:**609, 1980.

72. Reissmann, K.R.: Protein metabolism and erythropoiesis. I. The anemia of protein deprivation, Blood **23:**137, 1964.

73. Riggs, B.L.: Postmenopausal and senile osteoporosis: Current concepts of etiology and treatment, Endocrinol. Jpn. **26**(suppl.):31, 1979.

74. Riggs, B.L., and others: Calcium deficiency and osteoporosis: Observations in 166 patients and critical review of the literature, J. Bone Joint Surg. **49A:**915, 1967.

75. Riggs, B.L., and others: Treatment of primary osteoporosis with fluoride and calcium. Clinical tolerance and fracture occurrence, JAMA **243:**446, 1980.

76. Riggs, B.L., and others: Differential changes in bone mineral density of the appendicular and axial skeleton with aging. Relationship to spinal osteoporosis, J. Clin. Invest. **67:**328, 1981.

77. Roe, D.A.: Drug-induced nutritional deficiencies, Westport, Conn., 1976, AVI Publishing Co.

78. Saltin, B., and others: Physical training and glucose tolerance in middle-aged men with chemical diabetes, Diabetes **28**(suppl. 1):30, 1979.

79. Sartin, J., and others: The role of hormones in changing adaptive mechanisms during aging, Fed. Proc. **39:**3163, 1980.

80. Sidney, K.H., Shepard, R.J., and Harrison, J.E.: Endurance training and body composition of the elderly, Am. J. Clin. Nutr. **30:**326, 1977.

81. Siimes, M.A., Refino, C., and Dallman, P.R.: Manifestation of iron deficiency at various levels of dietary iron intake, Am. J. Clin. Nutr. **33:**570, 1980.

82. Silverstone, F.A., and others: Age differences in the intravenous glucose tolerance tests and the response to insulin, J. Clin. Invest. **36:**504, 1957.

83. Smith, E.L., Reddan, W., and Smith, P.E.: Physical activity and calcium modalities for bone mineral increase in aged women, Med. Sci. Sports Exerc. **13:**60, 1981.

84. Smith, R.W., Jr., and Rizek, J.: Epidemiologic studies of osteoporosis in women of Puerto Rico and southeastern Michigan with special reference to age, race, national origin and to other related or associated findings, Clin. Orthop. **45:**31, 1966.

85. Thomas, J.H., and Powell, D.E.: Blood disorders in the elderly, Bristol, 1971, John Wright & Sons, Ltd.

86. Timaffy, M.: A comparative study of bone marrow function in young and old individuals, Gerontol. Clin. **4:**13, 1962.

87. United States Department of Health, Education and Welfare: Ten-State Nutrition Survey 1968-1970. IV. Biochemical, DHEW Publication No. (HSM) 72-8132, Atlanta, 1972, Centers for Disease Control.

88. United States Department of Health, Education and Welfare: Diabetes and aging, DHEW Publication No. (NIH) 79-1408, Washington, D.C., 1979, U.S. Government Printing Office.

89. United States Department of Health and Human Services: Hematological and nutritional biochemistry reference data for persons 6 months-74 years of age: United States, 1976-1980, DHHS Publication No. (PHS) 83-1682, Washington, D.C., 1982, U.S. Government Printing Office.

90. Valberg, L.S., and others: Serum ferritin and the iron status of Canadians, Can. Med. Assoc. J. **114:**417, 1976.

91. Vaughan, J.: The physiology of bone, ed. 3, Oxford, 1981, Clarendon Press.

92. Whedon, G.D.: Effects of high calcium intake on bones, blood and soft tissues; relationships of calcium intake to balance in osteoporosis, Fed. Proc. **18:**1112, 1959.

93. Whedon, G.D.: Recent advances in management of osteoporosis, Adv. Exp. Med. Biol. **128:**597, 1980.

94. Whedon, G.D., and others: Mineral and nitrogen metabolic studies on Skylab orbital space flights, Trans. Assoc. Am. Physicians **87:**95, 1974.

95. Wintrobe, M.M., and others: Clinical hematology, ed. 7, Philadelphia, 1974, Lea & Febiger.

96. Woodford-Williams, E., and others: Red cell longevity in old age, Gerontol. Clin. **4:**184, 1962.

Chapter 9

Drugs and Nutritional Considerations in the Aged

Increasing chronic disease and physical discomfort result in wide use of both prescription and over the counter (OTC) drugs by older people. The long term effects of drug use on nutritional status are only beginning to be explored. Drug-food and drug-drug interactions may add to the negative effects of either OTC or prescription drugs.

Vitamin and mineral supplements and alcohol can act as drugs and if used in excess are detrimental to nutritional and physical health. On the other hand, nutrient supplementation has been suggested as a means of reversing degenerative changes in mental function in older individuals. The nutritional impact of drugs must be considered when making dietary recommendations for older clients.

DRUG USE BY THE AGED

Aspects of the Problem

The aged are particularly vulnerable to adverse nutritional effects from drug therapy.[32] Nutritional status may already be jeopardized by physiologic changes and less than optimum nutrient intake influenced by social and economic conditions. Chronic disease necessitates long term drug therapy that can contribute to gradual depletion of nutrient reserves. Multiple drug intake can lead to drug-drug interactions and compound nutrition difficulties. Moreover, the effects of most drugs have been validated on younger individuals who have different rates of drug absorption, metabolism, and excretion, based on differences in body composition and renal function.[3]

Older people living in the community and responsible for self-medication may have limited understanding of the role of the prescribed drug or make errors in use. Among 178 persons age 60 or over attending an outpatient clinic, 59% did not know why they were taking particular drugs or reported incorrect dosages, sequences, or drug combinations.[38] These factors further add to the possibility of drug overdose or nutritional consequences.

Extent of Drug Use

Older people are among the chief users of drugs in the United States.[31] Although they comprise 11% of the population, they consume 22% of all prescription drugs.[48] Cardiovascular preparations (i.e., digitalis, antihypertensive agents), tranquilizers, diuretics, and sedatives account for about half of all prescription drugs sold to older people.[49]

A 3-year follow-up of over 1700 persons age 65 and over living in the community suggests that 77% of older persons use at least one drug on a regular basis and drug use increases with age.[16] Those under age 70 used one to two different drugs, whereas those above age 84 used two to three. Drugs most commonly used were antihypertensive agents, vitamins, cardiovascular agents, and analgesics. In another community group 65% were taking one to three prescription drugs and 20% were taking four to nine prescribed drugs.[38] Use of OTC drugs was not reported.

Table 9-1. Types and examples of commonly used drugs

Type	Therapeutic Action	Example
Analgesic	Acts on central nervous system; relieves pain without causing sleep	Salicylates, narcotics, nonsteroidal antiinflammatory agents
Sedatives and tranquilizers	Acts on central nervous system; reduces level of excitement and relieves tension or anxiety; does not usually impair normal mental function	Chlorpromazine, barbiturates, chloral hydrate
Antidepressants	Stimulates the central nervous system by acting on the synapse; promotes mental and motor activity and general feeling of well-being	Amitriptyline, desipramine, nortriptyline, monoamine oxidase inhibitors
Antiinfective agents	Used to treat or prevent infection	Penicillin, tetracycline, neomycin, isoniazid, sulfonamides
Anticonvulsant	Prevents seizures or convulsions; used in treatment of epilepsy	Phenobarbitol, phenytoin
Cardiac drugs	Increases strength of contraction of the heart muscle	Digitalis derivatives
Antilipemics	Lowers blood lipid levels by increasing excretion of bile acids; may interfere with lipoprotein synthesis or excretion	Cholestyramine, clofibrate
Diuretics	Increases formation of urine with net loss of sodium and water	Mercurials, spironolactone, ethacrynic acid, furosemide, thiazides, triamterene
Antihypertensive agents	Acts to reduce blood pressure; may inhibit sympathetic stimulation or act as a vasodilator	Diazoxide, hydralazine, captopril

Data from references 6, 9, 31, and 32.

Common drug categories with examples are defined in Table 9-1. Drugs for treating arthritis and tuberculosis as well as anticonvulsants, cardiovascular agents, diuretics, and hormones are frequently prescribed for long term maintenance. Many drugs in these categories are capable of inducing vitamin or mineral deficiencies.

OTC drugs can be obtained without the advice or prescription of a physician.[40] Among the aged, analgesics are used most commonly for relief of headache, backache, and muscle pain.[40] Other OTC drugs include antacids, laxatives, sedatives, and vitamin or mineral supplements. It is assumed that all population groups use OTC drugs to some extent. However, women and older people of both

sexes have the highest user rates.[40] Expenditures for both prescription drugs and OTC items exceeded 8 billion dollars in 1979.[48]

NUTRITIONAL ASPECTS OF OVER THE COUNTER DRUGS

Supervision of Use

Unfortunately, OTC drugs, easily obtained and commonly used, are often perceived by the user to be without risk. As noted by Shomaker,[40] older people may increase the dose above that recommended if the desired effect is not achieved. Use of OTC drugs may not be reported to the physician, creating the possibility of a dangerous interaction with a prescription drug. Self-medication can have serious consequences for nutritional status.

Analgesics

Prolonged use of aspirin (acetylsalicylic acid) is believed to be a frequent cause of iron-deficiency anemia.[31] Intakes of 1 to 3 gm/day (three to nine tablets) can induce some degree of gastrointestinal blood loss in over two thirds of normal individuals.[31] (One tablet contains 5 grains or 324 mg aspirin.) This level of dosage is not unusual among individuals with arthritis or other chronic pain.

Plasma ascorbic acid levels were found to be abnormally low in patients with rheumatoid arthritis ingesting high doses of aspirin (12 or more tablets/day).[32] It has been suggested that aspirin blocks the movement of ascorbic acid into the platelets, leading to depletion of body stores. Aspirin also appears to interfere with folate utilization by competing for binding sites on folate transport proteins. This may accelerate folate excretion, however, further evidence is needed.[31]

Gastrointestinal Drugs

Laxatives such as petrolatum liquid, phenolphthalein, and bulk salts, although considered harmless by many people, carry risk of nutritional imbalance. Bulk formers that impede the reabsorption of water in the intestine[32] are high in sodium and can equal 250 mg per packet.[40] Mineral oil taken in excess retards gastric emptying and interferes with absorption of calcium and fat soluble vitamins. (Older people have reported using ½ cup of mineral oil per day.[40]) Chronic diarrhea brought on by laxative abuse can induce sodium depletion and hypokalemia, leading to renal damage.[8]

Baking soda, antacids, and liquid products for control of nausea and vomiting increase the pH of the stomach,[32,40] inactivating thiamin and hindering the absorption of iron and antibiotic medicines. Abuse of antacids containing aluminum hydroxide

has been implicated in the development of osteomalacia. Aluminum hydroxide combining with phosphates in the intestine results in phosphorus depletion with subsequent mobilization of bone mineral (see Chaper 8).[32]

Alcohol

Use of Alcohol. Few dietary surveys have reported intakes of alcohol. Iber and coworkers[21] using HANES data suggest that alcohol consumption is widespread, although more common among men than women. Alcohol ingestion peaks between ages 40 and 60 and then declines. In that report, highest intakes were 5% to 6% of total calories. Alcohol provided 6% and 3% of total calories among British men between ages 62 and 74 (n = 158) and 75 and 90 (n = 54), respectively.[25]

McGandy and associates[26] observed that alcohol consumption decreased with age among their middle to upper class male subjects. Average daily intake was 17 gm between ages 55 and 64 and only 8 to 9 gm between ages 65 and 99. Among 270 healthy aged in New Mexico, 46% of men and 41% of women consumed alcohol at least once over the 3-day record period.[13] Mean daily intake was higher for men than women (12 versus 6 gm) and also decreased with age.

Although a significant number of older people appear to consume alcoholic beverages regularly, the number of alcohol abusers is not known. Physical and emotional upset, loneliness, and bereavement all contribute to increased use of this drug.[21,54] Of 280 consecutive admissions of men age 65 or above requiring medical or surgical care in a veterans facility, 11% were alcoholics.[35] Others have estimated that 2% to 10% of persons above age 60 are alcohol abusers.[21] Incidence of abuse is higher (10% to 15%) among those admitted to nursing homes or clinics providing psychiatric or physical care.[54]

Chronic alcoholics often have multiple nutrient deficiencies caused by (1) general lack of food intake, (2) alcohol interference with nutrient absorption, and (3) toxic effects of alcohol on the pancreas, liver, and gastrointestinal tract.[31] These combined effects on nutritional status and general health may contribute to the increased percentage of alcohol abusers among older people admitted to long term care facilities.

Nutritional Aspects. Tolerance to alcohol decreases and adverse side effects increase with age, even in chronic alcoholics.[39] The risk of nutritional deficiency arising from use of other drugs is markedly increased by excessive use of alcohol or when prior alcoholism has depleted nutrient stores. Moreover, alcohol interacts with some drugs to exacerbate negative effects. Both alcohol and aspirin irritate the stomach mucosa and can lead to gastrointestinal bleeding. When both drugs are combined the anticoagulant effect of aspirin can result in serious hemorrhage.[39]

High intakes of alcohol decrease serum potassium levels. This presents a serious danger to the cardiac patient taking digitalis as both cardiac arrhythmias and digitalis toxicity can result (see Chapter 7). The insulin-dependent diabetic may become hypoglycemic following high alcohol intake as alcohol interferes with gluconeogenesis.[39]

Damage to the intestinal mucosa results in malabsorption of both vitamin B_{12} and folate. Poor zinc status with excessive zinc excretion is also associated with alcohol abuse.[32] Extreme urinary zinc excretion (1000 to 5000 μg daily) has been observed in alcoholics regardless of liver damage.[44] Although the mechanism by which this occurs has not been established, zincuria is also seen in pancreatic disease. Pancreatitis is common in alcoholic patients[31] and is believed to contribute to the general malabsorption syndrome sometimes observed.

Thiamin Deficiency. Alcohol interferes with thiamin absorption. At the low concentrations normally found in the intestine, thiamin is absorbed against a concentration gradient by an active transport mechanism requiring both oxygen and energy. Al-

though alcohol does not inhibit thiamin uptake by the mucosal cell, the vitamin is not released into the blood as a result of alcohol inhibition of the enzyme required for this step (Na-K ATPase).[21]

Thiamin absorption is impaired in alcoholics with or without liver disease[47] and returns to normal when alcohol use is discontinued (within an 8-week period).[47] The direct effect of alcohol on the absorption mechanism is confirmed by the observation that absorption is similarly depressed in normal subjects given alcohol prior to thiamin ingestion. As a result of ineffective absorption, thiamin deficiency is common among alcohol abusers. In one report nearly half of a group of chronic alcoholics (n = 50) had below normal red blood cell transketolase activity[21] as compared to only 2% of healthy adults (n = 1152).

Neurologic disorders such as Wernicke-Korsakoff syndrome with visual disturbances, abnormal gait (ataxia), mental confusion, and memory loss occur in thiamin deficiency regardless of associated alcoholism.[21,24] Degeneration of the peripheral nerves with loss of normal reflexes and burning sensations, weakness, and pain in the lower extremities are classic signs of inadequate thiamin. Clinical beri-beri with disturbed cardiac function, edema, and eventual cardiac failure has been described in experimental as well as accidental thiamin deficiency. As pointed out by Iber and coworkers,[21] cardiac disease, loss of memory, and loss of vibratory sense in the lower extremities, suggestive of thiamin deficiency, frequently occur with advancing age. The diagnostic problem is complicated further by the fact that older people regardless of alcohol abuse may have multiple vitamin deficiencies.[24]

Although aged alcoholics or individuals with poor thiamin intake (over at least 3 months) often respond to thiamin therapy, both behavior changes and cardiac symptoms in older people can result from a variety of disease conditions. Long term neurologic and psychologic follow-up of older people whose thiamin status was restored to normal is needed to provide information regarding both physiologic and behavior changes pertinent to thiamin problems in this age group.

Vitamin and Mineral Supplements

Level of Use. A large proportion of older people use vitamin and mineral supplements. This was true for 37% of older people studied in Rochester, New York,[23] 40% of rural aged in Pennsylvania,[15] and 59% of middle income older people in New Mexico.[13] Of the 44 rural Pennsylvanians using supplements, 19 had been so advised by their physician, 11 decided for themselves, and 3 had been advised by friends; others gave no particular reason.[15] The majority did not know why their doctor had prescribed supplements, and 80% did not know what was in the supplement.

The vitamin and mineral supplements used, however, do not necessarily correct existing dietary deficiencies. In Rochester, New York, 50% of those taking supplements already consumed more than the RDA for the seven vitamins and minerals evaluated.[23] Among those with diets supplying less than the recommended level of at least one nutrient, only one fourth selected a supplement containing the nutrient(s) in shortest supply; half were meeting some but not all of their shortages through supplements, and the remainder selected supplements containing nutrients already consumed in adequate amounts. An older woman living alone was deficient in calcium, iron, and the B complex vitamins but was taking supplements containing vitamins A and C.[23] In another study 66% were consuming less than 67% the RDA for calcium but few used calcium supplements.[15]

Among healthy aged in New Mexico, 95% of those taking a daily multivitamin preparation also used additional vitamin or mineral products.[13] The most common supplement was ascorbic acid and median intake was about 6 times the RDA among women, and 8 times the RDA among men. Ninety percent of the group already obtained at least 100% the RDA from food.

The nutrient supplemented at the highest level relative to recommended intake was vitamin E (median supplemental intake equaled 1800% the RDA); the nutrient supplemented at the lowest level was phosphorus (20% of the RDA). Supplements did, however, contribute toward meeting the recommended daily intake of vitamins B_6 and D and folic acid. For those not taking supplements, median intakes of those three vitamins were less than 67% the RDA. In the supplemented group median intakes ranged from 150% to 287% the RDA. As pointed out by Garry and coworkers,[13] limited information about the vitamin B_6 and folate content of foods may have contributed to the low calculated intakes; the fact remains, however, that 25% of the group appeared to consume less than 50% the RDA. This was also true for vitamin D. Although these individuals were not taking prescription drugs, such low levels of intake would present additional risk for people on medications known to interfere with nutrient absorption or metabolism.

Risks of Megavitamin Dosage. A panel of experts evaluating the potential danger of excessive ingestion of vitamins or minerals concluded that toxicities are unlikely to occur as a result of food intake except in those consuming the most unusual food pattern.[28] On the other hand, unwise consumption of vitamin and mineral preparations presents a real hazard.[28] Present legislation sets no maximum limits on the vitamin and mineral content of preparations available without prescription, with the exception of folic acid. Folic acid supplements may not contain more than 400 μg per capsule, although an individual is not limited in the number of capsules he chooses to ingest. Claims relating nutrient supplementation and optimum health, recovery from chronic disease, and an extended life span are particularly attractive to older people who fear deteriorating health.[14,42]

Although many people believe that large amounts of vitamin A are beneficial and can be ingested safely, the symptoms of chronic vitamin A toxicity such as loss of appetite, pain and tenderness of the long bones, loss of hair, liver enlargement, and abnormal skin pigmentation are well known. On the basis of available evidence, daily intakes of vitamin A in amounts above five times the RDA (25,000 IU) should be avoided.[12,28] Consumption of large amounts of vitamin E (more than 10 times the RDA) over prolonged periods without medical monitoring is equally hazardous.[28] Although information is limited, vitamin D is potentially toxic and intakes should approximate the RDA (5 μg daily); there is no convincing evidence that normal people are benefited by intakes above that amount.[12]

Despite the hazards of excessive intakes of the fat soluble vitamins some older people living in the community are reported to routinely consume supplements containing at least five times the recommended levels of vitamins A and D and 100 times the recommended level of vitamin E.[13] Vitamin D may have value in treating some bone disorders in older women; however, medical supervision is mandatory. Continued use of the reported dosages of vitamins A, D, and E could result in toxicity and should be discouraged.

A dietary level of 60 mg of vitamin C is recommended for adults of both sexes. Intakes of ascorbic acid far exceeding physiologic requirements (1 gm/day or more) have pharmacologic or druglike effects that are not related to the normal function of the vitamin.[12] At present there appear to be no particular benefits from such use and renal and bladder problems can result.

Ascorbic acid and the B complex vitamins (thiamin, riboflavin, and niacin) are frequently consumed at levels of 10 to 100 times the RDA on the assumption that extra amounts can be easily excreted. At present we do not know the maximum blood vitamin levels reached following ingestion of high potency supplements nor the period of time such levels are maintained. It is likely, however, that the kinetics of tissue disposal or excretion differ in older as compared to younger individuals based on reduced glomerular filtration rate and re-

nal tubular secretion of metabolites. The fact that the aged adult is more susceptible to drug overdose and toxicity than a younger adult lends credence to such an argument. Whether excessive ingestion of the water soluble vitamins carries the potential for toxicity in the older adult is not known but must be evaluated.

DRUG-NUTRIENT INTERACTIONS

Modes of Drug-Nutrient Interactions

Substances that interfere with the normal physiologic processes involving nutrients can adversely affect nutritional status. Drugs may interact at the point of ingestion, absorption, utilization, or excretion of nutrients.[31]

Ingestion. Food intake may decrease as a result of drugs that are unpleasant to the taste (i.e., potassium chloride liquid, chloral hydrate, or vitamin B complex liquids) or that depress appetite (antidepressants or thyroid preparations).[32] Many common drugs such as digitalis, narcotics, analgesics or clofibrate can cause nausea and vomiting. Gastric upset can be particularly severe with the antineoplastic drugs used in cancer chemotherapy. Some tranquilizers such as chlorpromazine have the opposite effect and stimulate the appetite, resulting in weight gain.[32]

Digestion and Absorption. Drugs may interfere with the secretion of digestive enzymes, alter gastrointestinal transit time and pH, adsorb or inactivate bile salts, or damage the intestinal mucosa and block nutrient uptake.[27] Long term therapy with corticosteroids can damage the exocrine pancreas causing decreased production and release of pancreatic enzymes and consequent incomplete digestion of the macronutrients. Colchicine used in the treatment of gout inhibits secretion of disaccharidases (sucrase, maltase, and lactase) in the gut.[32]

Other drugs interfere with nutrient binding to receptor sites, inflict cellular damage on the mucosa, or selectively block nutrient transport.[27] Tetracycline forms chelates with various minerals including calcium and magnesium, thereby blocking absorption.[32] Cholestyramine disrupts the formation of micelles and prevents the reabsorption of bile salts, thus decreasing absorption of the fat soluble vitamins.[32] Cholestyramine also binds to intrinsic factor preventing uptake of vitamin B_{12}, as does para-aminosalicylic acid.[32] Drugs often associated with malabsorption in older people include alcohol, cathartics, hypocholesterolemic agents (e.g., cholestyramine), antibiotics (neomycin, tetracycline), and the antitubercular agent para-aminosalicylic acid.[31]

Utilization and Excretion. Drugs may replace nutrients on carrier protein binding sites or form complexes with essential nutrients that are then excreted in the urine.[27] The antitubercular drug isoniazid and the antihypertensive agent hydralazine increase the excretion of vitamin B_6 in this manner.[31-32] Antivitamins are drugs or foreign chemicals that interfere with the metabolic conversion of a vitamin to its active form. Chemotherapeutic agents such as methotrexate lead to folic acid deficiency because they inhibit the enzyme responsible for the activation step.

Drugs may increase the rate of metabolism of certain vitamins by enhancing the production of catabolic enzymes or inhibiting controlling enzymes. Although the anticonvulsant phenytoin is believed to interfere with folate absorption, the folate depletion observed may also relate to enhanced activation and destruction of folate.[31-32]

Food-Drug Interactions

Foods or specific components in food can decrease the effectiveness or increase the hazards of drug therapy. Foods may delay, accelerate, or reduce the efficiency of drug absorption or alter the rate of excretion through shifts in urinary pH.[27] For example, the antibiotic tetracycline can form complexes with calcium salts that reduce absorption of the drug. The mechanisms of these effects are not the same for all drugs. While the absorption of some drugs may be delayed or impaired when taken with food, other drugs are irritating to the stomach mucosa and are better tolerated when taken immediately before or after meals (e.g., aspirin).[50] Drugs should not be mixed with fruit juice, milk, or other beverages unless so ordered.

Dietary status can alter drug metabolism. Enzyme systems that detoxify drug metabolites leading to their removal from the body decrease in activity when intakes of protein and such minerals as zinc and magnesium are deficient.[27] The effects of sedatives or tranquilizers are potentiated by simultaneous or proximate alcohol ingestion.[39]

Pharmacologically active substances present in foods can alter response to a drug taken at the same time. Tyramine-containing foods such as cheese or Chianti wine have this effect when taken along with monoamine oxidase inhibitors, resulting in a dangerous rise in blood pressure.[27] The nutritional and clinical implications of food and drug interactions are at this point only poorly understood.

Influence of Drugs on Nutritional Status

Vitamins and minerals are the nutrients most likely to be affected by drug use. Table 9-2 summarizes nutrients and drugs associated with problems in older people. The clinical significance of these interactions relates to the drug, the nutrient involved, and the individual.[31] Nutrient depletion is most likely to occur with a drug inhibiting nutrient absorption or a drug taken for an extended period of time. Use of a drug that acts as a vitamin antagonist or affects a nutrient such as folic acid that participates in a variety of metabolic processes will result in impaired biochemical function. Finally, nutritional effects of drugs will be more serious in individuals with preexisting subclinical malnutrition. Older individuals with marginal status who, as a result of chronic illness, are consuming multiple drugs over periods of years are at greatest risk of nutrient depletion.

Table 9-2. Examples of nutrients influenced by drugs

Nutrient	Drugs Interacting
Ascorbic acid	Adrenal corticosteroids, barbiturates, levodopa, salicylates, sulfonamides, tetracycline
Folic acid	Adrenal corticosteroids, alcohol, anticonvulsants, barbiturates, isoniazid, salicylates, sulfonamides, tetracycline, triamterene
Pyridoxine	Adrenal corticosteroids, anticonvulsants, diuretics, hydralazine, isoniazid, levodopa, sulfonamides
Vitamin A	Adrenal corticosteroids, colchicine, cholestyramine, clofibrate, petrolatum liquid
Vitamin B$_{12}$	Alcohol, anticonvulsants, barbiturates, cholestyramine, clofibrate, colchicine, para-aminosalicylic acid, phenobarbitol, potassium chloride, sulfonamides, triamterene
Vitamin D	Adrenal corticosteroids, anticonvulsants, barbiturates, cholestyramine, petrolatum liquid
Vitamin K	Anticoagulants, anticonvulsants, cholestyramine, petrolatum liquid, salicylates, tetracycline
Calcium	Aluminum hydroxide, anticonvulsants, cholestyramine, digitalis glycosides, mercurial diuretics, tetracycline, thiazide diuretics, triamterene
Iron	Alcohol, antacids (carbonate), cholestyramine
Potassium	Adrenal corticosteroids, colchicine, diuretics except spironolactone and triamterene, penicillin
Zinc	Alcohol, tetracycline, thiazide diuretics

Modified from Roe, D.A.: Handbook: Interactions of selected drugs and nutrients in patients, ed. 3, Chicago, 1982, American Dietetic Association.

Nutritional Intervention

Nutritional intervention is appropriate as a preventive or therapeutic measure for individuals at risk because of drug therapy. The first step should be determination of present nutrient intake through analysis of a diet history.[31] Many of those suffering from drug-induced malnutrition have diets that are marginal at best and do not meet the elevated requirements imposed by drug intake. If a person taking a drug that increases the requirement for folic acid has a diet low in fruits, legumes, and leafy vegetables and does not eat liver, nutrient depletion is likely to ensue. Unfortunately, dietary counseling is sometimes ineffective in reducing risk as food intake is dictated by long term habits as well as economic considerations. In individual clients, however, it is possible to obviate the risk of drug-induced deficiency by dietary modification.

Some writers believe that a daily vitamin-mineral tablet is justified for the older population in general.[4,51] Others maintain that, although therapeutic regimens including vitamin and mineral supplements are appropriate for people with observed deficiencies or those at risk, such prescriptions should be written only when necessary.[41]

In a study of 433 older patients admitted to health care facilities, 10% were taking specific vitamin or mineral supplements prescribed with no appropriate diagnostic indication; for 1% vitamins or minerals had not been prescribed when medical diagnosis indicated they should have been.[41] Seventeen percent were taking a standard multivitamin-mineral supplement. Vitamin B$_{12}$ and iron were most frequently prescribed without demonstrated need. Over 70% of those taking vitamin B$_{12}$ had no diagnosis of anemia. About half of the subjects had been living in the community; the others were admitted from other nursing facilities. Use of supplements was not evaluated on the basis of previous residence. When vitamin supplementation is indicated, intramuscular rather than oral administration may be more effective for those with suspected malabsorption.[2]

When nutrient supplements are prescribed it is essential that clients understand the level of dosage and the dangers of overdose. Excessive therapeutic doses of nutrients can interfere with the effectiveness of particular drugs. Seizures can increase in both number and frequency when high levels of folic acid are given to epileptics receiving anticonvulsants, although this is not consistent.[31] Another case in point is the relationship between levodopa (used to treat parkinsonism) and pyridoxine. While levodopa is a pyridoxine antagonist, supplementation with pyridoxine (10 to 25 mg) decreases drug effectiveness.[32] It is ironic that nutrient supplements tailored to meet the nutrient needs induced by specific drugs are not easily obtained,[31] although megavitamin and mineral preparations are advertised as therapeutic for a host of symptoms unrelated to nutritional deficiency.

Many factors contribute to the development of iatrogenic malnutrition in older people, and resolution of the difficulties will require considerable effort. Closer communication between the physician, nutritionist, and pharmacist could contribute to solutions to some of these problems.

DRUGS AND CLINICAL DISORDERS

Treatment of Hypertension

Dietary management has had only limited use in treatment of hypertension because of the proven effectiveness of oral diuretics and the commonly held belief that drastic sodium restriction and massive weight loss were necessary to achieve any significant drop in blood pressure. Wilber[53] summarized several studies indicating that weight control and sodium restriction are effective in controlling mild hypertension (diastolic pressure 95 to 109 mm Hg) either in combination with or as a complement to drug therapy. Of particular interest is the conclusion that achievement of desirable or near desirable weight was not required; moderate weight loss (about 5% to 6% body weight) led to a reduction in blood pressure regardless of beginning weight status.

Most hypertensive individuals are given oral diuretics. Thiazide and mercurial diuretics all increase urinary potassium excretion. A strong argument for sodium restriction in these situations is that potassium loss is directly proportional to sodium excretion, which increases with dietary intake.[53] As sodium intake rises, the level of potassium lost also rises. Nutrition intervention in these cases should include assistance with limiting sodium intake and, if indicated, moderate weight loss. Wilber[53] suggests limiting sodium intake to 75 mEq, accomplished by eliminating highly salted prepared foods from the diet and not salting at the table. This approach enhances the effectiveness of the oral diuretic and may eliminate the need for potassium supplements or the relatively expensive potassium-sparing diuretic combinations.

If potassium supplementation is required, current thinking points to potassium chloride as the compound of choice. According to Kassirer and Harrington,[22] the loss of sodium, water, and chloride as a result of diuretic therapy leads to enhanced secretion of hydrogen ions by the kidney tubule, subsequent metabolic alkalosis, and accelerated potassium loss. Correction of the potassium deficit requires correction of the chloride deficit as well.

The relative risk of hyperkalemia incurred by use of potassium supplements as compared to the risk of developing hypokalemia remains controversial. Hyperkalemia can lead to cardiac arrest and sudden death. Older people appear to be at greater risk of developing hyperkalemia with long term potassium chloride supplementation than younger people. On the other hand, an evaluation of the relative cost of 50 mEq of potassium per day[22] suggests that a potassium chloride liquid is more practical for an older individual than trying to obtain this amount of potassium from orange juice or bananas. The pharmaceutical would cost about half as much as the juice or fresh fruit.

Those authors[22] suggest that people on diuretics be monitored at 1- to 2-month intervals using serum potassium concentrations. Unless serum levels fall below 3.0 mEq/L, digitalis is also being administered, or symptoms characteristic of potassium deficiency develop, supplementation would not seem to be justified.[22] Limiting sodium intake and efforts at weight control may reduce the need for additional potassium.

Nutrition and Mental Status

Impairment of Mental Function. Mental confusion (delirium), dementia, and hallucinations have been described in classic deficiency of folic acid, thiamin, or vitamin B_{12}.[18,21,24] In a young individual a change in personality or sudden loss of awareness is investigated in relation to nutritional or physiologic status. Unfortunately, the expectation of such behavior in an older person may preclude such an evaluation. Dementia or impaired intellectual function usually develops slowly and symptoms may be noticed by the older individual as well as family and friends.[45] Inability to concentrate or remember recent events suggests that mental function is deteriorating. Delirium, on the other hand, most often occurs abruptly with reduced alertness, confusion, hallucinations, or emotional upset.[45] Physical symptoms may include a change in usual sleep pattern, overactivity, or flushed skin.

The older individual is extremely sensitive to changes in the internal environment that result from a variety of disorders. Adverse drug reactions or drug overdose can cause delirium or dementia.[45] Metabolic disturbances such as hyponatremia, hypokalemia, hyperthyroidism or hypothyroidism, dehydration, renal failure, or congestive heart failure lead to mental dysfunction. Bacterial infections such as pneumonia can cause delirium. Mental impairment relating to such disorders is reversible. It is estimated that about 10% to 20% of those with dementia can be successfully treated.[45] The remaining 80% suffer from Alzheimer's disease, characterized by degenerative changes in the neurons, or organic brain disease resulting from occlusion of the cerebral arteries.

Nutritional disorders most commonly associated with mental dysfunction are water and electrolyte and thyroid disturbances and vitamin deficiency. Potassium depletion and dehydration resulting in confusion, delirium, or apathy were discussed in Chapter 7. Portnoi[29] described a woman age 82 with thyrotoxicosis who became incoherent, incontinent, and unable to feed herself. On treatment her speech became fluent and she regained the ability to care for her personal needs. Thyrotoxicosis and hypothyroidism sometimes result in apathy or depression (see Chapter 3).

Vitamin B_{12} deficiency leads to mental impairment, which can be reversed if treated promptly (before neurologic damage has occurred). A typical case history was presented by Thomas and Powell[46] who treated a man 68 years of age who over a month's time became confused and then suddenly psychotic. On admission to the hospital his hemoglobin was 3.5 gm/100 ml and his blood smear consistent with pernicious anemia. He responded to vitamin B_{12} therapy and when discharged was mentally competent with a normal blood picture. He was still well, mentally and physically, 5 years later.

When an older person who has been responding normally begins to rapidly deteriorate in intellectual function or undergoes sudden changes in temperament or outlook, nutritional status and general medical condition should be evaluated. Recent drug use and intakes of potassium, thiamin, folate, and vitamin B_{12} are of particular importance. Although nutritional problems are generally not the sole basis of altered mental function, this aspect should be evaluated before assuming that observed changes are the result of degenerative changes.

Influence of Vitamin Status

Problems in Evaluation. Although the relationship between nutritional therapy and restoration of mental function is fairly clear in the case of well-defined disorders such as pernicious anemia or hypokalemia, the value of nutrient supplementation in either preventing or reversing mental deterioration not associated with a specific clinical disorder is still unresolved. Folic acid, vitamin B_{12}, ascorbic acid, and niacin have been administered to older patients in an effort to improve general well-being.[1,17,34,37] The first and most common problem associated with these reports is that both psychotropic drugs and vitamins were used in combination; therefore it is impossible to separate the effects of one from the other.[1,37] A second problem is the lack of a control, or placebo group, in studies involving hospital or nursing home patients.[17] The increased attention and mental stimulation associated with a clinical evaluation may in itself improve the outlook and orientation of a previously isolated individual. A third problem is the lack of specific criteria to define mental upset or disturbance.[34] As a result, it is difficult to compare one evaluation with another or to arrive at any firm conclusions.

Vitamin B_{12} and Folic Acid. In light of the known association between pernicious anemia and neurologic function, older people with dementia have been evaluated for vitamin B_{12} status. An often quoted study is that of Droller and Dossett[10] who examined the mental state and serum vitamin B_{12} levels of 69 older persons admitted to a geriatric facility, who had no organic basis for mental disturbance. None of the normal patients as compared with 55% of those with dementia and 28% of those described as confused had serum B_{12} levels below 180 pg/ml. Criteria used for mental assessment were not described.

In retrospect, however, it cannot be determined what was cause or effect. Mental impairment can result in poor food choices with lower intake of vitamin B_{12} and a subsequent drop in serum levels. Those authors[10] concluded that the symptoms observed were not of nutritional origin as all groups were similar in body weight. This overlooks the fact that confused older people could consume high levels of sweets, bread, and starches providing calories but lacking in vitamin B_{12}.

Subsequent evaluations have failed to confirm a relationship between serum vitamin B_{12} levels and mental status. A review of 80 hospital admissions (40 mentally normal and 40 with persistent mental confusion with no organic cause) found no differences in serum vitamin B_{12} in pairs matched for sex and age.[7] An evaluation of 533 persons age 65 and over in a Welsh community found no relationship between serum vitamin B_{12} or folate levels and mental impairment.[11] Scores on paired association tests of words and pictures (measuring both learning and recall) were not correlated with serum vitamin or hemoglobin levels.

Schulman[37] maintains that vitamin B_{12} deficiency cannot be considered the cause of mental disturbance unless symptoms are removed on vitamin therapy. Thirty-nine noninstitutionalized older persons with serum vitamin B_{12} levels below 150 pg/ml but no evidence of pernicious anemia were given either 1000 μg vitamin B_{12} or a placebo once per week for 6 weeks and assessed according to appetite, fatigue, sleep patterns, and general psychiatric state.[19] About one third improved in at least one category regardless of the injection received. Seven of 20 receiving vitamin B_{12} and 6 of 19 receiving placebo improved based on a psychiatric interview. Hughes and coworkers[19] concluded that repeated visits to the home by health and research personnel improved general well-being. Participation in the study appeared to be especially beneficial to those living alone as 11 of 24 women improved compared to 2 of 15 men. None of the men but eight of the women lived alone.

Inadequate nutrient intake with low serum folate has been reported in older people with organic and functional behavior disorders.[20,30,36] In those with senile dementia, poor food intake resulted from inability to care for their own needs and in some cases refusal to accept help.[36] Those who were depressed or apathetic often had poor appetites. In a comparison of 59 older psychiatric patients and

61 controls of similar age, 80% of the patients as compared to 30% of the controls had serum folate levels below 6 ng/ml.[36] Hurdle and Picton Williams[20] looked at serum folate levels in 72 persons (age 70 or above) evaluated for mental state on hospital admission. Incidence of serum folate levels below 5 ng/ml was 22% in those with minimal physical impairment and normal mental state, 38% in those with severe mobility problems but normal mental state, and 67% in those with no physical handicap but lacking in motivation. (Serum folate levels between 2.1 and 5.9 ng/ml are considered marginal.) Those authors concluded that individuals less concerned about their diet are more likely to be folate deficient.

Although mental disturbance or depression resulting in inadequate intake is the basis for low folate levels observed in some older people, the fact remains that severe folate deficiency (with associated anemia) can lead to mental impairment. If folate deficiency is the primary cause, the condition will be reversed when folate status improves.[18]

Multivitamin Supplements. Multivitamin supplements including ascorbic acid and the B complex (thiamin, riboflavin, niacin, pyridoxine, and pantothenic acid) have been administered to patients in long term care facilities in an effort to improve both physical and mental status; however, results are inconclusive.[1,5,17] In a double-blind evaluation of 132 aged psychiatric patients given a multivitamin supplement (vitamin C plus B complex) or placebo for 6 weeks, nonschizophrenic patients given the vitamins improved, as evidenced by reduced agitation and hyperactivity.[1] Patients were also given psychotropic drugs, although, according to those authors, drug therapy alone produced no behavioral effect. There was no indication of dietary intake over the test period or evaluation for possible vitamin deficiency prior to the test period. Therefore various factors including improvement of existing vitamin deficiencies or a synergistic effect between the drug and vitamins could have contributed to this result.

Recent work with ascorbic acid supplementation[33-34] has not confirmed a therapeutic effect on mood or psychologic outlook in institutionalized older perople.[33-34] A preliminary report suggested that 1 gm ascorbic acid daily for 28 days led to increased interest in the environment and participation in dressing and feeding activities.[33] Mean plasma ascorbic acid before supplementation was only 0.22 mg/100 ml.

Another double-blind trial carried on for 2 months with 94 patients resulted in weight gain and alleviation of physical signs of ascorbic acid deficiency (i.e., petechial hemorrhages) in those given the vitamin but no change in mental outlook or physical mobility.[34] As pointed out by Schorah and coworkers,[34] slight changes in mentally disturbed patients are difficult for nurses to detect over a short period of time. It may be necessary to use an outside evaluator who is less familiar with the patient and therefore more cognizant of change.

The weight gain associated with vitamin supplementation has not always been explained.[17,34] In a report in which all patients received a multivitamin supplement Hecht[17] suggested that weight gain was related to increased appetite and attention of the nursing staff to feeding procedures. Steffee[43] suggests that malnourished people who are confused and generally antagonistic to feeding become more interested in food after 5 to 10 days of nutritional therapy.

There is a need for controlled, systematic evaluation of vitamin therapy and mental status in older people. Present studies have been short term and have not always assessed the nutritional status of the individual at the outset. Both biochemical and behavioral data are pertinent.

The interaction or competition of one vitamin with another also needs to be considered. One report describing neurologic evaluation of older people[52] raises a concern about single or incomplete vitamin supplements. Independent-living older people consuming vitamin preparations not containing vitamin B_{12} had poorer neurologic performance as measured by vibratory sense threshold than those taking either a vitamin B_{12}–containing supplement or no vitamin supplement at all. Whether an abundance of one vitamin aggravates a limited supply of another has not been resolved. Therefore vitamin supplementation at levels above those generally recommended is inadvisable.

SUMMARY

Use of OTC and prescription drugs in treatment of chronic disorders can be deleterious to nutritional status. Laxatives and antacids result in malabsorption of phosphorus, iron, and the fat soluble vitamins; aspirin use can lead to blood loss. Thiamin deficiency resulting in mental and motor dysfunction frequently accompanies alcohol abuse. Vitamin and mineral supplements, often consumed at higher than recommended levels, do not always supply the nutrients lacking in the diet.

Prescription drugs can interfere with nutrient intake, absorption, or metabolism or enhance nutrient excretion. Drugs may compete for binding sites on carrier proteins, interfere with metabolic conversion of the vitamin to the active form, or enhance enzyme activity leading to increased vitamin destruction and turnover. Food-drug interactions jeopardize both nutritional status and drug effectiveness. For the older person consuming a poor diet and also consuming prescription drugs known to interact with nutrients, nutritional counseling is indicated. If the diet cannot be improved, supplementation within recommended levels is appropriate.

Although usually treated with diuretics, hypertension can be controlled with less extensive drug therapy if moderate sodium restriction and weight loss are also initiated. Such an approach might eliminate the need for potassium supplements with possible complications.

Nutrient intake and metabolic disease are sometimes related to loss of mental function. Acute dehydration, disturbances in sodium or potassium levels, hypothyroidism or hyperthyroidism, or vitamin B_{12} or folic acid deficiency can lead to changes in personality, disorientation, or dementia. Unfortunately, the expectation of such behavior in older people may preclude efforts at diagnosis.

Although individuals with clinical folate or vitamin B_{12} deficiency improve both physically and mentally on vitamin repletion, vitamin supplementation appears to have no beneficial effect on mental status in those with marginal or adequate vitamin B_{12} and folate levels.

REVIEW QUESTIONS

1. Name types of OTC drugs commonly used by older people to relieve gastrointestinal disturbances and general pain. What are the nutritional implications of their use?
2. What is the relationship between alcohol abuse and thiamin status? What are problems in diagnosis of thiamin deficiency in older alcohol users?
3. What are problems related to (a) selection of vitamin and mineral supplements and (b) abuse of vitamin and mineral supplements by older people?
4. Describe the mechanisms by which drugs may be detrimental to nutritional status. Name a common drug type associated with each.
5. Does available evidence justify nutrient supplementation in the case of (a) long term therapy with prescription drugs and (b) mental disturbance or dementia? Cite specific examples.

REFERENCES

1. Altman, H., and others: Behavioral effects of drug therapy on psychogeriatric inpatients. II. Multivitamin supplement, J. Am. Geriatr. Soc. **21**:249, 1973.
2. Baker, H., Frank, O., and Jaslow, S.P.: Oral versus intramuscular vitamin supplementation for hypovitaminosis in the elderly, J. Am. Geriatr. Soc. **28**:42, 1980.
3. Bender, A.D.: A pharmacodynamic basis for changes in drug activity associated with aging in the adult, Exp. Gerontol. **1**:237, 1965.
4. Brin, M., and Bauernfeind, J.C.: Vitamin needs of the elderly, Postgrad. Med. **63**:155, 1978.
5. Brin, M., Schwartzberg, S.H., and Arthur-Davies, D.: A vitamin evaluation program as applied to 10 elderly residents in a community home for the aged, J. Am. Geriatr. Soc. **12**:493, 1964.
6. Burgen, A.S., and Mitchell, J.F.: Gaddum's pharmacology, ed. 8, Oxford, 1978, Oxford University Press.
7. Buxton, P.K., and others: Vitamin B_{12} status in mentally disturbed elderly patients, Gerontol. Clin. **11**:22, 1969.

8. Cummings, J.H.: Progress report. Laxative abuse, Gut **15:**758, 1974.

9. DiPalma, J.R.: Basic pharmacology in medicine, ed. 2, New York, 1982, McGraw-Hill Book Co.

10. Droller, H., and Dossett, J.A.: Vitamin B_{12} levels in senile dementia and confusional states, Gerontol. Clin. **1:**96, 1959.

11. Elwood, P.C., and others: Haemoglobin, vitamin B_{12} and folate levels in the elderly, Br. J. Haematol. **21:**557, 1971.

12. Food and Nutrition Board: Recommended dietary allowances, ed. 9, Washington, D.C., 1980, National Academy of Sciences.

13. Garry, P.J., and others: Nutritional status in a healthy elderly population: Dietary and supplemental intakes, Am. J. Clin. Nutr. **36:**319, 1982.

14. Grotkowski, M.L., and Sims, L.S.: Nutritional knowledge, attitudes, and dietary practices of the elderly, J. Am. Diet. Assoc. **72:**499, 1978.

15. Guthrie, H.A., Black, K., and Madden, J.P.: Nutritional practices of elderly citizens in rural Pennsylvania, Gerontologist **12:**330, 1972.

16. Hale, W.E., Marks, R.G., and Stewart, R.B.: Drug use in a geriatric population, J. Am. Geriatr. Soc. **27:**374, 1979.

17. Hecht, A.: Effects of routine vitamin supplementation in the aged, J. Am. Geriatr. Soc. **17:**421, 1969.

18. Herbert, V.: The nutritional anemias, Hosp. Pract. **15:**65, 1980.

19. Hughes, D., and others: Clinical trial of the effect of vitamin B_{12} in elderly subjects with low serum B_{12} levels, Br. Med. J. **1:**458. 1970.

20. Hurdle, A.D.F., and Picton Williams, T.C.: Folic-acid deficiency in elderly patients admitted to hospital, Br. Med. J. **2:**202, 1966.

21. Iber, F.L., and others: Thiamin in the elderly, relation to alcoholism and to neurological degenerative disease, Am. J. Clin. Nutr. **36:**1067, 1982.

22. Kassirer, J.P., and Harrington, J.T.: Diuretics and potassium metabolism: A reassessment of the need, effectiveness and safety of potassium therapy, Kidney Int. **11:**505, 1977.

23. LeBovit, C., and Baker, D.A.: Food consumption and dietary levels of older households in Rochester, New York, Home Econ. Res. Rep. No. 25, Washington, D.C., 1965, U.S. Government Printing Office.

24. Leevy, C.M.: Thiamin deficiency and alcoholism, Ann. N.Y. Acad. Sci. **378:**316, 1982.

25. Lonergan, M.E., and others: A dietary survey of older people in Edinburgh, Br. J. Nutr. **34:**517, 1975.

26. McGandy, R.B., and others: Nutrient intakes and energy expenditure in men of different ages, J. Gerontol. **21:**581, 1966.

27. National Dairy Council: Diet-drug interactions, Dairy Council Digest, vol. 48, No. 2, Mar.-Apr., 1977.

28. National Nutrition Consortium: Vitamin-mineral safety, toxicity, and misuse, Chicago, 1978, American Dietetic Association.

29. Portnoi, V.A.: Thyrotoxicosis as a mimic of dementia and/or stroke-like syndrome, Postgrad. Med. **66:**219, 1979.

30. Read, A.E., and others: Nutritional studies on the entrants to an old people's home, with particular reference to folic-acid deficiency, Br. Med. J. **2:**843, 1965.

31. Roe, D.A.: Drug-induced nutritional deficiencies, Westport, Conn., 1976, AVI Publishing Co.

32. Roe, D.A.: Handbook: Interactions of selected drugs and nutrients in patients, ed. 3, Chicago, 1982, American Dietetic Association.

33. Schorah, C.J., and others: Clinical effects of vitamin C in elderly patients with low blood-vitamin-C-levels, Lancet **1:**403, 1979.

34. Schorah, C.J., and others: The effect of vitamin C supplements on body weight, serum proteins, and general health of an elderly population, Am. J. Clin. Nutr. **34:**871, 1981.

35. Schuckit, M.A., and others: A three year follow-up of elderly alcoholics, J. Clin. Psychiatry **41:**412, 1980.

36. Schulman, R.: A survey of vitamin B_{12} deficiency in an elderly psychiatric population, Br. J. Psychiatry **113:**241, 1967.

37. Schulman, R.: Vitamin B_{12} deficiency and psychiatric illness, Br. J. Psychiatry **113:**252, 1967.

38. Schwartz, D., and others: Medication errors made by elderly, chronically ill patients, Am. J. Public Health **52:**2018, 1962.

39. Seixas, F.A.: Drug/alcohol interactions: Overt potential dangers, Geriatrics **34:**89, 1979.

40. Shomaker, D.M.: Use and abuse of OTC medications by the elderly, J. Gerontol. Nurs. **6:**21, 1980.

41. Sorensen, A.A., Sorensen, D.I., and Zimmer, J.G.: Appropriateness of vitamin and mineral prescription orders for residents of health related facilities, J. Am. Geriatr. Soc. **27:**425, 1979.

42. Stare, F.J.: Megavitamins, Wis. Med. J. **80**(10):18, 1981.

43. Steffee, W.P.: Nutrition intervention in hospitalized geriatric patients, Bull. N.Y. Acad. Med. **56:**564, 1980.

44. Sullivan, J.F., and Lankford, H.G.: Urinary excretion of zinc in alcoholism and postalcoholic cirrhosis, Am. J. Clin. Nutr. **10:**153, 1962.

45. Task Force, National Institute on Aging: Senility reconsidered: Treatment possibilities for mental impairment in the elderly, JAMA **244:**259, 1980.

46. Thomas, J.H., and Powell, D.E.: Blood disorders in the elderly, Bristol, 1971, John Wright & Sons, Ltd.

47. Tomasulo, P.A., Kater, R.M., and Iber, F.L: Impairment of thiamin absorption in alcoholism, Am. J. Clin. Nutr. **21:**1341, 1968.

48. United States Department of Health and Human Services: Health, United States. 1980, DHHS Publication No. (PHS)81-1232, Hyattsville, Md., 1980, U.S. Government Printing Office.

49. United States Department of Health and Human Services: Drug utilization in office practice by age and sex of the patient: National Ambulatory Medical Care Survey, 1980, Advance data from Vital and Health Statistics, No. 81, DHHS Publication No. (PHS)82-1250, Hyattsville, Md., 1982, U.S. Government Printing Office.

50. Visconti, J.A.: Drug-food interactions. Nutrition in disease, Columbus, Ohio, 1977, Ross Laboratories.

51. Whanger, A.D.: Vitamins and vigor at 65 plus, Postgrad. Med. **53:**167, 1973.

52. Whanger, A.D., and Wang, H.S.: Clinical correlates of the vibratory sense in elderly psychiatric patients, J. Gerontol. **29:**39, 1974.

53. Wilber, J.A.: The role of diet in the treatment of high blood pressure, J. Am. Diet. Assoc. **80:**25, 1982.

54. Zimberg, S.: The elderly alcoholic, Gerontologist **14:**221, 1974.

Chapter 10

Nutritional Status in the Aged

Evaluation of nutritional status is difficult with all age groups and particularly so with older individuals because nutritional status, physical health, and the degenerative effects of the aging process are interrelated. It is not always possible to separate the influences of inadequate nutrition from changes resulting from physiologic aging and degenerative disease. Standards developed for use with young individuals may not be appropriate for the aged. Finally, when clinical or biochemical deficiencies are observed, it is difficult to determine whether they represent poor dietary intake or problems in nutrient absorption or utilization. Each of these issues should be considered when evaluating the nutritional status of older people.

GENERAL CONSIDERATIONS

Definitions

Conclusions relating to nutritional health are influenced by both the individual being evaluated and the particular methods used. Christakis[23] developed the concept of nutritional status, which includes both collection and evaluation of biochemical, dietary, and clinical information about an individual or group. In the broadest sense, an evaluation of nutritional status takes into consideration related factors that contribute to the observed findings. (e.g., Why does the individual eat or not eat certain foods? Are prescription drugs interfering with the absorption of ingested nutrients?) The terms *nutritional status* and *nutrition survey* are not inter-changeable. The latter is nonspecific and can mean different things.[82] Nutrition surveys may involve only one method of collecting information, such as a food intake record, or a variety of methods, as does the evaluation of nutritional status. Surveys that include information on (1) general health, (2) food availability as related to economics or transportation, and (3) food preferences can provide a base of information for developing a nutrition intervention program, such as congregate or home-delivered meals.[23]

Among the aged, vitamin or mineral deficiencies seldom develop abruptly; instead they evolve slowly over a period of time as a result of limited intake, impaired absorption, or excessive excretion.[59] Marginal deficiency is characterized by gradual nutrient depletion and personal lack of well-being, associated with impairment of certain biochemical functions.[16] Depression, tiredness, weight loss, or decreased appetite can have many causes and are not necessarily recognized as nutrition problems, particularly in the aged for whom such characteristics may erroneously be considered to represent normal aging. Nutritional deficiencies are difficult to diagnose and treat in that symptoms and cure are neither explicit nor finite.[6] Because chronic malnutrition varies in severity a single indicator is inadequate for diagnosis, as it will be more sensitive at one level of malnutrition (e.g., marginal or severe) and less sensitive at another.[44-45] Using several indicators will allow a more reasonable diagnosis.

Evaluation of nutritional status is a complex procedure requiring (1) professional time for planning, implementation, and evaluation; (2) funds for supplies or hiring additional personnel if project is large-scale; (3) appropriate facilities and equipment; and (4) the cooperation of individuals being evaluated.[23] Therefore available resources must be considered carefully when selecting methods for evaluation of a client or target group.

Purpose of Evaluation

The goal of the nutritional evaluation will determine the procedures to be carried out. Types of evaluations range from simple screening to determine individuals at risk to an in-depth study of a person with an absorption or metabolic problem.[23] The questions to be answered regarding either the individual or group should be carefully formulated before any evaluation is begun. Too frequently dietary records are being collected before anyone has determined what is to be done with them.

Level of Cooperation Required. Older people often have reservations regarding participation in nutritional assessment. They may be embarrassed to admit that food intake is inadequate, particularly if this is the result of limited income.[92] An older person with limited education may have difficulty understanding what is expected if directions are complicated. Finally, a person may not wish to be inconvenienced and therefore ignore instructions, for example, eating the usual breakfast before what is supposed to be a fasting blood test. The ability and desire of the client to cooperate must be considered carefully when a protocol is developed.

When participants in a community program are to be examined, the cooperation of the sponsoring agency is required. A screening program to seek out individuals at risk at a local senior center will need the approval of the administrators of the center. If the senior center is affiliated with a government agency, such as the state office on aging, official approval must be granted by that unit. In no case can a project be undertaken without the consent of all parties involved.

Informed Consent. When evaluation of nutritional status is a component of medical care and initiated by the individual's physician, it is with the consent of the client. At other times a university, government agency, or non-profit community agency may undertake a nutrition survey as part of a research, intervention, or planning program. In that case informed consent of the participants must be obtained.[98] Individuals should be informed as to who is conducting the survey, how the information will be used, and exactly what will be expected of them.[98] Participants must be guaranteed confidentiality and the right to withdraw from the study at any time. An example of a consent form is given on p. 252.

Most community evaluations involve only fairly routine procedures including recording food intake, measuring height and weight, or procuring a blood sample. An individual found to have a nutritional problem should receive dietary counseling and be referred to other agencies or services as indicated. Protection of the privacy of the individual is paramount. This is especially critical in local nutrition intervention programs when participants and evaluators may know each other. If a dietary questionnaire includes income, health status, family situation, or other items of a personal nature, it must be clear that the individual has the right to refuse to answer such questions.[64,98]

Human Resources. Nutritional assessment will require professional or lay interviewers for obtaining dietary information, health personnel to perform anthropometric or clinical measurements, and laboratory personnel with suitable equipment to both procure and analyze blood samples.[23] An in-depth evaluation including a physical examination by medical staff usually requires admission to a hospital or clinic. Procedures requiring less supervision may be carried out in an ambulatory setting or in the client's home.

Cost of Evaluation

Dietary Evaluation. The total cost of a dietary evaluation includes the salary of the interviewer as well as travel expenses incurred visiting the client.[104] When working with a congregate meal program, clients can be interviewed at the meal site, thereby decreasing expense. In a hospital situation travel time is eliminated. In addition to time spent with the clients, costs include training of interviewers and evaluation of the diet record obtained.

Biochemical Evaluation. Biochemical assessment is both time consuming and costly. If the client is not able to travel to the hospital or laboratory, a home health nurse can visit the home to obtain a blood sample. If analysis is to include only a routine automated procedure, such as hemoglobin, cost will be minimal. If many complicated biochemical assays for vitamins or enzymes are included, costs will escalate rapidly. When resources are limited, biochemical evaluation may not be feasible.

ASSESSMENT OF NUTRITIONAL STATUS

Components of Assessment

Evaluation of nutritional status requires various types of information[23,51,59,89]:

Dietary
  Record of usual food intake
  Food preferences
  Meal and snacking pattern
  Prescribed diet, if any
  Use of nutritional supplements
Socioeconomic
  Living situation (alone or with someone)
  Facilities for food preparation
  Shopping habits
  Economic situation
Physical and clinical
  Body weight relative to standard
  Triceps skinfold thickness and muscle circumference
  Dental situation
  Clinical signs of vitamin or mineral deficiency
  Presence of chronic disease
  Use of drugs
  Use of alcohol or tobacco

Biochemical
  Blood vitamin levels
  Iron and hematologic status
  Blood lipid status
  Glucose tolerance (if indicated)
  Urinalysis (presence of glucose, ketones, protein, occult blood)
  Urine vitamin levels

Dietary records indicating both present and previous food intake as well as general practices relating to food shopping, preparation, and selection are most commonly used. Food records provide information regarding either primary deficiencies or the lack of nutrients in the diet. Secondary deficiencies become apparent only on clinical or biochemical evaluation.[59-60] Impaired absorption resulting from prescription drugs, laxative abuse, or increased requirements brought about by blood loss through the gastrointestinal tract are examples of conditions leading to secondary deficiency in the older individual.

Dietary evaluation can provide insight as to a potential problem; if intake of a nutrient is extremely low the probability of developing a deficiency is rather high. However, in the older person with physiologic impairment and chronic disease, nutritional adequacy cannot be determined on the basis of dietary information alone. Unfortunately, adequate intake is frequently assumed to reflect absence of deficiency.

Methods of Dietary Evaluation

An accurate record of either prior or present food intake is extremely difficult to obtain, because the method selected to record food choices may at the same time influence those choices.[48,93,104] The goal is to obtain a true picture of the food pattern of the individual. The purpose of the evaluation and time and expertise available, as well as the characteristics of the individual client, will determine the method selected. Unfortunately, evaluations of current methods have been conducted primarily with younger persons. Information regarding their validity and reliability with older age groups is limited.[31]

Dietary History. A detailed record of food intake over previous weeks or months minimizes the variation of day to day intake. With older people a health history including use of over the counter and prescription drugs as well as socioeconomic characteristics and food preferences should be included. A format for collecting this information is given on pp. 253-256.

Although the diet history is highly informative, it requires a well-trained and experienced professional interviewer, which makes it less appropriate for use in a community nutrition program if a dietitian or nutritionist is unavailable. Use in a clinical situation will depend on the time available, as the interview usually requires at least an hour.[10,18,103] This method may be particularly useful with an older client who has recently been placed on a therapeutic diet or developed a physiologic problem that has led to a change in food patterns.[69] The diet history will provide a perspective on both previous and present food intake.

Weighed Food Intake Record. Although the weighed record provides the most accurate representation of food intake, it is inappropriate for the general evaluation of clients.[50] Ohlson and coworkers[72] successfully used this technique with 18 older women in a series of nutrient balance studies; however, extensive training and constant supervision were required. Even though weighing of foods and liquids may be relatively easy for younger people, poor coordination and failing eyesight can make it extremely difficult for older individuals. In a nutrition survey of 200 English aged living at home, about half were able to undertake some weighing of food; however, only one fourth of the records were considered reliable on the basis of a daily visit by an observer.[62] This method also influences food choices, as the women studied by Ohlson and coworkers[72] consumed less food when it had to be weighed beforehand.

Written Food Intake Record. The written food record has been used successfully with older people in the United States[24] and Great Britain[19] and is considered to provide a good estimate of food con-

sumed. Ideally, the client should agree to cooperate for at least 3 days; however, this may not be possible if arthritis or other physical problems make writing difficult. Before approaching an older client about keeping written records one should be sensitive to the fact that very limited education or English as a second language may prevent participation.

The recording process can influence food choices both quantitatively and qualitatively. An individual may eliminate his usual snack of an oatmeal-raisin cookie if it must be described according to diameter and type. MacLeod[62] pointed out that clients should be instructed to record foods consumed as snacks, as her subjects considered those items unimportant and not really foods.

Food Frequency Form. Although food frequency questionnaires administered by interview or in written form are increasing in use, this method has not been evaluated with older clients. Unless portion sizes are recorded the usefulness of the information obtained is limited. I recall an older client who indicated that she had milk at least four times each day. The serving turned out to be approximately two tablespoons, added to each cup of coffee; her total milk for the day was one-half cup providing about 150 mg calcium. Use of a food frequency form does presume some ability to recall previous food intake. (A sample format is given on pp. 257-259.

24-Hour Recall Record. Use of the recall method with older clients has been criticized on the basis of its dependence on recent memory[21] and the fact that the variability of the diet from day to day makes a single record limited in usefulness.[35] Although nonprofessionals can obtain a 24-hour recall record, they must be trained in seeking additional information when memory appears to be faltering.[21] Fomon[32] has described the items most frequently overlooked by both interviewers and clients (see p. 260.). A 24-hour recall record does have the advantage of being quickly administered (20 to 30 minutes), leading to a high rate of participation by those approached.[103]

Although the 7-day weighed record is most accurate, it is not practical for use in clinical or community situations. A diet history is not applicable to large groups if trained interviewers are not available and time is limited. As a result, 24-hour recall records have been commonly used with older clients.[36,42,63]

Because most people do not consume the same foods each day, a 24-hour recall record for a given day will probably contain significantly more or less of a particular nutrient than was consumed the day before or the day after and may not represent the general quality of the diet.[7,11-12,35] A record obtained on a day when the diet was considerably better than usual can lead to the erroneous conclusion that the nutrient intake of the individual is adequate. Therefore a 1-day food record whether obtained in recall or written form is inadequate for evaluation of an individual.[35] Data collected with older people, however, suggest that 24-hour records do provide a valid estimate of the nutrient intake of groups of 50 or more.[72] Consequently, this method would be appropriate for the evaluation of a client group.[17,69,103]

Variability of Diet Records

Socioeconomic Factors. The day of the week on which a single diet record is obtained will influence the estimated intake, as intake patterns on weekend days can differ from those on weekdays.[22] Although the older individual may no longer be employed, food intake may change on a weekend day if family comes to visit or if the older parent is invited out. Sunday dinner is still a special meal in many homes. The older person who is consuming very monotonous meals on a daily basis, as a result of a special diet or limited resources, may splurge on a weekend day with a relative or friend.

Nutrient intake on a particular day may also be influenced by attendance at a congregate meal program or delivery of a meal to the home.[58] In either case a record including such a meal can be significantly higher in nutrient quality than when all food consumed came from the individual's personal resources (see Chapter 12). When evaluating such a client, records should be obtained on both participation and nonparticipation days.

Diet Components. The variability of the diet is influenced by the distribution of nutrients in particular foods.[34,43] Among English aged (n = 200) vitamin-containing foods were consumed irregularly, so that a 7-day record was required to obtain a reliable estimate of intake of vitamins A, C, and D.[62] Dark green or deep yellow vegetables, or liver may be consumed only occasionally. Use of a highly fortified cereal (1 ounce = 10 mg iron) would produce significant differences in iron intake, if not included every day.

Individual Habits. Roberts and coworkers[79] suggested that dietary patterns are more consistent among older people because meals are less frequently missed and food sprees less common than among younger individuals. Following a special diet that allows few options will decrease day to day variability. If income is limited or the diet composed of a few staple items, the individual will eat the same foods each day. Ostfeld[73] described an older man who ate only bread and stewed tomatoes three times each day and an aged woman who lived on canned vegetable soup. Although these individuals are exceptions, nearly one fourth of the 382 aged persons evaluated had highly consistent diet patterns.

For six women, ranging in age from 68 to 80, daily variability over a 4-month period was an individual characteristic.[34] The percent variability based on mean nutrient intake was calculated for 11 nutrients. The highest variability for six nutrients occurred in the diet of one individual. Vitamin A, thiamin, riboflavin, and ascorbic acid varied most from day to day.

Application of the 24-Hour Recall Record

Dependence on Memory. A study conducted some years ago questioned the use of the recall record with older people who may be unable to remember all foods consumed.[21] Older institutionalized individuals were, on initial inquiry, less likely to mention all foods consumed than a younger institutionalized group. When the menus for the previous day were read, the older group added nearly twice as many calories to the recall record as the younger group. It is important to recognize, however, that these data were obtained with institutionalized individuals who are not representative of the general population. Campbell and Dodds suggest that a food checklist be used along with a recall record to obtain a more reliable estimate of food intake.

Women seem to provide more accurate descriptions of food eaten than men,[105-106] which could relate to their involvement in meal preparation. If mealtime is a high point in an otherwise monotonous day, the recall of foods consumed could be more complete.

Food Consumed Versus Food Recalled. A recent study evaluated the ability of independent-living older people to recall both the quantity and the type of food consumed in the previous 24-hour period.[63] Food intake reported by 76 participants in a congregate meal program was compared with that observed by trained personnel at the noon meal. The older subjects were not aware that actual food intake was being recorded.

Mean nutrient intake computed by the two methods differed for calories only. Reported intake contained fewer calories than observed, although for 25% of the participants the difference was less than 40 kcal. Recalled and observed intakes of protein, vitamins, and minerals were not significantly different. Of importance, however, is the proportional relationship between recalled and observed intakes. For example, does a 10% increase in observed intake result in a 10% increase in reported intake? For calories, protein, and vitamin A this was not a constant relationship. Individuals tended to exaggerate their level of intake when they consumed small amounts. Conversely, those consuming large quantities underestimated actual intake.

This phenomenon may be particularly important when two groups of older people are being compared. Because of the tendency of people to mentally compensate for high or low intakes, the actual difference in nutrient intake between two groups is likely to be greater than the reported difference. This is especially pertinent if the true differences are small. The inability of the 24-hour recall method to demonstrate a difference in nutrient intake when indeed there is one has serious implications for the evaluation of nutrition programs; an improvement in nutrient intake, brought about by the program, may not be observed.[36]

Application of Written Food Records

As a tool for dietary evaluation, the written record avoids the problem of people forgetting foods consumed. Conversely, an individual may make an effort to consume a better diet on a day when keeping a record. Among older women in Michigan (age 51 to 77), a 3-day written record compared reasonably with a 7-day weighed record (considered the best possible estimate) in revealing general nutrient intake.[72] Although 3- or 4-day written records have limitations because of day to day variability and nutrients found in only a few foods, it is a reasonable compromise between a 1-day record, of little value for an individual, and the generally preferred 7-day written record.[26,36,69]

Problems arise with both validity and individual cooperation in a 7-day written record. With older participants in a congregate meal program, written food records were generally accurate on the basis of observed versus recorded intake; however, the validity deteriorated as the week progressed.[36] Records for days 1 and 2 were consistent with observed intakes for all nutrients with the exception of protein. By days 5 through 7, estimates for only three nutrients (thiamin, ascorbic acid, and vitamin A) were valid. Individuals with a higher level of education (greater than 9 years of schooling) were more likely to complete records for all 7 days.

Requiring a 7-day record may decrease both participation by people with limited education and the reliability of information obtained. Because of the relationship between education and income people with limited education are particularly vulnerable to nutrient deficiencies and therefore should be included in dietary evaluations. It would be of greater benefit to both the client and the nutrition program being evaluated to reduce the days of recordkeeping and increase participation by people at risk.

Identification of Aged at Risk

When working with large numbers of older people (e.g., congregate or home-delivered meals program) and resources are limited, a detailed dietary assessment of all participants will not be feasible. Instead, the priority will be identification of those at high risk. Initial screening could be handled by a nonprofessional, such as a volunteer who delivers the meal to the home or works at the senior center. The following information correctly identified persons with inadequate diets among 264 English aged living at home[19]:

1. Seven or less hot meals per week
2. Some degree of physical disability relating to mobility or use of the hands
3. Very limited amount of money spent for food per week (Standard might be that recommended by the USDA for the Thrifty Food Plan.)

People who met all three criteria were getting less than two thirds the recommended intake of at least one nutrient. Social class, living alone, or psychiatric problems were not significantly associated with malnutrition. Individuals meeting the three criteria listed above should be targeted for further evaluation.

Despite known limitations, a 24-hour recall appears to be at least as effective as a diet history in identifying people with deficient intakes. MacLeod,[62] in a study with older Britons, compared three dietary methods: (1) a 7-day weighed record (assumed to provide an accurate record of intake), (2) a 24-hour recall record, and (3) a diet history. The latter methods were evaluated according to

Table 10-1. Identifying older persons with inadequate intakes

	Percentage Correctly Identified by	
	Dietary History	24-Hour Recall
Calories (kcal)	52	70
Protein	40	58
Vitamin A	41	68
Vitamin C	51	77
Calcium	65	50
Iron	67	78

Modified from MacLeod, C.C.: Methods of dietary assessment. In Carlson, L.A., ed.: Nutrition in old age, Symposia of the Swedish Nutrition Foundation X, Stockholm, 1972, Almqvist & Wiksell.

their value in predicting inadequate intakes evident in the 7-day record (Table 10-1). For critical nutrients, with the exception of calcium, the 24-hour recall was more effective than the diet history. Older people are known to overestimate their milk consumption on dietary records[71-72]; however, in this study fewer people were low in calcium than any other nutrient.

The recall record appeared to have predictive value for calories, vitamins A and C, and iron, which are frequently problem nutrients for older persons. At the same time, 22% to 32% of those low in these nutrients were not identified by the recall record and even less were identified by the diet history. This points to the need for a reliable evaluation tool that can be completed within a limited amount of time.

Many methods exist for the assessment of dietary intake; however, all have problems relating to validity, reliability, or extended cooperation.[91] When trained interviewers are available, a 24-hour recall or 1- to 3-day written record coupled with a short diet history, including food likes and dislikes, socioeconomic situation, and health status, can provide a reasonable estimate of intake. Although food frequency lists have not been validated with older age groups, such a record coupled with a short diet history may also allow a reasonable judgment of dietary adequacy. Nonprofessionals can be trained to administer a food frequency or simple screening tool.

Evaluating the Quality of the Diet

The method selected for evaluating dietary records will depend on the facilities, staff time, and funds available, as well as the purpose of the evaluation. For research purposes or sophisticated program evaluation diet records can be coded for computer calculation of nutrient content using tapes of food nutrient content available from the USDA. Private firms provide nutrient calculations of diet records for a fee, but they should be carefully reviewed beforehand and validity affirmed on the basis of a diet record of known nutrient content.[49] Nutrient content of diet records can also be calculated using a programmable pocket calculator.[83]

Diet records must be evaluated both qualitatively and quantitatively. The problem with using the RDA for assessing the nutritional adequacy of the diet relates to the differences among individuals.[33,61] An intake less than 100% that recommended is not necessarily deficient, although a diet meeting 100% of the recommended level for each nutrient should be the goal. However, an older person with impaired absorption as a result of medications may be clinically deficient despite an intake meeting the standard. Because of the margin of safety calculated within the RDA, an intake two thirds of the recommended level has been considered adequate for most people and used as a criterion in evaluating diet records.[42,43] An older client consuming less than 67% of the RDA should be considered at risk and provided with counseling and nutritional support. An older person with special problems, however, may not be nutritionally secure at 67% of the RDA. For this reason biochemical and clinical measurements are required to accurately assess the nutritional status of an individual.

The diet record can be evaluated according to the number of servings of specified foods.[13] Evaluation based on the various food groups has been found to be sufficiently sensitive to assess changes occurring in food intake as a result of nutrition education or intervention programs.[13] This implies that a deterioration in the quality of the diet could also be observed; such a deterioration could occur in an older person having increasing difficulty in mobility or adjusting to a prescribed diet.

The fact remains, however, that foods classified within the same food group can have markedly different nutrient contents. The nutrients for which these methods of evaluation are least reliable are zinc, iron, and vitamin B_6.[43] Although one consumes the correct number of suggested servings, intake might not meet recommended levels. Iron is distributed among many different food items; few foods with the exception of liver or highly fortified cereals are high in iron. Vitamin B_6 is found in legumes, fish, poultry, and meat.[33] In contrast, one can obtain the total daily requirement of ascorbic acid from a 4-ounce glass of citrus juice.

A recent modification of the basic four food guide has identified foods known to be good sources of those nutrients frequently low in the American diet including vitamin E, vitamin B_6, magnesium, zinc, and iron[55] (Table 10-2). The suggested intake of dairy foods is the same as generally recommended. Protein foods are defined according to animal or vegetable origin. Legumes are good sources of vitamin B_6, magnesium, and zinc. Nuts, leafy greens, and oils contribute vitamin E. Whole grain products contain at least twice the levels of vitamin E, vitamin B_6, folacin, and particular trace elements as contained in refined and enriched products. King and coworkers[55] also suggest variations of the basic pattern for those who choose to limit or omit milk, meat, or legumes from their diet or who require low cost menus.

The modified basic four is a simple yet nutritionally sound means of evaluating a diet record when more complex methods are prohibitive. This

Table 10-2. Modified basic four food guide

	Number of Servings*	Total Servings
Milk and milk products		2 servings
Protein foods		4 servings
Animal protein	2 servings	
Legumes and/or nuts	2 servings	
Fruits and vegetables		4 servings
Vitamin C–rich	1 serving	
Dark green	1 serving	
Others	2 servings	
Whole grain cereal products		4 servings
Fat and/or oil		1 serving

*Common serving sizes are 3 oz. meat, poultry, or fish; 2 eggs; ¾ cup cooked legumes, cereal, or pasta; 1 oz. nuts or dry cereal; 1 cup milk; ¾ cup cooked or 1 cup raw leafy greens; 1 slice bread; 1 tablespoon vegetable oil or wheatgerm.

Modified from the *Journal of Nutrition Education*, King, J.C., and others: Evaluation and modification of the Basic Four Food Guide, **10:**27, 1978, © Society for Nutrition Education.

method takes into account vitamin B_6, folate, magnesium, and zinc, nutrients frequently low in the diets of older people.

Interviewing the Older Individual

Success in obtaining valid dietary information from an older individual is dependent on the interviewer.* This person must be well trained in techniques of obtaining food information and in the specific method being used. A feeling of trust is essential if the interview or any further attempt at counseling is to be successful.[92,102]

Preparing for the Dietary Interview. The interviewer must be well informed regarding the common food preferences of the client group and general food availability in the locality. This includes a basic idea of the ingredients of local mixed dishes and the special favorites of any ethnic group.[39] The interviewer must also become familiar with the food stores in the area, checking the choices available and pricing. This is particularly important

*References 10, 18, 39, 75, 84, 102.

when working with older people whose options are limited because of lack of transportation.

The interviewer should conduct practice interviews with the record form being used[64] and learn to clarify both items and serving sizes consumed. It is equally important, however, that the older client not be ''led by suggestion'' when describing what he or she had to eat.[10,18,64] If an individual reports eating a slice of bread further information required would include the (1) thickness (e.g., regular, thin-sliced), (2) type (e.g., white, whole wheat), and (3) spread if any (e.g., margarine, jam).[64] In the case of mixed dishes such as tuna-noodle casserole or beef stew it will be necessary to define the relative proportion of the various constituents (see p. 260).[36,39,63] A protocol has been developed for training dietary interviewers.[64]

Cups, bowls, and glasses of known volume can aid in determining the liquid quantity consumed because the client can point to the shape of the container and level to which it was filled. An advantage of working with a person in his home is that serving dishes are available for describing the quantity consumed. A small ruler for describing thickness can help in obtaining an accurate description of foods.[67] Food models, representing a serving of known household measure, are available from commercial manufacturers. A frame of reference can be valuable for odd-shaped items, such as a pork chop or wedge of pie. One disadvantage of food models is the tendency for the client to identify the food model as the size of the portion consumed.

Food models do improve the estimates of food consumed.[67] Respondents are less frustrated when able to refer to a food portion than when forced to describe totally in words what they had to eat. Since many adults tend to underestimate the food consumed, the use of visual aids can increase the validity of a record.

Attitude of Interviewer. The reliability of the record obtained depends on the rapport developed between interviewer and client. If the client perceives a judgmental attitude he will be less likely to present an honest picture of the true situation, particularly if circumstances are less than favorable.[84,92,102] The client is put at ease by a friendly, relaxed interviewer. Considering the difficult circumstances under which many impoverished aged are forced to live, it may be necessary to develop this rapport in homes that are unbearably hot in summer, unheated in winter, cluttered, unclean, or unpleasant in odor.

When selecting interviewers to work with older clients one should consider their attitude toward the aged. Negative attitudes hinder rapport with the older person and can bias subjective evaluations.[75] Unfavorable attitudes may reflect only limited contact with this age group. In one situation interviewers became less critical of clients' ability to cope as they continued their activities with older people.

Potential interviewers may question both the ability and willingness of older people to cooperate in an interview. In a midwestern community 75% of older persons approached participated in a social services interview; 10% were too ill to cooperate and 15% refused for other reasons.[47] For those who were lonely, the interview was an opportunity to have company. Individuals with higher incomes and better educations were generally more cooperative. Low income persons may have had unpleasant experiences in previous interviews with government or social service workers.[92] The perceived attitude of the interviewer toward the aged client will be a significant factor in encouraging participation.

Physical Setting for the Interview. The location and circumstances under which an interview takes place will influence its value for both the interviewer and client. In an institutional setting, a senior center, or a congregate meal site finding a spot of relative privacy is essential. Visiting a client at home can provide an indication of the cooking and storage facilities available for food preparation.

It is essential to allow adequate time for the exchange of information.[85,102] Even an individual with impaired speech following a stroke usually has some means of communication and can write words that cannot be pronounced.[84] If sight or hearing is poor conversation can be facilitated by sitting facing the client. It may be necessary to print the questions for the hearing impaired or read aloud to the partially blind. With sufficient time and patience, institutionalized persons above age 80 can be successfully interviewed regarding their dietary preferences or problems.

CLINICAL ASPECTS OF NUTRITIONAL ASSESSMENT

Clinical assessment may include (1) anthropometric measurements, (2) dental examination, and (3) physical examination with emphasis on tissues particularly responsive to nutrient deficiency.[38,51,59] Evaluation of findings is sometimes difficult as existing standards are not always appropriate for older age groups.

Anthropometric Measurements

Anthropometric measurements most commonly used in evaluation of nutritional status include (1) standing height, (2) body weight, (3) triceps skinfold thickness (upper arm), and (4) arm circumference taken at the point that triceps skinfold thickness is measured.[23,51] There is no discomfort involved and the client need not disrobe; therefore these measurements could be completed at a congregate meal site or senior center. A screen of some kind, placed in a corner of the room, offers some privacy and reduces interruption. For homebound people reliable scales that include a height meter are available in models easily transported. Equipment and procedures for measurement are described in detail in reference 54. Standards for evaluation of anthropometric measurements were given in Chapter 3.

Dental Examination

An indication of dental condition should be included in the assessment of every older person.[23,51] If professional dental personnel are not available recorded information will be limited to loss of teeth, availability and adequacy of either partial or complete dentures, and pain in the mouth. If possible, evaluation should include level of oral hygiene, existence of periodontal disease, and number of teeth that are decayed, missing, or filled (D-M-F).

Physical Examination

Clinical signs of deficiency with associated nutrients and differential diagnosis are outlined in

Table 10-3. Physical signs and differential diagnosis

Physical Sign	Related Nutrient(s)	Differential Diagnosis
Face or skin		
Nasolabial seborrhea	Niacin, riboflavin, pyridoxine	Poor personal hygiene
Xerosis	Essential fatty acids, vitamin A	Aging, loss of skin lubricants, environmental exposure
Follicular hyperkeratosis	Essential fatty acids, vitamin A	"Goose flesh," aging?
Eyes		
Circumcorneal injection	Riboflavin	—
Conjunctivae xerosis	Vitamin A	—
Lips		
Cheilosis	Niacin, riboflavin	Exposure to sun or cold, ill-fitting dentures
Angular fissures	Niacin, riboflavin, iron, vitamin B_6	Ill-fitting dentures
Gums		
Spongy, bleeding	Ascorbic acid	Periodontal disease, build-up of tartar near gum line, ill-fitting dentures, dilantin toxicity
Tongue		
Glossitis (magenta tongue)	Folic acid, niacin, riboflavin, vitamin B_{12}, pyridoxine, iron	Food irritants, antibiotic administration, uremia
Papillae atrophy	Niacin, folic acid, vitamin B_{12}, iron	Ill-fitting dentures, aging process, food irritants
Extremities		
Bilateral edema	Protein, sodium	Congestive heart failure, liver disease, renal failure
Absence of neural reflexes	Thiamin, vitamin B_{12}	Aging process

Modified from references 51, 81, and 86.

Table 10-3. Physical changes occurring with age and common practices of older people must be considered in clinical evaluation. Wearing of dentures, especially if poorly fitted, can lead to inflammation of the tongue or gums or fissures at the corners of the mouth (cheilosis).[27,81] Atrophy of the sebaceous glands of the skin and less efficient replacement of epidermal cells lost at abrasion points (elbows and knees) may contribute to skin problems.[51]

The subjectivity of the evaluator can influence interpretation of physical symptoms.[15] Sandstead and coworkers[81] described an older banker with a rash on his forearms, perifollicular hemorrhages, and transient pain who was found after considerable deliberation to have scurvy. Little attention had been directed toward his diet because it was assumed he would not have a deficiency disease. When used in conjunction with dietary and biochemical data, clinical methods can help identify nutrient problems.[25]

BIOCHEMICAL ASPECTS OF NUTRITIONAL ASSESSMENT

Selection of Biochemical Measurements

Both physiologic changes associated with normal aging as well as chronic disease leading to secondary nutrient deficiencies need to be considered when selecting methods for biochemical assessment. Plasma or serum nutrient levels generally reflect recent intake[5] but can be maintained at the expense of body stores, even though intake has become inadequate (see Chapter 6). Functional tests of enzyme activity identify both the problem and its relative magnitude.[5,16,23] Unfortunately, such analyses are both highly sophisticated and costly.

Urine nutrient content may be of limited value in the assessment of older people, although this requires further study. With fasting or random urine samples vitamin level is expressed per gram of creatinine.[5,51,60,74] This standard may not be appropriate for the older individual when muscle mass and creatinine excretion decline.[14] Loading tests, which evaluate vitamin saturation on the basis of nutrient content of the first urine voided in the morning or the vitamin level excreted over a specific period of time, do not always take into account the slowed kidney response in the aging individual. Whenever possible, tests that minimize age-related influences should be selected. Current work is focusing on hair and saliva as test substances for evaluating trace mineral status.[40] The influence of age on the appropriateness of these samples is not known.

Procurement of Samples

Blood Sample. To obtain a blood sample clients can be transported to a hospital laboratory or a home health nurse who is experienced in this procedure can visit a congregate meal program, senior center, or homebound individuals. Although fasting blood samples are most useful[23] because postprandial fluctuations are avoided, they cause more inconvenience for the client. Many older people use prescription drugs to be taken the first thing in the morning with breakfast. Individuals may not feel well enough to travel to the collection site with no food beforehand. One compromise is a breakfast consisting of one or two slices of bread or toast, plain jelly (no butter or margarine), and black coffee or tea (with sugar if desired). These food items have no significant effect on commonly used blood and enzyme measurements.[24] This breakfast is not appropriate, however, if tests are to include glucose tolerance.

Urine Sample. Clients asked to collect either a 24-hour urine specimen or the first voiding in the morning should be given full directions as well as a suitable container that has been treated with a preservative.[51] Disposable devices to simplify urine collection for women are available at hospital supply companies. Urine samples are screened for glucose, ketones, protein, and occult blood.

Table 10-4. Guidelines for biochemical assessment of adults

Nutrients (units)	Criteria for Evaluation		
	Deficient	Marginal	Acceptable
Blood			
Hemoglobin (gm/100 ml)			
Males	<12.0	12.0-13.9	≥14.0
Females	<10.0	10.0-11.9	≥12.0
Hematocrit (packed cell volume in %)			
Males	<37	37-43	≥44
Females	<31	31-37	≥38
Serum albumin (gm/100 ml)	<2.8	2.8-3.4	≥3.5
Serum protein (gm/100 ml)	<6.0	6.0-6.4	≥6.5
Serum ascorbic acid (mg/100 ml)	<0.1	0.1-0.19	≥0.2
Plasma vitamin A (μg/100 ml)	<10	10-19	≥20
Plasma carotene (μg/100 ml)	<20	20-39	≥40
Serum iron (μg/100 ml)			
Males	<60	—	≥60
Females	<40	—	≥40
Transferrin saturation (%)			
Males	<20.0	—	≥20.0
Females	<15.0	—	≥15.0
Serum folacin (ng/ml)	<2.0	2.0-5.9	≥6.0
Serum vitamin B_{12} (pg/ml)	<100	—	≥100
Plasma vitamin E (mg/100 ml)	<0.2	0.2-0.6	>0.6
Red blood cell transketolase			
TPP-effect (ratio)	>25	15-25	<15
Red blood cell glutathione reductase			
FAD-effect (ratio)	≥1.2	—	<1.2
Urine			
Thiamin (μg/gm creatinine)	<27	27-65	>65
Riboflavin (μg/gm creatinine)	<27	27-79	≥80

Modified from Christakis, G., ed.: Nutritional assessment in health programs, Washington, D.C., 1973, American Public Health Association.

Standards for Evaluation of Biochemical Tests

Criteria currently used in evaluation of biochemical measurements are given in Table 10-4. It must be recognized that these standards are based on research conducted with young adults and may not be appropriate for the aged.[14] Tissue and fluid nutrient levels, site and form of nutrient storage, and nutrient excretion patterns may change as a function of normal aging in healthy, well-nourished older people. A synergistic effect of the aging process and chronic disease could result in changes in accepted patterns. Although several clinicians have raised the possibility of an age-related decline in hemoglobin levels (see Chapter 8), no criteria specific to older people have been developed. This is a topic requiring immediate and extensive research and reflection.

INTEGRATION OF DIETARY, BIOCHEMICAL, AND CLINICAL EVALUATION

Christakis[23] pointed out that older people bear the lifelong effects of physiologic aging and disease and cannot be considered to be the same as younger age groups. Nutrient relationships common in younger people may be extremely complicated in an older population. Factors relating to both the individual evaluated and the methods used contribute to the inconsistencies observed. Both dietary and clinical records are subject to error. Biochemical standards may not be suitable. Physical signs thought to relate to nutritional deficiency may have a different origin. As a result, compiled dietary, biochemical, and clinical data can lead to indefinite conclusions.[60-61,76,100]

Nutrient Relationships

In older people dietary and serum nutrient levels are more closely related than are either dietary or serum levels and clinical observations[37,41,68,88]; however, agreement differs according to nutrient. Although dietary and serum levels of ascorbic acid are positively related in older individuals,* the association between dietary and serum vitamin A is less well understood.[29,37,94] Urinary excretion of thiamin and riboflavin are reasonably consistent with reported intakes,[94] although relationships between dietary intake and red blood cell enzyme levels are less well defined.[80]

Chronologic factors, individual variability, and metabolic relationships contribute to these differences.[61,76] A dietary record traces recent intake, whereas biochemical levels reflect past weeks or months. The exchange of nutrients between serum

*References 2, 8-9, 29, 68, 94.

or plasma and storage sites is unclear, leading to uncertainty in interpretation.

Chronologic Pattern

Clinical assessment is most representative of long term patterns of intake. Physical symptoms do not appear for some time after intake has fallen below adequate levels, but they may still remain long after optimum intake has been restored.[3,30,76,88]

A long term double-blind study of 80 institutionalized aged indicated that clinical lesions do respond to improved dietary intake.[41,88] Before supplementation with thiamin, riboflavin, niacin, pyridoxine, and ascorbic acid 90% had both biochemical and clinical signs of vitamin deficiency. After 3 months biochemical levels returned to normal in 85% of those receiving vitamins but remained the same or deteriorated in 87% of those given the placebo.

Clinical improvement, however, required continued supplementation for a year or more, suggesting that the healing process proceeds slowly long after biochemical deficiencies have been corrected. Studies reporting that clinical symptoms in the aged do not respond to vitamin therapy[3,4] may have been discontinued before improvement became obvious. Nutritional rehabilitation is a long term procedure and may require vitamin intakes above the RDAs.

ASSESSMENT OF INSTITUTIONALIZED AGED

Standards for Care

Present federal regulations governing patient care and review in long term care facilities receiving Medicare reimbursement address nutritional care.[56,99] In contrast to patients in acute care facilities, patients may remain in a nursing home for months or years; therefore continued assessment of the diet in light of changes in the food preferences or health condition of the patient is essential.[77] This requires the participation and effective communication of a multidisciplinary team including the physician, nurse, and dietitian. Other professionals, such as a dentist, social worker, physical therapist, or psychiatrist, may provide expertise as needed.[65]

The Patient Care Plan

Developing a Plan. The patient care plan is a plan of action developed to restore or maintain the individual at an optimum level of function.[1,56,90] The first step in development of a care plan is patient assessment to establish needs, priorities, and goals. The types of information required are similar to those for aged in the community (see p. 163). If the newly admitted patient is unable to provide background information, the social worker may obtain nutrition-related information from family members.[90] Pertinent problems to be identified include inadequacy of present or past food intake, food allergies, and use of medications known to interfere with nutrient absorption or metabolism.[1]

When present needs and problems have been identified future goals should be established. Steps to be taken to achieve the established goals and the individual or service responsible for implementation must be defined. A final component is the procedure for evaluating patient progress and readjusting both treatment and goals as necessary.[65] (Examples of patient care plans can be found in reference 1.)

Screening for Nutrition Problems. The normal weight patient who accepts a wide variety of foods and is able to feed himself may not require further assessment unless indicated by additional factors (e.g., recent surgery or blood loss, heavy use of medications, severe mental or emotional stress, signs of dehydration, or edema).[1,85] The individual who (1) is either gaining or losing weight, (2) has elevated nutrient requirements because of wound healing or pressure sores, or (3) is following a prescribed diet severely limited in either type or quantity of food requires further evaluation.[1]

In-Depth Nutritional Assessment. Although the individual or family may provide helpful information concerning previous intake or food preferences, present food intake should be monitored for further evaluation.[1,77] A form listing the menu items with a space to enter the approximate percentage consumed is more suitable than subjective comments, such as "patient doesn't eat."

Mindful of the need to develop efficient methods of obtaining dietary information in extended care facilities, Caliendo[20] evaluated the validity of a 24-hour recall record (based on 18 food groups) with 89 older patients. Food items recalled were compared with food items consumed, as recorded from examination of the tray following the meal. Eggs, meat, milk, cereal, soup, and low vitamin A vegetables had the greatest degree of association between the two records. Main items were more accurately recalled. Cereal was in the highest association group whereas low vitamin C fruits served at breakfast had the lowest degree of association.

Older patients may require further training in the method, because milk consumed at breakfast, usually eaten with cereal, was seldom recalled although the cereal itself was mentioned. Although the recall method did not provide a valid representation of the food items consumed by these patients, exploration of the technique should be continued. Factors such as health status, sex, or educational level may have a bearing on the ability of patients to provide dietary information.

A recent evaluation suggests that serum albumin is a predictor of malnutrition among the aged as values below 4 gm/100 ml were uncommon among healthy individuals regardless of age.[66] Mean values in malnourished aged were 2.5 and 2.6 gm/100 ml for men and women, respectively. One advantage was the lack of overlapping values between the malnourished and the healthy groups. Ninety-eight percent of the healthy had levels above 3.5 gm/100 ml, whereas about half of the malnourished were below 2.5 gm/100 ml. Arm muscle circumference and hemoglobin levels were less effective in distinguishing healthy from malnourished. Mitchell and Lipschitz[66] point to the need for appropriate control values and methods for evaluating older people.

Continuous Evaluation. Long term patients should be evaluated regularly to determine the effectiveness and appropriateness of the plan of care.[1,77] A change in physical condition or the addition or deletion of a particular drug can require a modification of the diet plan. A patient may stop eating because of gastrointestinal distress or chewing problems.

Evaluation procedures must include monitoring of all patients along with periodic consideration of individual patients.[1] Monitoring activities could include (1) visiting patient units at meal time, (2) routine checking of returned trays, and (3) measuring body weight on a monthly basis. Unexpected changes in body weight or regular return of food on the tray signals the need for individual reassessment.

The time interval for periodic review of each patient will depend on physical condition and dietary problems. If the patient is stable review at monthly or quarterly intervals may be sufficient if monitoring procedures are continued.[1] For the patient who is critically ill, in a period of rehabilitation, or adjusting to a new diet, daily or weekly review is indicated.

NUTRITIONAL STATUS OF AGED IN THE UNITED STATES

Until recently, minimal attention was directed toward older age groups by government or public health agencies or research groups. Existing reports usually focused on limited numbers of individuals residing in a particular community[28,42,78] or region,[57,71] or participating in a specific program.[24,52,58,63] Methods and evaluation criteria differed for each.

Two recent studies standardized methods so that regional, ethnic, and income groups could be compared. The Ten-State Nutrition Survey 1968-1970,[94-95] focused on individuals considered to be particularly vulnerable to poor nutrition because of income or ethnic group. The on-going Health and Nutrition Examination Survey (HANES) included a randomized sample representative of all ethnic, racial, and income groups nationwide.[53,96-97] In both studies, however, the numbers of participants age 60 and above were limited.

Ten-State Nutrition Survey 1968-1970

The Ten-State Survey[94-95] revealed severe nutrition problems in the aged, with the highest incidence among low income groups. In low income ratio states over half of those surveyed had incomes below the poverty level. In high income ratio states over half had incomes above the poverty level. Evaluation included dietary, biochemical, and clinical methods.

Although poor iron status was recognized to some degree among all groups, the problem was less serious among older whites with higher incomes. Older blacks in all income groups had lower intakes of iron and riboflavin. Spanish-Americans differed according to income and place of residence. Those residing in low income ratio states (southern states) were more likely to be deficient in vitamin A whereas those in high income ratio areas (northern states) had generally adequate levels. Obesity was particularly prevalent among women.

In the Ten-State Survey mean caloric intake was below standard for all older groups, with the majority consuming less than the recommended level. Over half of the men had intakes below 2000 kcal, and half of the women had less than 1500 kcal. Dietary iron, protein, and thiamin were related to total caloric intake. Blacks and Spanish-Americans had lower energy intakes than whites, and high income ratio groups had slightly higher intakes. Limited calorie intake contributed to the serious iron problem observed among low income blacks. Fifteen percent of low income black men and 32% of low income black women had hemoglobin levels below 12.0 gm/100 ml. Impaired iron absorption or utilization as well as intake could contribute to the iron problem observed among all groups.

Ascorbic acid and riboflavin status (reflected in both dietary and biochemical observations) depended on specific food choices rather than total food intake. Men are less likely to consume fruits and vegetables than women; lower serum ascorbic acid levels could reflect smoking habits among aged men or sex-related differences in ascorbic acid metabolism (see Chapter 6). Limited use of dairy products by blacks, possibly related to lactose intolerance, could contribute to poor riboflavin status.

Income as well as food patterns differed between Spanish-Americans in high income ratio states (primarily of Puerto Rican background) and those in low income ratio states (primarily of Mexican background). Total calories influenced to some extent vitamin A intake; however, fruit and vegetable sources of vitamin A tend to be expensive and not commonly included in the Mexican-American meal pattern. Nearly 13% of this ethnic group had serum vitamin A below 20 μg/100 ml. The widespread identification of nutritional problems points to the need for constant surveillance of vulnerable groups.

Health and Nutrition Examination Survey 1971-1974

HANES[53,96-97] has evaluated the nutritional status of the general population. Because of the limited numbers of subjects age 60 and above, biochemical data for both sexes were pooled. Although a high proportion had nutrient intakes below 100% of the RDA (Table 10-5), considerably less had biochemical levels in the deficient range.[53]

Problems identified in the Ten-State and HANES surveys reflect both the different populations and reference standards used. According to HANES

Table 10-5. Relationships between dietary and biochemical measurements in older people*

	Percentage of Persons Below Established Standards	
	White	**Black**
Protein		
Dietary protein	36	50
Total serum protein	10	3
Serum albumin	2	3
Vitamin A		
Dietary vitamin A	65	64
Serum vitamin A	<1	<1
Thiamin		
Dietary thiamin	60	72
Urinary thiamin/ creatinine ratio	8	20
Riboflavin		
Dietary riboflavin	43	61
Urinary riboflavin/ creatinine ratio	2	7
Iron		
Dietary iron	61	75
Hemoglobin	7	27
Hematocrit	15	34
Serum iron	3	7

*Includes both men and women, age 65 to 74 years.

Modified from Kerr, G.R., and others: Relationships between dietary and biochemical measures of nutritional status in HANES I data, Am. J. Clin. Nutr. **35**:294, 1982.

(Table 10-5), 10% of white aged are low in serum protein and 20% of black aged are low in urinary thiamin; these figures point to problems not suggested by the Ten-State Survey. This could reflect higher reference standards used in evaluating HANES data, although the higher incidence of deficient serum protein levels in whites than blacks is unexplained in light of higher protein intakes among whites.

Low serum vitamin A, noted among Spanish-Americans in the Ten State Study, was not a problem identified by HANES. Although the majority of blacks examined had riboflavin intakes below the RDA, only 7% had excretion levels below standard. Riboflavin status was not a general problem in the Ten-State Survey although riboflavin deficiency was more common among blacks than whites. Both iron intake and hematocrit levels reported in HANES confirm a serious iron problem in the black population.

Although HANES represents a population lower in risk than the Ten-State Survey, nutrition problems still exist. Furthermore, the difference between numbers of people with intakes below standard and biochemical values below standard suggests that (1) serum or urinary nutrient levels are being maintained at the expense of body stores, (2) the nutrient requirements of these people are less than those proposed, or (3) dietary records obtained do not reflect true intake.

Although it is understood that individual requirements may be less than 100% of the RDA, a significant number of older people are consuming less than 67% of the RDA (Table 10-6) for one or more nutrients. More than one third of men had inade-

Table 10-6. Percentage of older persons with inadequate dietary intakes*

Nutrient	Men	Women
Calories	36	51
Protein	12	13
Vitamin A	56	58
Vitamin C	34	32
Calcium	44	56
Iron	14	35
Thiamin	21	26
Riboflavin	12	18
Niacin	25	33

*Intakes below two thirds of the RDA.

Data from United States Department of Health, Education and Welfare: Dietary intake source data. United States, 1971-74. DHEW Publication No. (PHS) 79-1221, Hyattsville, Md., 1979, U.S. Government Printing Office.

quate levels of calories, calcium, vitamin A, and ascorbic acid. Significant numbers of women reported low intakes of those nutrients as well as niacin and iron. In the HANES study 13% of persons above age 60 had fissures of the tongue,[14] a possible indicator of niacin deficiency.

Regression analysis of the HANES data[53] confirms that socioeconomic variables of race, sex, age, income, and place of residence are more valuable predictors of biochemical status than a 1-day dietary record. For serum vitamin A, 26% of the variation among individuals was explained by the characteristics given above; only 1% related to recorded dietary intake. Although this calculation included all age groups, it reinforces the important influence of life-style and living situation on nutrient intake.

The Ten-State and HANES surveys confirm other reports evaluating smaller groups of aged. A recent summary of dietary studies pointed to low intakes of energy and calcium, the nutrients most likely to be deficient in this age group.[70] Although protein intake has usually been adequate, it may decrease as protein foods represent a major portion of the food dollar. Vitamins A and C are more of a problem among men and institutionalized subjects.[78,87] Iron and the B vitamin complex are consumed at less than desirable levels by many older people.

SUMMARY

Evaluation of nutritional status requires dietary, biochemical, clinical, and anthropometric information. Although a dietary record provides an estimate of food consumption, it does not indicate whether nutrients are being absorbed and metabolized. Impaired absorption or utilization, resulting from prescription or over the counter drugs, alterations in the gastrointestinal tract, or chronic problems such as gallbladder disease, becomes evident on biochemical and clinical evaluation.

Current methods of collecting food intake information include 24-hour recall record, dietary history, weighed or written food record, and food frequency checklists. Although a 1-day record provides a reasonable estimate of the nutrient intake of a group, it is not appropriate for assessment of an individual. A diet history, although reliable, requires a lengthy interview and a highly trained interviewer. Food frequency records, unless coded for portion size, do not estimate true nutrient intake. A 3-day record is a reasonable compromise between a 1-day record, of little value because of day to day variability, and a 7-day record that provides a reliable estimate of food intake but lowers participation of those with limited education.

Procurement of a blood sample requires highly trained personnel and extensive cooperation on the part of the client. When possible biochemical measurements should focus on functional parameters such as red cell enzyme activity indicating long term status, rather than serum or urine levels reflecting recent intake. Clinical parameters can be difficult to interpret in older people because physical signs frequently associated with nutrient deficiency may be age related. As a result, dietary, clinical, and biochemical records do not always agree.

Institutionalized older people, because of chronic disease, high use of prescription drugs, and problems in feeding or chewing, are especially vulnerable to poor nutritional status. Developing a nutritional care plan in cooperation with medical and nursing personnel and monitoring progress and food intake on a regular basis is essential to ensure patient satisfaction and optimum nutrition.

Both the Ten-State Nutrition Survey and HANES suggest that many older people are consuming diets containing less than 67% of the RDA, although fewer have biochemical deficiencies. Older people may require lower levels of nutrients than younger people. An alternative explanation is that blood levels are being maintained at the expense of body stores.

The evaluation of the nutritional status of an older individual is a difficult task, dependent on procedures and standards developed with younger people in mind. Valid methods that are simple and easy to use and require limited resources to complete are urgently needed.

REVIEW QUESTIONS

1. What types of measurements must be performed to adequately define the nutritional status of an individual?
2. What methods have been used to obtain dietary information from older people? Discuss the advantages and limitations of each method.
3. How would you explain the lack of agreement that sometimes exists between dietary, clinical, and biochemical findings in older individuals?
4. Develop a protocol for both routine and in-depth assessment of nursing home patients.
5. Within the older population, which groups are most vulnerable to poor nutritional status? Which nutrients are most likely to be deficient?

REFERENCES

1. American Dietetic Association: Patient nutritional care in long-term care facilities. A handbook for consultant dietitians and dietetic service supervisors, Chicago, 1977, American Dietetic Association.
2. Andrews, J., Brook, M., and Allen, M.A.: Influence of abode and season on the vitamin C status of the elderly, Gerontol. Clin. **8**:257, 1966.
3. Andrews, J., Letcher, M., and Brook, M.: Vitamin C supplementation in the elderly: A 17-month trial in an old person's home, Br. Med. J. **2**:416, 1969.
4. Andrews, J.D.: Clinical signs and their true relationship to vitamin C deficiency. In Exton-Smith, A.N., and Scott, D.L., eds.: Vitamins in the elderly, Bristol, 1968, John Wright & Sons, Ltd.
5. Arroyave, G.: Biochemical evaluation of nutritional status in man, Fed. Proc. **20**:39, 1961.
6. Austin, J.E.: The perilous journey of nutrition evaluation, Am. J. Clin. Nutr. **31**:2324, 1978.
7. Balogh, M., Kahn, H.A., and Medalie, J.H.: Random repeat 24-hour dietary recalls, Am. J. Clin. Nutr. **24**:304, 1971.
8. Bates, C.J., Burr, M.K., and St. Leger, A.S.: Vitamin C, high density lipoproteins and heart disease in elderly subjects, Age Ageing **8**:177, 1979.
9. Bates, C.J., and others: Long-term vitamin status and dietary intake of healthy elderly subjects. 2. Vitamin C, Br. J. Nutr. **42**:43, 1977.
10. Beal, V.A.: The nutritional history in longitudinal research, J. Am. Diet. Assoc. **51**:426, 1967.

11. Beaton, G.H.: Evaluation of nutrition interventions: Methodologic considerations, Am. J. Clin. Nutr. **35** (suppl.):1280, 1982.

12. Beaton, G.H., and others: Sources of variance in 24-hour dietary recall data: Implications for nutrition study design and interpretation, Am. J. Clin. Nutr. **32**:2546, 1979.

13. Bowering, J., and others: Evaluating 24-hour dietary recalls, J. Nutr. Educ. **9**:20, 1977.

14. Bowman, B.B., and Rosenberg, I.H.: Assessment of the nutritional status of the elderly, Am. J. Clin. Nutr. **35**(suppl.):1142, 1982.

15. Bransby, E.R., and Hammond, W.H.: Reliability of the clinical assessment of ''nutritional state,'' Br. Med. J. **2**:330, 1951.

16. Brin, M.: Erythrocyte as a biopsy tissue for functional evaluation of thiamin status, JAMA **187**:762, 1964.

17. Burk, M.C., and Pao, E.M.: Methodology for large-scale surveys of household and individual diets, Home Economics Res. Rep. No. 40, Agricultural Research Service, Washington, D.C., 1976, U.S. Government Printing Office.

18. Burke, B.S.: The dietary history as a tool in research, J. Am. Diet. Assoc. **23**:1041, 1947.

19. Caird, F.I., Judge, T.G., and MacLeod, C.: Pointers to possible malnutrition in the elderly at home, Gerontol. Clin. **17**:47, 1975.

20. Caliendo, M.A.: Validity of the 24-hour recall to determine dietary status of elderly in an extended care facility, J. Nutr. Elderly **1**(2):57, 1981.

21. Campbell, V.A., and Dodds, M.L.: Collecting dietary information from groups of older people, J. Am. Diet. Assoc. **51**:29, 1967.

22. Chalmers, F.W., and others: The dietary record: How many and which days? J. Am. Diet. Assoc. **28**:711, 1952.

23. Christakis, G., ed.: Nutritional assessment in health programs, Washington, D.C., 1973, American Public Health Association.

24. Clarke, R.P., Schlenker, E.D., and Merrow, S.B.: Nutrient intake, adiposity, plasma total cholesterol, and blood pressure of rural participants in the (Vermont) Nutrition Program for Older Americans (Title III), Am. J. Clin. Nutr. **34**:1743, 1981.

25. Dann, W.J., and Darby, W.J.: The appraisal of nutritional status in humans with special reference to vitamin deficiency diseases, Physiol. Rev. **25**:326, 1945.

26. Darby, W.J.: The influence of some recent studies on the interpretation of the findings of nutrition surveys, J. Am. Diet. Assoc. **23**:204, 1947.

27. Darby, W.J., and Milam, D.F.: Field study of the prevalence of the clinical manifestations of dietary inadequacy, Am. J. Public Health **35**:1014, 1945.

28. Davidson, C.S., and others: The nutrition of a group of apparently healthy aging persons, Am. J. Clin. Nutr. **10**:181, 1962.

29. Dibble, M.V., and others: Evaluation of the nutritional status of elderly subjects, with a comparison between fall and spring, J. Am. Geriatr. Soc. **15**:1031, 1967.

30. Disselduff, M.M., and Murphy, E. La C.: Leucocyte vitamin C levels in elderly patients with reference to dietary intake and clinical findings. In Exton-Smith, A.N., and Scott, D.L., eds.: Vitamins in the elderly, Bristol, 1968, John Wright & Sons, Ltd.

31. Exton-Smith, A.N.: Epidemiologic studies in the elderly: Methodological considerations, Am. J. Clin. Nutr. **35** (suppl.):1273, 1982.

32. Fomon, S.J.: Nutritional disorders of children. Prevention, screening and follow-up, DHEW Publication No. (HSA) 77-5104, Washington, D.C., 1977, U.S. Government Printing Office.

33. Food and Nutrition Board: Recommended dietary allowances, ed. 9, Washington, D.C., 1980, National Academy of Sciences.

34. Fry, P.C., Fox, H.M., and Linkswiler, H.: Nutrient intakes of healthy older women, J. Am. Diet. Assoc. **42**:218, 1963.

35. Garn, S.M., Larkin, F.A., and Cole, P.E.: The real problem with 1-day diet records (letter), Am. J. Clin. Nutr. **31**:1114, 1978.

36. Gersovitz, M., Madden, J.P., and Smiciklas-Wright, H.: Validity of the 24-hour dietary recall and seven-day record for group comparisons, J. Am. Diet. Assoc. **73**:48, 1978.

37. Gillum, H.L., and Sailer, F.: Nutritional status of the aging. V. Vitamin A and carotene, J. Nutr. **55**:655, 1955.

38. Goodhart, R.S.: The diagnosis and management of malnutrition in office practice, Med. Clin. North Am. **45**(6):1533, 1961.

39. Goodman, S.J.: Assessment of nutritional impact of congregate meals programs for the elderly, Ph.D. thesis, University Park, 1974, Pennsylvania State University.

40. Greger, J.L., and Sickles, V.S.: Saliva zinc levels: Potential indicators of zinc status, Am. J. Clin. Nutr. **32**:1859, 1979.

41. Griffiths, L.L.: Biochemical findings of the Farnborough survey. In Exton-Smith, A.N., and Scott, D.L., eds.: Vitamins in the elderly, Bristol, 1968, John Wright & Sons, Ltd.

42. Guthrie, H.A., Black, K., and Madden, J.P.: Nutritional practices of elderly citizens in rural Pennsylvania, Gerontologist **12**:330, 1972.

43. Guthrie, H.A., and Scheer, J.C.: Validity of a dietary score for assessing nutrient adequacy, J. Am. Diet. Assoc. **78**:240, 1981.

44. Habicht, J.P.: Some characteristics of indicators of nutritional status for use in screening and surveillance, Am. J. Clin. Nutr. **33**:531, 1980.

45. Habicht, J.P., Lane, J.M., and McDowell, A.J.: National nutrition surveillance, Fed. Proc. **37**:1181, 1978.

46. Hankin, J.H., and Huenemann, R.: A short dietary method for epidemiologic studies. 1. Developing standard methods for interpreting seven-day measured food records, J. Am. Diet. Assoc. **50**:487, 1967.

47. Havighurst, R.J.: Problems of sampling and interviewing in studies of old people, J. Gerontol. **5**:158, 1950.

48. Houser, H.B., and others: Dietary intake of nonhospitalized persons with multiple sclerosis, J. Am. Diet. Assoc. **54**:391, 1969.

49. Hunt, I.F., and others: Nutrient estimates from computerized questionnaires vs. 24-hour recall interviews, J. Am. Diet. Assoc. **74**:656, 1979.

50. Jain, M., and others: Evaluation of a diet history questionnaire for epidemiologic studies, Am. J. Epidemiol. **111**:212, 1980.

51. Jelliffe, D.B.: The assessment of the nutritional status of the community, Geneva, 1966, World Health Organization.

52. Justice, C.L., Howe, J.M., and Clark, H.E.: Dietary intakes and nutritional status of elderly patients: Study in a private nursing home, J. Am. Diet. Assoc. **65**:639, 1974.

53. Kerr, G.R., and others: Relationships between dietary and biochemical measures of nutritional status in HANES I data, Am. J. Clin. Nutr. **35**:294, 1982.

54. Keys, A.: Recommendations concerning body measurements for the characterization of nutritional status, Hum. Biol. **28**:111, 1956.

55. King, J.C., and others: Evaluation and modification of the Basic Four Food Guide, J. Nutr. Ed. **10**:27, 1978.

56. Kocher, R.E.: Monitoring nutritional care of the long-term patient, 1. Policies and systems that support the on-going evaluation of care, J. Am. Diet. Assoc. **67**:45, 1975.

57. Koh, E.T., Myung, S.C., and Lowenstein, F.W.: Comparison of selected blood components by race, sex, and age, Am. J. Clin. Nutr. **33**:1828, 1980.

58. Kohrs, M.B., O'Hanlon, P., and Eklund, D.: Title VII Nutrition Program for the Elderly, J. Am. Diet. Assoc. **72**:487, 1978.

59. Krehl, W.A.: The evaluation of nutritional status, Med. Clin. North Am. **48**:1129, 1964.

60. Krehl, W.A., and Hodges, R.E.: The interpretation of nutrition survey data, Am. J. Clin. Nutr. **17**:191, 1965.

61. Leverton, R.M.: Rose's foundations for nutritional evaluation, J. Am. Diet. Assoc. **37**:553, 1960.

62. MacLeod, C.C.: Methods of dietary assessment. In Carlson, L.A., ed.: Nutrition in old age, Symposia of the Swedish Nutrition Foundation X, Stockholm, 1972, Almqvist & Wiksell.

63. Madden, J.P., Goodman, S.J., and Guthrie, H.A.: Validity of the 24-hour recall: Analysis of data obtained from elderly subjects, J. Am. Diet. Assoc. **68**:143, 1976.

64. Madden, J.P., Goodman, S.J., and Thompson, F.E.: Recording the 24-hour dietary recall, Department of Agricultural Economics and Rural Sociology, University Park, 1974, Pennsylvania State University.

65. Matthewson, G.H.: Current concerns of the consultant dietician, 3. Contributing information to patient care plans, J. Am. Diet. Assoc. **63**:45, 1973.

66. Mitchell, C.O., and Lipschitz, D.A.: The effect of age and sex on the routinely used measurements to assess the nutritional status of hospitalized patients, Am. J. Clin. Nutr. **36**:340, 1982.

67. Moore, M.C., Judlin, B.C., and Kennemur, P.McA.: Using graduated food models in taking diet histories, J. Am. Diet. Assoc. **51**:447, 1967.

68. Morgan, A.F., Gillum, H.L., and Williams, R.I.: Nutritional status of the aging. III. Serum ascorbic acid and intake, J. Nutr. **55**:431, 1955.

69. Morgan, R.W., and others: A comparison of dietary methods in epidemiologic studies, Am. J. Epidemiol. **107**:488, 1978.

70. O'Hanlon, P., and Kohrs, M.B.: Dietary studies of older Americans, Am. J. Clin. Nutr. **31**:1257, 1978.

71. Ohlson, M.A., and others: Dietary practices of 100 women from 40 to 75 years of age, J. Am. Diet. Assoc. **24**:286, 1948.

72. Ohlson, M.A., and others: Nutrition and dietary habits of aging women, Am. J. Public Health **40**:1101, 1950.

73. Ostfeld, A.M.: Nutrition and aging. In Ostfeld, A.M., and Gibson, D.C., eds.: Epidemiology of aging, DHEW Publication No. (NIH) 75-711, Bethesda, Md., 1977, U.S. Government Printing Office.

74. Pearson, W.N.: Biochemical appraisal of nutritional status in man, Am. J. Clin. Nutr. **11**:462, 1962.

75. Pihlblad, C.T., Rosencranz, H.A., and McNevin, T.E.: An examination of the effects of perceptual frames of reference in interviewing older respondents, Gerontologist **7**:125, 1967.

76. Plough, I.C., and Bridgforth, E.B.: Relations of clinical and dietary findings in nutrition surveys, Pub. Health Rep. **75**:699, 1960.

77. Poleman, C.M.: Monitoring nutritional care of the long-term patient, 2. Experiences at the Mercy Health and Rehabilitation Center, Auburn, N.Y., J. Am. Diet. Assoc. **67**:47, 1975.

78. Rawson, I.G., and others: Nutrition of rural elderly in southwestern Pennsylvania, Gerontologist **18**(1):24, 1978.

79. Roberts, P.H., Kerr, C.H., and Ohlson, M.A.: Nutritional status of older women: Nitrogen, calcium, and phosphorus retentions of nine women, J. Am. Diet. Assoc. **24**:292, 1948.

80. Rutishauser, I.H., and others: Long-term vitamin status and dietary intake of healthy elderly subjects. 1. Riboflavin, Br. J. Nutr. **42**:33, 1979.

81. Sandstead, H.H., Carter, J.P., and Darby, W.J.: How to diagnose nutritional disorders in daily practice, Nutr. Today **4**:20, 1969.

82. Schaefer, A.E.: Assessment of nutritional status: Food intake studies. In Beaton, G.H., and McHenry, E.W., eds.: Nutrition: A comprehensive treatise, vol. III, Nutritional status: Assessment and application, New York, 1966, Academic Press, Inc.

83. Schlaepfer, L.V., and Shmerling, D.H.: The use of a programmable pocket calculator in clinical dietetics, Res. Exp. Med. **174**:267, 1979.

84. Schmidt, M.G.: Interviewing the old old, Gerontologist **15**(6):544, 1975.

85. Shapiro, L.R.: Streamlining and implementing nutritional assessment: The dietary approach, J. Am. Diet. Assoc. **75**:230, 1979.

86. Sinclair, H.H.: The assessment of human nutriture, Vitam. Horm. **6**:102, 1948.

87. Stiedemann, M., Jansen, C., and Harrill, I.: Nutritional status of elderly men and women, J. Am. Diet. Assoc. **73**:132, 1978.

88. Taylor, G.F.: A clinical survey of elderly people from a nutritional standpoint. In Exton-Smith, A.N., and Scott, D.L., eds.: Vitamins in the elderly, Bristol, 1968, John Wright & Sons, Ltd.

89. Todhunter, E.N., and Darby, W.J.: Guidelines for maintaining adequate nutrition in old age, Geriatrics **33**:49, 1978.

90. Treadwell, D.D.: Planning the nutrition component of the long-term care, J. Am. Diet. Assoc. **64**:56, 1974.

91. Trulson, M.F.: Assessment of dietary study methods, J. Am. Diet. Assoc. **30**:991, 1954.

92. Tryon, R.: How to reach and work with the poor, Ross Timesaver, Ross Laboratories, Columbus, Ohio, **15**(3):1, June-Sept., 1975.

93. Turner, D.: The estimation of the patient's home dietary intake, J. Am. Diet. Assoc. **16**:875, 1940.

94. United States Department of Health, Education and Welfare: Ten-State Nutrition Survey 1968-1970. IV. Biochemical, DHEW Publication No. (HSM)72-8132, Atlanta, 1972, Centers for Disease Control.

95. United States Department of Health, Education and Welfare: Ten-State Nutrition Survey 1968-1970. V. Dietary, DHEW Publication No. (HSM)72-8133, Atlanta, 1972, Centers for Disease Control.

96. United States Department of Health, Education and Welfare: Preliminary findings of the first Health and Nutrition Examination Survey, United States, 1971-1972. Dietary intake and biochemical findings, DHEW Publication No. (HRA)74-1219-1, Rockville, Md., 1974, U.S. Government Printing Office.

97. United States Department of Health, Education and Welfare: Dietary intake source data. United States, 1971-74. DHEW Publication No. (PHS)79-1221, Hyattsville, Md., 1979, U.S. Government Printing Office.

98. United States Department of Health and Human Services: Final regulations for amending basic HHS policy for the protection of human research subjects, effective July 27, 1981, CFR 46, Bethesda, Md., 1981.

99. United States General Services Administration, Office of the Federal Register: Code of federal regulations, Federal health insurance for the aged and disabled, Skilled nursing facilities, Public Health **42**:400, Fed. Register, vol. 39, No. 12, Jan. 17, 1974.

100. Wadsworth, G.R.: Nutrition surveys: Clinical signs and biochemical measurements, Proc. Nutr. Soc. **22**:72, 1963.

101. Wisconsin Department of Health and Social Services: Nutrition screening and assessment manual, Madison, 1980.

102. Young, C.M.: The interview itself, J. Am. Diet. Assoc. **35**:677, 1959.

103. Young, C.M.: Dietary methodology. In Food and Nutrition Board, eds.: Assessing changing food consumption patterns, Washington, D.C., 1981, National Academy of Sciences.

104. Young, C.M., and Trulson, M.F.: Methodology for dietary studies in epidemiological surveys. II. Strengths and weaknesses of existing methods, Am. J. Public Health **50**:803, 1960.

105. Young, C.M., and others: A comparison of dietary study methods. I. Dietary history vs. seven-day record, J. Am. Diet. Assoc. **28**:124, 1952.

106. Young, C.M., and others: A comparison of dietary study methods. II. Dietary history vs. seven-day record vs. 24-hr. recall, J. Am. Diet. Assoc. **28**:218, 1952.

Chapter 11

Food Selection Patterns Among the Aged

Although food intake is a biologic process, it has great social and emotional significance as well.[5] In the older person food patterns reflect lifelong attitudes and habits as influenced by the changing environment. To better understand the influence of life-style, health, and economic status on food choices, these factors have been identified and evaluated in older individuals. They include the following:

Psychologic
Loneliness
Bereavement
Social isolation
Food aversion
Symbolism of food
Mental awareness
Feelings of self-worth
Food faddism
Nutrition knowledge
Physiologic
Loss of appetite
Loss of taste
Dental problems
Prescribed diets
Chronic disease
Food intolerance
State of health
Physical disability
Degree of physical exercise
Socioeconomic
Age
Sex

Level of income
Cooking facilities
Daily schedule
Retirement/leisure time
Level of education
Distance to food store
Availability of transportation
Availability of familiar foods

Although each is considered singly, all act in combination. The older woman who has enjoyed food preparation and prided herself on "cooking from scratch" may no longer be able to do so if worsening arthritis makes it difficult to move about the kitchen. Possible alternatives for her are reliance on heat-and-serve items requiring little preparation, home-delivered meals, and relocation to another living situation. If a spouse is present, he may be able to take over food responsibilities. Helping older people solve their food problems often involves seeking alternatives and doing things differently than was the usual practice.

The later years can be characterized as a period of continual adjustment to new situations.[22] Loss of income and death of a spouse are beyond the older person's control and can lead to drastic changes in life-style and personal satisfaction.[82] Alternatively, retirement allows time for participation in hobbies or rewarding community service. Changes in living situation can be detrimental to food intake and nutritional status. Although factors such as living alone or having less money to spend on food do lead to poor nutrient intake in *some* older people, this is not true of *all* older people. The stereotype of the older person subsisting on tea and toast is not substantiated by survey data from the United States or Great Britain. Although there are individuals who do follow this pattern, it is *not typical* of this age group. For most there are positive aspects of the diet to serve as a foundation for any further improvement required.

CHANGES IN LIFELONG FOOD PATTERNS

For older people life is more a continuation of previous habits than a change.[83] Patterns associated with pleasant experiences are continued. Changes in food availability, however, can modify the dietary pattern. A recent article in a popular magazine for senior citizens reflected on childhood memories of awaking to the aroma of hot cereal on cold winter mornings.[75] The cornmeal cereal previously enjoyed may no longer be on the market. On the other hand, oranges, formerly enjoyed once a year as a Christmas treat by children in cold climates, are now available all year round. The diet of the older client therefore reflects both traditional patterns and the general food supply. Contrary to popular opinion, older people do try new foods and adapt to changing food situations such as a prescribed diet. The mere fact of their survival points to their ability to select a reasonably adequate diet

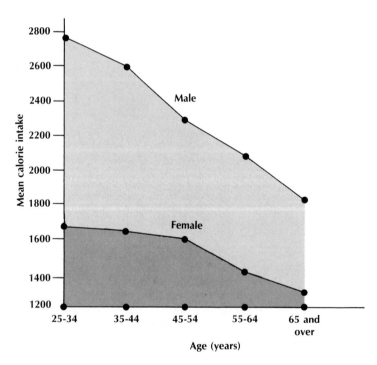

Fig. 11-1. Age-related changes in energy intake by age and sex. (Data from United States Department of Health, Education, and Welfare: Dietary intake source data. United States, 1971-1974, DHEW Publication No. [PHS] 79-1221, Hyattsville, Md., 1979, U.S. Government Printing Office.)

over a period of years.[83] Advancing age, however, does lead to changes in food intake.

Age

Normal aging brings about a decrease in both energy requirements and the quantity of food consumed.[25-26,36,79] According to recent HANES data mean daily intake decreased by about 900 kcal in men and 300 kcal in women between 25 and 65 years old[89] (Fig. 11-1). Decreases in calorie intake influence the quantity of other nutrients consumed. Dietary analysis of 2200 women in the North Central region ranging in age from 30 to 90 years suggested that daily intake declined by 85 kcal, 4 gm protein, 30 mg calcium, and 194 IU vitamin A per decade.[79] Over a 60-year period, this results in loss of about 500 kcal, 24 gm protein, 180 mg calcium, and 1200 IU vitamin A from the daily diet. Although energy needs decrease, requirements for protein and the micronutrients remain the same. The greater decrease in caloric intake among the North Central as compared to the HANES women (500 versus 300 kcal)[79,89] probably relates to the age (90 years) of the oldest North Central women. The oldest group in HANES was 65 to 74 years of age.

In general older persons decrease their energy intake by consuming less of all foods normally eaten rather than selectively reducing intake.[26,60] The detrimental effect on diet quality was apparent in two groups of women with mean ages of 72 and 81, and calorie intakes of 2074 and 1674, respectively.[26] Protein intake decreased from 63 to 48 gm, calcium from 924 to 760 mg, and iron from 11.3 to 8.0 mg as calorie intake declined. Reducing food intake without adjusting the dietary pattern to increase nutrient density contributes to poor health.[60]

Meat, poultry, and dairy products, sometimes considered to be high calorie foods on the basis of fat content, are also good sources of protein, iron, the B complex vitamins, zinc, and calcium. Diets of older women were significantly improved in cal-

cium, riboflavin, and protein when dairy products were consumed on a daily basis.[28] Whole grain products add valuable vitamins and trace minerals. Foods that contain primarily carbohydrate and fat and few other nutrients (e.g., sweet baked items, soft drinks, crackers, alcoholic beverages) should be the first to be deleted from the diet. Food preparation methods that add additional calories in the form of fat or rich sauces should be avoided.

Both men and women age 75 or above tend to have poorer diets than those age 65 to 74.[25,47] Energy intakes of those above age 75 often range from 1000 to 1200 kcal per day.[72] This group is also lower in income than those age 65 to 74 and has more physical disabilities, which can interfere with meal preparation (see Chapter 1). The influence of educational level on diet in the very old also warrants examination. In a survey of retired college employees the group over age 80 had the highest proportion of good diets.[11] This may reflect the enhanced survival of those of higher socioeconomic class or with optimum nutrient intake (see Chapter 2). Evaluation of nutrient intake in specific age cohorts beyond age 65 should be included in future national surveys.

Health Considerations

Medical advice or belief that a particular food is good or bad for health leads to changes in food consumption and preparation. About 50% of participants at a Boston senior center changed their diet in some way for health reasons.[17] Elimination of fatty or fried foods was most common, followed by a decrease in highly spiced foods. Gastrointestinal upset may have prompted avoidance of fat or highly spiced items. Publicity in the popular press toward prevention of cardiovascular disease could influence older individuals to limit their fat intake, substitute polyunsaturated for saturated fat, and broil rather than fry foods. Perceived health benefit was a stronger determinant of food choice than convenience, price, or prestige value for 194 aged Canadians.[45] These findings support the idea that nutrition education can be effective in helping older people modify their food patterns.[45]

General Trends

Changes occurring in agriculture, food preservation, and food processing over the past 30 years have multiplied the food forms now available to the consumer. Frozen orange juice, unheard of during the early adult years of people now above age 60, is a common item. TV dinners and instant mashed potatoes used by young and old consumers are fairly recent additions to the cultural food pattern.[15]

Changes in the food choices of the general population were paralleled in 28 Michigan women who provided food records in both 1948 and 1972.[72] When interviewed in 1972 they ranged in age from 64 to 90 years. Whole milk and cream were the usual dairy choices in 1948; by 1972 all but one used low fat or skim milk, and cream had disappeared from the diet records. Ice milk, a popular item at the time of the resurvey, was not available in 1948. In 1972 participants consumed less fat as well as a different type of fat, shifting from butter to margarine. Meats were stewed or broiled rather than fried. Over the 24-year period consumption of bread, cereals, and vegetables declined, as it did in the general population. In contrast to younger age groups these women *decreased* their intakes of sweets and baked products high in sugar and fat. Changes in food habits were attributed to health as well as general food availability.

Healthy Boston aged, 51 to 97 years of age, were asked to recall any major changes in their use of milk, eggs, meat, and fish after reaching adulthood.[17] Although about 50% reported no change in milk-drinking habits, the remainder were divided. About 25% began drinking more milk for health reasons or because it was easily accessible. The decrease in milk intake reported by others related to living situation or health. Intestinal upset was not given as a reason for change. Health reasons could relate to the fat content of whole milk.

Although eggs were popular because they are versatile to prepare, about 10% decreased egg consumption because of cholesterol content. Fish and meat were eaten less frequently after age 60, with cost and living alone following the loss of a spouse given as factors. Nearly half had meat less frequently than in earlier years. Although some of the participants commented that meat was not good for older people, no one admitted having chewing problems.[17]

Although it has been assumed that food habits formed early in life are not changed, it is apparent that older persons are faced with changing living situations and resources, and food patterns must be adapted accordingly. Any change in food habits has nutritional implications. Changes for health reasons should have a positive effect on nutrient intake. Infrequent use of meat or fish without replacement of other sources of protein, iron, and the B complex vitamins can result in serious malnutrition. Increased use of highly processed items to simplify meal preparation will decrease intakes of fiber and trace minerals. Among independent-living aged in Kansas, the greater the number of reported changes in the customary diet pattern, the lower the nutritional score.[15] Physical disability, economic problems, and social isolation contribute to changes that can reduce dietary quality. On the other hand, adoption of newly marketed food items by this age group suggests that nutritious foods not used previously may be accepted if they are introduced in a positive way.

PSYCHOLOGIC ASPECTS OF FOOD SELECTION

Adaptation to Changing Role

Cultures vary in the role assigned to those considered to be "old."[10] In some societies elders are accorded a position of honor. In this country older people are viewed less favorably. When an individual reaches the critical age (usually 60 or 65), he must adapt to a new set of expectations. This is in contrast to physiologic changes that occur slowly over a period of years, allowing gradual adaptation.[10]

Loss of primary role has a psychologic impact on the older adult.[38] For a man, retirement, whether voluntary or compulsory, changes his role as bread-winner-worker, which can result in loss of self-esteem. Since the husband is now home during the day, he may become involved in meal planning and food preparation. Although this can lead to conflict, it also means that another person is available to help with food responsibilities if the wife does not enjoy meal preparation or is in poor health.

For the woman who has enjoyed her role as wife and mother two events can be critical.[38] If she associated meal planning with nurturance of children, motivation toward these activities may be lost when the last child leaves home. Howell and Loeb[38] suggest that poor eating patterns can in some older women be traced to this period of life. A later loss for the woman comes with the death of her husband. When living alone she may resort to foods easy to prepare.

The supposition that retirement increases the husband's influence on food decisions was confirmed in 82 retired couples who were compared with couples in other stages of the life cycle.[67-68] Not only did retired husbands participate to a greater extent in food-related decisions, but the level of participation had nutritional implications. The greater his involvement in both meal planning and actual food purchase, the better the diet. Women who expressed dissatisfaction with their traditional role consumed poorer diets and could have had less commitment to meal planning and preparation. This study has important implications for nutrition education. Although food programs are often directed toward women, leaders should make an effort to involve men who (1) may be less bored with food activities and therefore more receptive and (2) strongly influence the food decisions within a retired family.

Feeling of Self-Worth

Food is a symbol of love and security for people of all ages.[92] Good food, well-prepared, conveys the message that a person is important and that someone cares about him.[8] Complaints about food, particularly in an institutional setting, may be a plea for attention. The older individual lacking sufficient or appropriate food experiences severe deprivation in the psychologic as well as the physical sense.[92] Feelings of worthlessness could lead to loss of interest in food and subsequent changes in nutrient intake. Among older midwestern couples and single women living alone, diet quality was not affected by self-esteem.[68] Those individuals, however, appeared to have adequate financial resources to meet their needs and may not be representative of low income aged with multiple problems.

Level of Social Interaction

Throughout life eating is a social activity.[83] Typical examples are the birthday party, the wedding breakfast, and family sharing at the evening meal. Loss of spouse or friends results in loss of eating companions for the older individual, who may find himself eating alone for the first time in his life. Loneliness contributes to the malnutrition observed in some older persons. Among 418 rural aged those with low morale scores had many problems with their diet, although specific nutrient intakes were not reported.[46] Morale was evaluated on the basis of personal well-being, loneliness, and attitude toward aging. Health and economic problems were also common and no doubt contributed to both low morale and diet problems in this group.

It is important to differentiate between isolation and desolation. According to Troll,[83] isolates are those who are content living alone and may have done so most of their lives. The desolates, on the other hand, live alone but are both lonely and unhappy. Physical isolation may be far less important than frequency of communication or exchange of messages. An individual who lives with other people but is ignored is far more lonely than the person who lives alone but has a daily telephone conversation with a friend or child.[83] Older persons who were satisfied with the degree of attention (in the form of visits or telephone calls) received from family members had fewer complaints about food and were better able to adjust to a prescribed diet.[46] Emotional dissatisfaction may be expressed in the form of food-related problems.

Health professionals working with community nutrition programs must be prudent in identifying individuals who could benefit from such a program. Some isolated aged are content with rather limited social interaction and have satisfying lives. Although they should be invited to participate, they may not choose to become active. Others with limited social contact may welcome the opportunity. Despite his loneliness, the shy individual may require special encouragement to join a program.[38]

Sherwood[77] describes a particular form of isolation existing among aged in low socioeconomic, urban settings. These individuals live in fear of being robbed or physically harmed, and they avoid going out even to shop for food. For those in single rooms with no kitchen privileges, meals may consist mainly of bread and sweet rolls and coffee or tea.[1]

Food Preferences

Food preferences are molded by ethnic, cultural, and religious backgrounds. Older people prefer foods associated with pleasant experiences[12] or related to home or place of origin.[38] Preferred foods may have been given as special treats or served on holidays or special occasions.[8] Age-appropriate behavior influences food selection.[12,38] Low milk consumption can symbolize rejection of a food associated with childhood and dependency.[8] For lonely aged food cravings may reflect the need for emotional gratification. In my experience one older woman regularly ate bread spread with butter and sprinkled with several teaspoons of sugar.[72] Although traditionally linked to particular ethnic groups, ''soul food'' in a broad sense may be any

food that has emotional significance.[9] When planning a diet for an older client it is pertinent to both recognize and respect individual food preferences. Such an approach is more likely to produce a diet that will be followed rather than accepted politely and then ignored.

Mental Awareness

Mental disorders in the older client can result in confusion, irritability, acute depression, or in extreme situations, true dementia. Those with organic brain syndrome may forget to eat or be unable to differentiate between breakfast, lunch, and dinner. If they are not able to prepare food, meals may consist totally of bread and jam or all prepackaged foods, thus limiting nutrient intake both quantitatively and qualitatively.

Individuals with neurologic or psychiatric disorders who live in their own homes often have severely low caloric intakes resulting in body wasting.[13,51] Sometimes severe paranoia relating to perceived harm from the ingestion of food causes the person to stop eating. One individual with chronic lung disease associated food intake and spasms of coughing.[13] Frail aged with swallowing problems may have a fear of choking. Chronic indigestion leads to the belief that all food is unsuitable. Discontinuing regular meals results in a downhill spiral that further jeopardizes both mental and physical health.

Blass[7] described the eating problems of older people with Alzheimer-type senile dementia. These patients are no longer aware of how to use a knife and fork or how to lift a cup or food item to the mouth. They may spread butter on their palm instead of the bread. For individuals living at home, relatives can be unaware of the cause of their behavior. A person who handles his food but does not eat it may be thought to be dissatisfied with the food served; no one may realize that he does not know how to eat.

In a clinical situation the aged patient with dementia who must be fed should be weighed regularly. Among 64 patients (age 60 to 101) in an extended care facility, 58% lost weight and 31% gained weight over a period of 6 to 48 months.[56] Weight loss ranged from 1 to 39 pounds; half of those losing weight lost 6 to 20 pounds. In four patients losses equaled nearly 30% of their admission weight. Ambulatory patients with or without brain damage were more likely to gain than lose weight. Although disinterest in food and feeding problems no doubt contribute to the low calorie intake of those with dementia, the increased risk of the nonambulatory remains to be clarified. Whether the ambulatory are more likely to receive food from visitors or other sources requires further evaluation.

PHYSIOLOGIC ASPECTS OF FOOD SELECTION

Physical changes occurring as a result of both normal aging and degenerative disease influence food habits. Loss of appetite or diminished taste sensitivity makes eating less pleasurable. A modified diet that eliminates favorite foods reduces interest in eating. Physical disability restricting food shopping and meal preparation limits food choices. Physiologic changes also affect psychologic outlook and level of social activity, making it sometimes difficult to identify the true cause of observed changes.

Sensory Aspects of Food Selection

Appetite. The majority of older persons living in the community describe their appetite as good to excellent.[17] Among 100 aged living alone, 67% rated their appetite as good and 25% rated their appetite as fair.[40] Less than 10% of older households (n = 283) in Rochester, New York,[47] reported general lack of appetite, although that group was more likely to have diets containing less than 67% of the RDA for at least one nutrient. (Smoking habits were not evaluated in these reports.) Poor appetite among institutionalized aged can reflect dissatisfaction with the food service or need for

attention.[36] People with chewing or multiple health problems are more likely to have poor appetites.[36,39] Anorexia is a common side effect of many prescription drugs used in treating chronic diseases, which may explain the reduced appetites reported by some aged[63] (see Chapter 9).

Scores on a life satisfaction rating (LSR), evaluating degree of adjustment to aging, were related to appetite in 60 older women residing either at home or in a nursing home.[36] All but five were ambulatory and all were able to feed themselves. In general, nursing home residents expressed more dissatisfaction than those living at home. Those with LSR scores above the mean rated their appetites as good and consumed more calories (1600 versus 1200). (Caloric intake was estimated from a graph.) Although appetite was reduced in dissatisfied nursing home patients, depression did not influence food intake among aged couples or single women living in the community.[68] Dissatisfaction or hopelessness may be more acute in an institutionalized group. This finding underscores the need to monitor food intake in extended care facilities (see Chapter 10).

Taste and Smell. Early work established that taste sensitivity to all four modalities (sweet, sour, salty, and bitter) declines after age 55.[16,33] This loss occurs in both sexes and is accelerated in heavy smokers.[42] Food technologists are currently using amino acids to improve both food flavor (sweetener) and quality.[70] Older people (mean age = 78) had taste detection thresholds for amino acids 2.5 times higher than those of young adults (mean age = 21). There were no differences between sexes; all persons tested were nonsmokers. Loss of taste has been related to observed decreases in both the number of tongue fungiform papillae and the number of taste buds per papillae. People at age 70 have 70% fewer taste buds than young adults.[41]

Reduced levels of testosterone and estrogen resulting in slowed cell division have been postulated as contributing to loss of taste.[70] Since taste bud receptor cells turn over every 10 days, a change in mitotic activity could reduce the number of receptor cells. Sensory cells within the taste bud have fingerlike projections that touch the surface of the tongue and respond to the chemical components in food.[41] Impulses produced by the taste cell are passed along afferent fibers to the central nervous system. When new cells are formed, a connecting synapse must be developed. Age-related changes in this process may also contribute to reduced taste perception.

Wearing of dentures or use of certain prescription drugs may contribute to reduced taste. Nutritional status may influence taste since vitamins A and B_{12} and folic acid are required for cell division within the taste apparatus[41]; poor zinc status, however, has not been shown to be a primary cause of decreased taste sensitivity in older people (see Chapter 7).

Perceived taste is a function of both taste and smell.[69,71] Healthy aged are less able to differentiate between food odors and correctly identify a test substance as compared with younger individuals. How changes in taste and odor influence the older person's selection and enjoyment of food has not been evaluated. In practice, the tendency to use generous quantities of salt may be an effort to strengthen this flavor when sensitivity has declined. Although an intense degree of sweetness becomes unpleasant in younger people, there is no similar response among aged people who have distorted taste perception. This may explain why some older people crave high sugar items.[41]

Dental Problems. Pathology of the soft tissues of the mouth is common in older people despite the absence of subjective symptoms. In a series of 785 veterans (age 45 to 97), 81% had oral lesions relating to ill-fitting dentures, nutrient deficiency, or the aging process.[6] Although the most common dental problem is loss of teeth, mastication may also be hindered by the wearing down of the occluding surfaces of the teeth in those retaining their natural teeth. Nizel[59] observed a decreased

Table 11-1. Dental status of persons age 65 to 74

Edentulous (both jaws)	46%
Edentulous (one jaw)	15%
Requiring immediate treatment (denture repair, periodontal disease or extraction)	61%
Requiring full denture	25%

Modified from United States Department of Health, Education and Welfare: Basic data on dental examination findings of persons 1-74 years. United States, 1971-1974, DHEW Publication No. (PHS) 79-1662, Hyattsville, Md., 1979, U.S. Government Printing Office.

range of movement of the jaws in some older people.

Data from a recent National Health Survey point to the existing dental needs of many aged[88] (Table 11-1). Periodontal disease results in loosening and eventual loss of teeth. Economic problems prevent some from seeking professional services for repair or replacement of dentures.[24] Nutrients sometimes affected by dental problems are protein, ascorbic acid, and vitamin A, since meat and some fruits and vegetables might be omitted from the diet if mastication is painful or difficult.[17,26,50]

Studies of both urban[47] and rural aged[35,65] suggest that chewing problems do not significantly influence intakes of these nutrients. A comparison of hemoglobin, serum folic acid, and serum vitamin B_{12} levels in 582 aged subjects who had either satisfactory dentures or no teeth and no dentures revealed only one significant difference.[4] Hemoglobin levels were higher in women with dentures (13.3 versus 12.7 gm/100 ml); however, this could also reflect an age difference, as women with dentures were younger (74.7 versus 76.4 years).

An evaluation of 58 residents of a veterans home before and after they were fitted with dentures revealed no differences in the frequency of eating protein foods, vitamin C–rich foods, or cooked dark green and yellow vegetables.[3] These men did increase servings of crisp raw vegetables and decrease servings of breads and cereals after being fitted with dentures. Wearing of dentures allowed greater selection within food groups because certain meats, raw vegetables and fruits, and nuts could now be consumed. An equally important finding was their greater enjoyment from eating when chewing was easier.

The lack of striking differences in foods consumed by efficient or nonefficient masticators could mean that food is swallowed before it is properly chewed. Individuals with poorer ability to chew or lacking teeth do not chew their food longer than those better able to masticate food.[58] Although not significant, incidence of gastric distress was more frequent among hospital patients with chewing problems,[57] suggesting the need for further evaluation of this question.

Providing quality nutrient sources requiring only limited chewing should be a priority in menu development. Dairy products, eggs, and well-cooked chicken and fish are good sources of high quality protein. Fruit juices and cooked vegetables can provide vitamins A and C. Many fresh fruits such as apples, melons, or bananas can be eaten by those who are partially or completely edentulous if the fruit is ripe, peeled, and cut into small pieces. Ground meats may be necessary in some cases. Pureed food should be considered only when all other possibilities have been exhausted.

Physical Health

Physical Disability. As pointed out in Chapter 1, a significant number of older people living in the community have some limitation in activity that can affect both food procurement and preparation. If limited in either vision or movement the older person may not be able to shop for groceries; therefore all food supplies must be delivered. Preparing vegetables can be difficult for one whose hands are crippled with arthritis; moving about the kitchen requires special effort for a person who must grasp a cane or walker. Poor eyesight can interfere with reading a nutrition label or package directions for preparation.

Unfortunately, there has been little nutritional evaluation of people with physical disability who live at home. Lonergan and associates[51] observed that several aged British women with failing vision and osteoarthritis of the hands and joints had poor calorie intakes (1000 kcal or less) and low skinfold thicknesses. Among long term patients in a geriatric facility,[53] poor protein status and below normal skinfold thicknesses were the result of poor energy intake prior to admission. Undernutrition was especially evident among those with severe arthritis. One fourth of all older people with activity limitations have arthritis.[87] These individuals may require special services such as home-delivered meals or a homemaker aide (see Chapter 12).

Older women in Kansas (n = 102) increased their use of frozen pot pies, frozen dinners, canned soups, and packaged mixes in an effort to simplify meal preparation,[15] although this is not a consistent pattern among older homemakers. Convenience foods are frequently viewed as more expensive and poorer in flavor than homemade.[66] Increased use of highly processed foods can have a detrimental effect on intakes of trace minerals and enhance intakes of sodium and fat. Nutrition education should focus on wise selection of convenience foods. Finally, there should be continuing effort on the part of food technologists to develop convenience items high in nutritional quality.

Prescribed Diets. Chronic diseases such as diabetes, cardiovascular problems, or gallbladder disorders frequently include a dietary prescription. It has been estimated that 18% to 43% of older individuals are following a special diet with restricted intakes of sodium, fat, cholesterol, calories, or carbohydrates.[11,39,47,80] Weight reduction is the most common problem among those referred for nutrition counseling.[80]

In an outpatient geriatric arthritis program nearly 25% of the 680 participants were following a special diet.[80] Of concern are the sources of the diets followed (Table 11-2). About one fifth had obtained their diet information from someone other

Table 11-2. Number of older persons obtaining special diets from various sources

Type of Diet	Source of Diet		
	Doctor or Nurse	Dietitian	Other
Weight reduction	13	7	18
Bland, low residue	26	5	5
Low sodium	14	5	2
Diabetic	16	10	6
Low cholesterol, low fat	11	2	1

Modified from Templeton, C.L.: Nutritional counseling needs in a geriatric population, Geriatrics **33**:59, 1978.

than a health professional. Nearly half of those attempting to lose weight had planned their own diet, consulted a friend, or used another nonprofessional source. Low calorie diets, poorly planned and lacking in essential vitamins and minerals, were a problem in older Rochester households.[47] Sugar, potatoes, and alcohol were avoided by men attempting to lose weight, although some women were still consuming cookies, cake, and other sweets while deleting nutrient-dense foods.[50] High fat, high protein, low carbohydrate diets popularized by the media place a heavy solute load on the kidney and may lead to loss of potassium and electrolyte imbalance.

Diets believed to either prevent or alleviate arthritis, if continued over long periods, are dangerous to health.[49,80] Some older people have eliminated milk, citrus fruit, or bread from their diets on the basis that these foods cause arthritis.[80] One patient was advised to avoid meat, milk, cheese, and bread, and reduce her intake of butter and eggs.[49] She continued to follow this diet for 10

years and when brought in for examination had developed both anemia and osteomalacia.

This points to the importance of continued follow-up of an aged person who has been placed on a modified diet. Although the plan may be designed for short-term treatment or be tentative based on the patient's response, the individual may continue to follow the diet when it is no longer appropriate. Diets severely restricted in fat can result in linoleic acid deficiency if a good source (unsaturated vegetable oil) is not included daily. Low residue bland diets deleting acid and fibrous fruits and vegetables and whole grain breads and cereals compromise intakes of vitamins A and C, iron, the trace minerals, and fiber.

Prescribed diets may have a *positive* influence on nutrient intake if foods high in calories and low in nutrient density are limited or deleted. Among older households in Rochester, New York, those following special diets (with the exception of weight reduction diets) selected food more wisely than did the group as a whole.[47] No diabetic consumed less than two thirds the recommended level of calories, protein, or the seven vitamins and minerals evaluated. The Exchange Lists for Meal Planning[2] developed by the American Dietetic Association and American Diabetes Association can be used in developing modified diets that include a variety of foods.

Deleting favorite foods from the diet or limiting use of salt, thereby altering flavor, reduces the pleasure associated with eating. Boykin[9] emphasizes an individual approach in developing a diet for an older person, recognizing the need to consider favorite foods based on the lifetime pattern even if they are inappropriate for the diet prescribed. How often and under what conditions such foods might be included in the diet should be based on a nutritional and health assessment in consultation with the patient's physician. Preparing a diet plan is a useless exercise if cooperation of the older client and his family is not achieved. Including the client in the decision-making process allows development of a diet that will be accepted and followed.

Food Tolerance. Some older individuals become increasingly sensitive to digestive upset and abdominal distress (see Chapter 4). Consequently, gas-forming, spicy, or fat-containing foods will be consumed seldom, if at all. The potential loss of linoleic acid from the diet has been mentioned; persons with low fat intakes absorb the fat soluble vitamins less efficiently. A common complaint is intolerance of gas-forming foods such as legumes, which are good sources of dietary fiber. In a survey of older Michigan women 17% avoided dried cooked beans, 9% avoided onions, and 5% avoided cabbage.[39] In those diets, however, 21% of the total fiber was supplied by cooked vegetables and 19% by bread. Avoidance of particular vegetables therefore does not necessarily lead to reduced fiber intake. In the relatively healthy individual food intolerance should not seriously affect the nutrient quality of the diet.

SOCIOLOGIC ASPECTS OF FOOD SELECTION

Life-style and living situation influence both eating pattern and food habits. Retirement from regular employment increases leisure time and sometimes leads to a change in residence. Death of a spouse may initiate or increase participation in a congregate meal program. Such factors should be considered when counseling the older client.

Living Situation

People continuing to live in their own homes usually have adequate facilities for food storage and preparation including a working stove, oven, and refrigerator. The type and size of appliance will affect use. With rising utility costs older people may hesitate to heat their conventional oven for one item such as a baked potato. A small electric appliance that can function as an oven is a wise investment for the person living alone or cooking for only two. An older style refrigerator with a very small freezer compartment presents problems for one who shops only infrequently. Food storage and preparation facilities are sometimes less than adequate in senior housing apartments with little or no counter space, limited storage area, and an apartment-sized refrigerator with little freezer space.

Individuals who rent a room with no access to kitchen facilities are forced to eat in restaurants or elsewhere. They may attempt to heat some foods on a hotplate in their room or use a heating coil for hot water for soup or beverages. Doughnuts, rolls, and similar items may form a major portion of the diet.[1] In urban locations it is difficult to find restaurants serving nourishing meals at low or moderate cost. These individuals should be directed to Title III-C congregate meal programs (see Chapter 12) or similar community projects. Nutrition education should focus on nutrient-dense food items that can be safely stored and eaten without refrigeration.

Food Shopping

Physical limitations, lack of transportation, and the changing locations of supermarkets present problems in food shopping. Seventy percent of older people reported problems with food shopping while only 20% had difficulty with meal preparation after food was brought into the home.[32] Poor eyesight makes it difficult to see items on the shelf.[55] Using a cane interferes with pushing a market basket. Supermarkets with bright glaring lights and long aisles present difficulties for those less physically adept.[76] Neighborhood grocery stores where a telephone call could bring delivery of a food order are disappearing rapidly.

If an automobile is not available for food shopping, the older person must ride the bus or walk to the store.[37,76,81] Sidewalks covered with ice and snow may preclude walking to the grocery store or carrying bundles home. In rural areas people can be shut in for days or even weeks during the winter months. Inability to shop frequently can limit intakes of perishable items such as dairy foods, fruits, vegetables and meats, particularly for those with inadequate storage space.[65] When groceries must be carried, lightweight dehydrated foods and packaged mixes may be selected rather than fresh, frozen, or canned ingredients, which are heavier.

Older people forced to shop at a store within walking distance are at a decided disadvantage. In rural areas if there is a store within walking distance, it is usually a general store with a limited variety of items and package sizes. In addition to poor selection, prices tend to be higher.[65] Urban aged have a similar problem as inner city supermarkets are closed because of poor profit margins and the growth of suburban malls. Independently owned grocery markets are frequently replaced by self-service convenience stores with higher prices.[78] A study of older shoppers revealed that 20% of those who walked to the store lived at a distance of eight or more blocks.[76] As illustrated in Fig. 11-2, walking to the store and carrying heavy bags presents severe limitations for those who must use a cane. Research evaluating the influence of shopping patterns on the nutritional adequacy of the diet is not presently available.

Community projects to aid in food shopping have included subsidized transportation to the supermarket. On those days a supermarket may provide assistance by packaging small units such as one chicken leg or two or three pieces of assorted fruit. Helping older people with shopping might be encouraged for those seeking worthwhile volunteer activities.

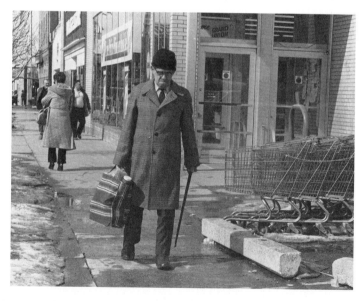

Fig. 11-2. Carrying groceries from the store is a difficult task for many older people.

Life-Style and Leisure Time

Number of Meals. Because the daily schedule is less rigid following retirement, many older people move away from the traditional pattern of three meals a day.[14,47,61-62] Among 680 Michigan aged (above age 55) 81% had three meals, 17% had two meals, and 3% had one meal each day.[80] Frequently, breakfast and lunch are combined. Of 47 older persons interviewed in Ithaca, New York (age 60 to 93), none had breakfast daily.[14] In a USDA survey about half of the older participants had their main meal at noon.[61] This has important implications for both home-delivered meal programs[18] and the Title III-C congregate meal program,[62] which serve at noon. Another common pattern is a late morning brunch and a second meal in late afternoon.[72] Decreasing the number of meals each day may represent an effort to control calorie intake. This is not always successful, however; in a study of 28 Michigan women the individual with the highest caloric intake (2153 kcal) consumed only two meals each day, but each contained substantial portions of food.[72]

Snacking. Snacking or eating between meals is popular among older people and frequently occurs in the evening.[14,47] About half of 504 New York aged reported snacking regularly.[14,47] A common snack of both men and women is coffee.[61] In general, however, men tend to choose more nutritious snacks than women.[47] Favorite items for men include milk and fruit as well as sweet baked items; women are more likely to select sweet baked goods. Beer and wine are other frequent snacks. Snacking can have a positive effect on the nutrient content of the diet; for one group snacks supplied more calcium than foods consumed with meals, and ascorbic acid from snacks equaled that consumed at breakfast.[47]

For retired people snacking is related to leisure time activity. The more hours of television they watch daily, the greater is the percentage of their total calories contributed by snacks.[14] Television viewing in the evening has been positively related to both fat and calorie intakes among 47 New York aged.[14] In those individuals the overall quality of the diet deteriorated as the proportion of calories from snacks increased. On the average 14% of all calories (range = 6% to 52%) came from snack foods. (Snack foods included sweet baked items, crackers, fruit drinks, soft drinks, potato chips, and candy.) For many older people, particularly those with limited mobility or no transportation, television is a favored pastime. In the study described people watched television about 5 hours each day. Since this does present an ideal environment for snacking, emphases in nutrition education should be the selection of nutritious snacks and planning for these items in the total daily meal pattern.

Social Activity

For the older individual food fulfills social as well as physiologic needs.[77] Although it is true that a person eating alone may not feel motivated to prepare adequate meals, available evidence does not support the common generalization that older individuals in one person households have poorer diets than those in households of two or more. Those with greater social participation have in some cases better diet scores, possibly relating to the variety of foods consumed.[17,34] A subsample of Boston aged who lived and ate their meals alone had a more limited variety of foods (53 versus 71) than those living with spouse or other family and were more likely to have below recommended levels of vitamin A, thiamin, riboflavin, and niacin.[17] Seven of the 10 had only a hotplate or a room with kitchen privileges, and this group was 8 years older than those living in a family situation. Therefore age with accompanying physical disability, poverty, and inadequate cooking facilities may also have contributed to the differences in dietary quality.

Socioeconomic status influences both social participation and nutrition in older people living alone.[14,34,52] Urban aged with higher incomes entertained at meals and ate in restaurants with friends more frequently than those with limited incomes and had higher intakes of iron, calories, B complex vitamins, protein, and ascorbic acid.[34] Low income aged in Vancouver had few visitors at mealtime (75% had one or less per month).[48] Frequency of visitors at mealtime may differ according to local expectations of host and guest. Toronto aged had mealtime visitors on a regular basis and served food items that they usually ate themselves (e.g., macaroni and cheese, tomato soup, frozen fish fillets).[45] There is no doubt that company at meals can have a positive influence on food intake, particularly for those who may not be motivated to cook for themselves.

A report from Dublin comparing aged who (1) lived with relatives, (2) lived alone and attended a day club providing a meal at noon, or (3) lived alone and received meals on wheels suggests that physical disability contributes to poor nutrient intake in aged living alone.[93] Those living with relatives met recommended intakes of protein, iron, and ascorbic acid, although calcium was low (239 mg). Diets of meal club participants contained more calcium (447 mg) but less ascorbic acid (32 mg). Although meals on wheels recipients had intakes similar to club attenders on delivery days, their diets consisted of bread and tea on weekends.[18,93]

The individual living alone who is confined to the home or has difficulty moving about may not have adequate food on nondelivery days or on sick days. If there is no one else in the household and a neighbor or support person is unavailable, the individual forced to remain in bed will have nothing to eat or drink. Such a situation can result in dehydration as well as malnutrition (Chapter 7). Ehrlich[23] described the isolation of older persons living in hotels and rooming houses in the inner city (single room occupancy) with no cooking facilities, very little income, and in some cases no friends. Meals often consisted of donuts and coffee. Presently, there is no information concerning the food intake and nutritional status of this group nor estimates of their number.[90]

A recent dietary and biochemical evaluation of 150 single and married men and women in Vancouver found no differences in levels of hemoglobin or transferrin, plasma vitamins (A, C, and E), or urinary vitamins (thiamin, riboflavin, and niacin) on the basis of household size.[48] Only one married man had low transferrin saturation; all other values were within normal ranges. Based on Canadian standards more single women than married women had inadequate intakes of protein (7% versus 0%), and niacin (33% versus 22%). More married women were inadequate in calcium (41% versus 16%) and thiamin (27% versus 16%). Single men tended to be low in iron, vitamin C, and niacin; married men were low in calcium and niacin. Single persons consumed more dairy products, which could relate to the lack of preparation required. About half of all persons interviewed did not eat fruits and vegetables, although this did not relate to ability to chew.

In general, single persons do not always have poorer diets than married persons of the same sex.[11,48,68] Cooking facilities, age, and physical disability contribute when differences are observed. Women living alone are more likely to be older than those living with a spouse, and they generally have lower incomes. Among women education is positively related to quality of diet.[68] An area for further study is the food pattern of widows versus single women. The individual accustomed to eating alone may be less vulnerable to inadequacy in later years than one for whom it is a new experience.

Sex

Single older men tend to have poorer diets than single older women.[25,47,65] Although these men are usually not accustomed to food preparation, other factors such as education, income, or food preferences may enter in. Single men consume few fruits and vegetables with consequent poor intakes of vitamins A and C,[40,65] although they drink generous quantities of milk providing riboflavin and calcium.[47] The greater vulnerability of older single men, particularly those above 75 years of age, is illustrated by a British study that found 41% of single men above age 75 to have low skinfold thicknesses as compared to only 22% of men of similar age living with relatives.[25]

ECONOMIC ASPECTS OF FOOD SELECTION

Women and minority groups are most likely to be poor (see Chapter 1), and this influences food patterns in various ways. First, the level of income will determine how much money can be spent for food. Second, the low income individual is less likely to own a car to simplify grocery shopping and is more likely to live in either the inner city or a rural area where food is more expensive. Therefore the buying power of the money available is reduced.

Food Budget

Older households spend a larger proportion of their total income on food than younger households (21.5% versus 16.9%).[30] Because the per capita income of older people is less, increasing the percentage spent for food may still not provide equivalent food dollars. Older people do spend less of their food dollar on food away from home (less than 20% as compared to 30% among younger families).[30] When older persons do eat outside of their homes on a regular basis, they often select a Title III-C congregate meal program requiring only a donation. The social life of younger people often revolves around eating in commercial restaurants; older individuals are more likely to eat at each others' homes or meet at a church or senior center for a pot luck social. Limiting the amount of money spent at restaurants may represent a conscious effort by older people to use their food dollars to best advantage. Lack of transportation or physical disability also interferes with eating outside the home.

In general, older households apportion their food dollars among the food groups in about the same way as younger households. Older people spend about 1% to 2% less on red meats, dairy products, nonalcoholic beverages, and prepared foods and about 3% to 4% more on fruits and vegetables than do other households.[29] This suggests that older families continue their established eating patterns rather than making radical changes. Vegetables, particularly potatoes, are a staple in many older households.[74] The inflation of the past decade did lead some older persons to reduce their intakes of meat and protein foods.[37]

Level of Income and Nutritional Adequacy

Both national[89] and regional surveys[35] suggest a relationship between income and nutritional adequacy. In the Ten State Survey (see Chapter 10) aged from low income ratio states had a higher incidence of inadequate iron, protein, and vitamin intakes. Low income older persons consume less food[89] and the items selected differ from those with higher incomes. In a national survey of single person households, low income aged spent a greater portion of their food money on cereals and baked products than those of higher income.[74] Low and high income older women spent about the same percentage of their food money on meat, fish, poultry, and eggs (32.6% versus 30.1%), although low income women bought fewer fruits and vegetables. Low income older men spent more money on protein foods and less on fruits and vegetables than higher income men. In real dollars low income women and men spent 15% and 30% less, respectively, on food than their higher income counterparts.

These data suggest that low income aged try to use wisely the food money available, focusing on nutrient-dense protein foods although this may be at the expense of fruits and vegetables. Bread and cereals add bulk at relatively low cost if total food is limited. Low income aged spent less of their food money on prepared foods, which may reflect an effort to control cost.

It is easier to obtain a nutritionally adequate diet as the food money available increases. Older households in Rochester, New York,[47] were grouped according to spending levels suggested by the USDA food plans.[86] Sixty-one percent on the low budget had diets containing less than two thirds the RDA for at least one nutrient; in contrast only 2% with a liberal budget failed to obtain at least 67% of the RDA for all nutrients evaluated. Nevertheless, wise selection is still a factor, as 33% on the low budget consumed 67% of the RDA for all nutrients and 6% met 100% of the RDA.

It is difficult to separate the effects of income,

education, and ethnic group on food intake. Kohrs and coworkers[44] found that intakes of total fat, protein, thiamin, and niacin were higher among aged with more than 12 years of school as compared to 8 or fewer years of school. Older people with less education are more likely to have lower incomes and at the same time may have fewer sources of information. The individual with limited reading ability has less opportunity to learn about diet selection.

Both income and ethnic group influence food selection[89] (Fig. 11-3). Calories decrease with income in both black and white women, although

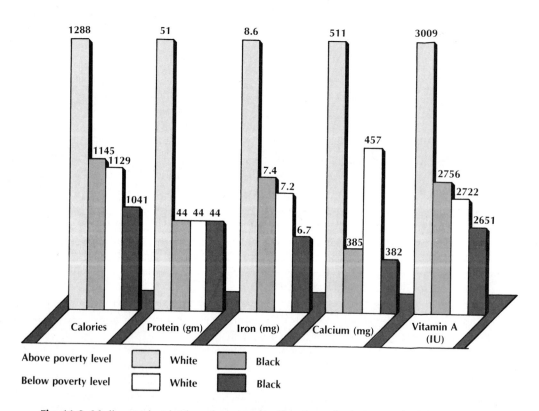

Fig. 11-3. Median nutrient intakes of women age 65 and over by income and ethnic group. (Data from United States Department of Health, Education, and Welfare: Dietary intake source data. United States, 1971-1974, DHEW Publication No. [PHS] 19-1221, Hyattsville, Md., 1979, U.S. Government Printing Office.)

blacks consume less food regardless of income. The similarity in protein intake between both income groups confirms the earlier suggestion that older people recognize the importance of protein foods. Differences in consumption of calcium-rich dairy foods relate to ethnic preferences as well as income. Iron intake would decline if vegetable proteins (lower in cost) were substituted for meat, fish, or poultry, and breads and cereals were replaced with sweet baked products.

Vitamin A calculated per 1000 kcal was higher among those with lower incomes. White women above the poverty level consumed 2332 IU (vitamin A)/1000 kcal, whereas black women below the poverty level consumed 2539 IU/1000 kcal, suggesting efforts in food selection. Iron intake per 1000 kcal was 6.7 and 6.4 mg in high and low income groups, respectively. The nutritional vulnerability of low income women in general and black women in particular is emphasized by the fact that median intakes are about two thirds the RDA for iron and vitamin A and less than half the RDA for calcium. Therefore 50% of those surveyed were consuming less than these amounts.

Influence of Food Stamps

Food assistance programs that increase buying power can improve the quality of the diet. Unfortunately, eligible older persons are less likely to participate in food stamp programs than eligible younger persons; 40% of eligible nonparticipants are age 65 or over.[30,73] Older persons may be less

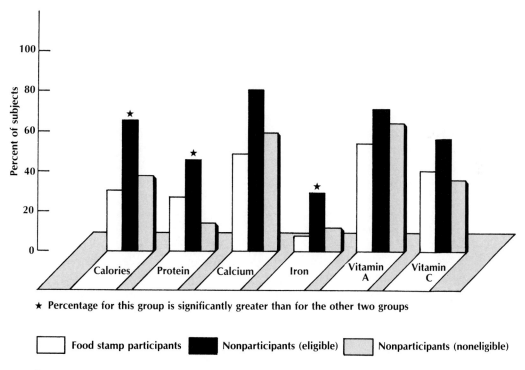

★ **Percentage for this group is significantly greater than for the other two groups**

☐ Food stamp participants   ■ Nonparticipants (eligible)   ▨ Nonparticipants (noneligible)

Fig. 11-4. Influence of food stamps on percent of persons consuming less than two thirds the RDA. (Data from Guthrie, H.A., Black, K., and Madden, J.P.: Nutritional practices of elderly citizens in rural Pennsylvania, Gerontologist **12**:330, 1972.)

well informed concerning available programs, may lack transportation to the appropriate office, or may choose not to apply because of pride. Efforts to ease these problems have included processing food stamp applications by mail or telephone for those lacking transportation. This also eliminates the embarrassment of having to appear at the county assistance or welfare office. Although consideration has been given to providing cash payments rather than food stamps, the fact remains that cash could be used for pressing needs other than food such as fuel, housing, or medical expenses.[73]

Guthrie and coworkers[35] compared the nutrient intakes of (1) aged food stamp recipients, (2) eligible aged nonrecipients, and (3) noneligible aged. Intakes of key nutrients did not differ between the food stamp recipients and those of higher income; however, low income households declining food stamps had poorer diets (Fig. 11-4). Nutrients significantly reduced were those found in meat, poultry, and fish, items limited on a low cost budget.

A USDA evaluation of 854 older persons either receiving or eligible to receive food stamps suggests that men and people age 75 and over benefit most from food stamps.[85] Intakes of protein, calcium, magnesium, and vitamin A did not differ between participating and nonparticipating women age 65 to 74; those receiving food stamps had higher intakes of vitamin B_{12}, although both groups met at least 100% of the RDA (182% versus 126%). Mean intakes of vitamin B_6 ranged from 51% to 59% of the RDA among all women evaluated. Men age 75 or over not receiving food stamps met less than 67% of the RDA for calories, magnesium, and vitamin B_6 and only 71% of the RDA for vitamin A. Men of similar age receiving food stamps met at least three fourths the RDA for all nutrients except vitamin B_6.

Magnesium and vitamin B_6 were particularly low in all diets. This could indicate use of more highly processed bread and cereal products and less use of vegetables, meat, poultry, and fish. Food selec-

tion patterns might be improved further by nutrition education programs directed toward these groups.

FOOD APPLICATIONS FOR SPECIAL NEEDS

Older people who are seriously ill or recovering from illness are sometimes not able to feed themselves. This can be a temporary situation with self-feeding resumed as strength is regained. In the case of stroke or chronic neurologic disorder such as parkinsonism, some degree of paralysis or incoordination can be permanent and interfere with the normal motions required for self-feeding.

Helping the Physically Impaired

An individual's attitude toward both food and mealtime is more likely to be positive if self-feeding is possible. Achieving this level of independence supports both physical and mental well-being. Problems in self-feeding may be caused by weakness in the hand or arm making it difficult to lift a cup or spoon. Partial paralysis can limit range of motion or make it difficult to flex the fingers and hand to grasp a cup or fork.[43]

Utensils for Self-Feeding. Various devices have been developed to help disabled individuals feed themselves.[43,54] In many cases only a slight modification of existing utensils will facilitate food handling. Special aids are often available from local hospital supply companies or can be ordered by mail. (See Selected Resources at the end of this chapter.)

Cups. Lightweight plastic cups are easier to handle when filled with liquid than glass or china cups. A cup with a partial lid or small opening (plastic travel cup) will prevent spills for those with abrupt movements and poor coordination. A stretch-knit coaster slipped onto the bottom of a glass or an adhesive-backed bathtub safety tread attached around the sides provides a nonslippery surface for grasping.[43]

Forks and Spoons. Utensils with extra-thick bamboo or plastic handles are easier to grasp if flexing the fingers is difficult. An inexpensive solution is placing a foam rubber curler over the handle of a standard utensil, as the foam surface increases the friction and aids in holding. For those unable to grasp, a cuff with a pocket holding a standard utensil can be slipped over the hand. A swivel spoon or extra long handle is helpful when motion is limited.[43]

Plates and Bowls. A suction device to prevent the dish from moving or a plate with a broad edge to push food against will help those with limited motor skills. Because self-feeding can require considerable time, a plastic dish with a lower compartment filled with hot water will keep food at a palatable temperature.[43,54] For the older individual who is returning to his own home, meal preparation must also be resumed. Resources for use in helping the handicapped regain skills for simple meal preparation are provided at the end of this chapter.

Facilitating Self-Feeding. Relearning feeding skills can be a long and difficult process. Careful selection of food served and a positive approach will facilitate progress and encourage effort.

Types of Food for Self-Feeding. A soft diet rather than pureed foods is not only more palatable but requires less skill in eating. Foods should not be cut into many small pieces; fewer motions are required to eat fewer medium-sized pieces.[54] Finger foods require less effort and energy for eating. Ideas for making difficult items into finger foods include putting ground meat in a roll, folding a pancake in half so it can be picked up, serving an egg hard cooked (must be peeled), or cutting an orange in halves or quarters to be eaten out of the rind. An easy to eat meal might include a sandwich (avoiding soft fillings that tend to fall out), soup served in a mug, apple slices (peeled and cored), and a carton of milk with a straw.[21,54]

Environment for Self-Feeding. Attention and praise provide incentive for continuing a painful and frustrating activity. Having the individuals in a self-feeding program sit at a table facing each other promotes both social interaction and mutual support as patients become helpful to each other.[19,20] Reducing the general noise level so that patients may more easily converse with staff members and each other contributes to a positive meal environment.[19] Sensitizing staff members to avoid negative outbursts such as scolding a self-feeding patient who has accidentally spilled food is essential for a rehabilitation program to be a success.[20]

The individual regaining self-feeding skills eats very slowly, particularly at the beginning of the rehabilitation program as muscle coordination is developing. Sufficient time to complete the meal should be planned before the tray is removed.[21,54]

Feeding the Chronically Ill

Preserving the dignity of the individual who has to be fed will influence his receptivity to the food offered. The emotional empathy between the individual performing the feeding and the patient is critical. Miller[56] described an 83-year-old woman with a bone fracture, parkinsonism, and organic brain syndrome who weighed 91 pounds on admission to an extended care facility. She was described as difficult to feed, and over the next 4 months she lost 20 pounds. When a particular nurse developed and carried out a feeding program including self-feeding whenever possible, the patient gained 9½ pounds in 3 weeks. An important consideration for a patient who will accept only a limited amount of food is the nutrient density of what is fed. Eight tablespoons of ice cream will provide more than twice the calories in 8 tablespoons of corn.

When a patient is consistently losing weight one factor may be the behavior of the patient. Feeding can be difficult with a patient who is mentally or emotionally disturbed.[56] The individual may refuse to swallow, take food in and then spit it out, or push away the food and the spoon. When an individual is unable to feed himself and refuses to be fed, intervention in the form of gastric tube feeding or intravenous feeding becomes necessary.

When a patient tires easily, helping him into a comfortable, sitting-up position encourages cooperation. (Patients should not be fed in a supine position.) Foods should be soft, easily chewed, and free of lumps. Sufficient time must be allowed for chewing and swallowing; foods should not be forced. Sips of water should be offered frequently. Frequent small feedings throughout the day may be more successful than three large meals.[27] Foods should be served in small amounts so they remain the proper temperature.[21,56]

Frail aged have problems both masticating and swallowing food (see Chapter 4). Fear of choking leads to rejection of food, particularly if it is being forced into the mouth too rapidly. Food aspiration can occur in forced feeding.[31]

Patient feeding and rehabilitation must be a cooperative effort between the nurse and dietitian.[64] Feeding patients who cannot feed themselves is a time-consuming process. The rehabilitation required to help a disabled patient relearn self-feeding skills demands careful planning and supervision. The dietary intake of patients with feeding problems should be monitored carefully. Collaborative effort involving nursing and physical therapy will be necessary if each patient is to reach the maximum level of independence possible.[21]

DIETARY PATTERNS: IMPLICATIONS FOR NUTRITION EDUCATION

In general most older people regularly consume some protein foods (meat, fish, poultry, and eggs); over 90% of low income aged (854 persons nationwide) had at least one serving on a 24-hour recall record.[85] Mean intake was about 6½ ounces. Breads and cereals are popular and most studies agree that these items are consumed daily. In a recent report, about one fifth of low income persons age 75 or above had a ready to eat cereal on the day of the interview.[84] Contrary to popular opinion only about one third had a sweet baked product.

Consumption of fluid milk is low in aged men and women. Although over three fourths report using milk on a daily basis, this represents only 250 to 300 mg calcium equivalent or about 1 to 1½ cups of milk per day.[85] Dark green and deep yellow vegetables are consumed in low amounts, particularly among men. Although three fourths of low income aged had at least one vegetable daily, less than 10% of men and 20% of women had a good source of vitamin A. With the exception of men age 75 or over, three fourths reported having citrus fruit or juice on a regular basis.

Regardless of limited budgets older people appear to consume foods from the meat group on a regular basis. These items coupled with servings of enriched bread and ready to eat cereals should provide adequate iron, although iron absorption in older people is not well understood. Encouraging use of legumes and whole grain products would add to intakes of trace minerals such as zinc, magnesium, and chromium, which are usually lost in processing. Although frankfurters and luncheon meats were reported by less than 20% of low income aged interviewed by USDA,[84] protein foods lower in sodium and fat and providing more protein for less cost (see Chapter 5) should be emphasized.

Incorporating dairy products into the daily meal pattern is essential if intakes of calcium and riboflavin are to be adequate. These items also contribute vitamins A and D and protein and should be a priority in nutrition education. Finally, many older persons are not consuming adequate amounts of dark green or deep yellow vegetables. This may relate to cost or problems in preparation of fresh vegetables. Frozen vegetables with no added sodium could be an alternative to fresh, particularly in the winter months. Implementation of nutrition education will be discussed in Chapter 13.

SUMMARY

Adaptation to changes in life-style, health, and economic status can bring about changes in eating patterns. Increasing age and decreasing calorie requirements result in consumption of less food and can lead to nutritional inadequacy. Older persons do change their food patterns according to general food trends and product availability and therefore can be receptive to nutrition education.

Depression, loneliness, and diminished feelings of self-worth can lead to disinterest in food. Social activity is positively related to quality of the diet. Patients with organic brain syndrome who cannot feed themselves frequently exhibit weight loss and should be monitored closely. Efforts at rehabilitation of those patients with loss of motor skills or partial paralysis should include self-feeding.

Physical changes in taste and smell, loss of teeth, and physical disability can adversely affect nutrient intake. A person who is confined to his home and dependent on others for food delivery or unable to move about easily within the home to carry on meal preparation is forced to depend on convenience items and can have limited intakes of fresh produce or dairy products. Prescribed diets or drugs used in treatment of chronic disease can result in diminished appetite and problems in food selection. Snacking is an important component of the food pattern of many older people; therefore nutrition education should stress snack items high in nutrient density.

Low income older people have diets poorer in nutritional quality than higher income older persons. Food stamps do make a significant nutritional contribution to the diets of older recipients; eligible nonusers tend to have diets containing inadequate levels of many nutrients.

Although older people living alone may have poor diets, this is not always the case. Since such individuals are typically women with a limited income and advanced in age ($\geq$ age 75), factors other than eating alone contribute to the problem. Men living alone and persons above age 75 are at particular risk of dietary inadequacy.

REVIEW QUESTIONS

1. How does social isolation or living alone influence nutrient intake in older persons? What other factors may influence nutrient intake in these individuals? Cite research findings to justify your conclusion.
2. Which nutrients are most likely to be present in less than desirable amounts in a low income diet? Do low income aged make wise food choices? Develop a 2-week food shopping list for an older client within the budget limits of the USDA thrifty food plan.
3. How may (a) physical disability, (b) modified diets, (c) loss of taste, and (d) ill-fitting dentures influence food intake and dietary adequacy? Give examples.
4. Develop a plan for a self-feeding rehabilitation program to be implemented in an extended care facility. Include recommendations for food items to be served, self-feeding implements to be made or purchased, and procedures to be followed.
5. Mr. K. is 78 years old, lives alone, and is edentulous. He has a refrigerator with no freezer compartment and does his cooking on a two-burner hotplate. Because of his heart condition he takes diuretics regularly and his physician has advised him to avoid salt and foods high in sodium. Develop a nutritional care plan for Mr. K. including sample menus, recipe ideas, shopping hints, and referral to available nutrition programs.

REFERENCES

1. Abrams, M.: The SRO elderly from the perspective of a hotel owner. In The invisible elderly, Washington, D.C., 1976, National Council on the Aging.
2. American Diabetes Association, American Dietetics Association: Exchange lists for meal planning, New York, 1976, American Diabetes Association, American Dietetics Association.
3. Anderson, E.L.: Eating patterns before and after dentures, J. Am. Diet. Assoc. **58**:421, 1971.
4. Bates, J.F., Elwood, P.C., and Foster, W.: Studies relating mastication and nutrition in the elderly, Gerontol. Clin. **13**:227, 1971.
5. Beeuwkes, A.: Studying the food habits of the elderly, J. Am. Diet. Assoc. **37**:215, 1960.
6. Bhaskar, S.N.: Oral lesions in the aged population: A survey of 785 cases, Geriatrics **23**:137, 1968.
7. Blass, J.: Food selection in the aged, Int. J. Obes. **4**:377, 1980.
8. Blumenthal, G.: Emotional aspects of feeding the aged, J. Am. Diet. Assoc. **32**:829, 1956.
9. Boykin, L.S.: Soul foods for some older Americans, J. Am. Geriatr. Soc. **23**:380, 1975.
10. Boykin, L.S.: Problems of the older person in obtaining adequate nutrition, Aging, No. 311-312, p. 4, Sept.-Oct. 1980.
11. Brown, E.L.: Factors affecting food choices and intake, Geriatrics **31**:89, 1976.

12. Busse, E.W.: How mind, body, and environment influence nutrition in the elderly, Postgrad. Med. **63**:118, 1978.

13. Chinn, A.B.: Some problems of nutrition in the aged, JAMA **162**:1511, 1956.

14. Clancy, K.L.: Preliminary observations on media use and food habits of the elderly, Gerontologist **15**:529, 1975.

15. Clarke, M., and Wakefield, L.M.: Food choices of institutionalized vs. independent-living elderly, J. Am. Diet. Assoc. **66**:600, 1975.

16. Cooper, R.M., Bilash, I., and Zubek, J.P.: The effect of age on taste sensitivity, J. Gerontol. **14**:56, 1959.

17. Davidson, C.S., and others: The nutrition of a group of apparently healthy aging persons, Am. J. Clin. Nutr. **10**:181, 1962.

18. Davidson, F., and Butler, A.: 1. Diets of elderly men and women receiving meals on wheels, J. N.Z. Diet. Assoc. **25**:5, June 1971.

19. Davies, A.D.M., and Snaith, P.A.: Mealtime problems in a continuing-care hospital for the elderly, Age Ageing **9**:100, 1980.

20. Davies, A.D.M., and Snaith, P.A.: The social behaviour of geriatric patients at mealtimes: An observational and an intervention study, Age Ageing **9**:93, 1980.

21. Deibel, A.W.: Feeding elderly patients, JPN Ment. Health Serv. **10**:35, Jan.-Feb. 1972.

22. Donahue, W.T.: Psychologic aspects of feeding aged, J. Am. Diet. Assoc. **27**:461, 1951.

23. Ehrlich, P.: Study of the invisible elderly: Characteristics and needs of St. Louis downtown SRO elderly. In The invisible elderly, Washington, D.C., 1976, National Council on the Aging.

24. Epstein, S.: Dental care and the aging, Perspect. Aging **5**:14, 1976.

25. Exton-Smith, A.N., Chrm., Panel on Nutrition of the Elderly: A nutrition survey of the elderly, Reports on Health and Social Subjects No. 3, London, 1972, Her Majesty's Stationery Office.

26. Exton-Smith, A.N., and Stanton, B.R.: Report of an investigation into the dietary of elderly women living alone, London, 1965, King Edward's Hospital Fund for London.

27. Ford, M.G., and Neville, J.N.: Nutritive intake of nursing home patients served three or five meals a day, J. Am. Diet. Assoc. **61**:292, 1972.

28. Fry, P.C., Fox, H.M., and Linkswiler, H.: Nutrient intakes of healthy older women, J. Am. Diet. Assoc. **42**:218, 1963.

29. Gallo, A.E., and Boehm, W.T.: Food purchasing patterns of senior citizens, Nat. Food Rev. **4**(3):42, 1978.

30. Gallo, A.E., Salathe, L.E., and Boehm, W.T.: Senior citizens: Food expenditure patterns and assistance, Agricultural Economics Report No. 426, Washington, D.C., 1979, U.S. Department of Agriculture.

31. Gelperin, A.: Sudden death in an elderly population from aspiration of food, J. Am. Geriatr. Soc. **22**:135, 1974.

32. Gibson, M.J.: Nutrition programs for the aging: How effective are they, Aging Int. **9**(4):17, 1982/1983.

33. Glanville, E.V., Kaplan, A.R., and Fischer, R.: Age, sex, and taste sensitivity, J. Gerontol. **19**:474, 1964.

34. Grotkowski, M.L., and Sims, L.S.: Nutritional knowledge, attitudes, and dietary practices of the elderly, J. Am. Diet. Assoc. **72**:499, 1978.

35. Guthrie, H.A., Black, K., and Madden, J.P.: Nutritional practices of elderly citizens in rural Pennsylvania, Gerontologist **12**:330, 1972.

36. Harrill, I., Erbes, C., and Schwartz, C.: Observations on food acceptance by elderly women, Gerontologist **16**:349, 1976.

37. Heltsley, M.E.: Coping: The aged in small town, U.S.A., J. Home Econ. **68**:46, 1976.

38. Howell, S.C., and Loeb, M.B.: Nutrition and aging: A monograph for practitioners, Gerontologist **9**(suppl.):1, 1969.

39. Johnson, C.K., and others: Health, laxation, and food habit influences on fiber intake of older women, J. Am. Diet. Assoc. **77**:551, 1980.

40. Jordan, M., and others: Dietary habits of persons living alone, Geriatrics **9**:230, 1954.

41. Kamath, S.K.: Taste acuity and aging, Am. J. Clin. Nutr. **36**:766, 1982.

42. Kaplan, A.R., Glanville, E.V., and Fischer, R.: Cumulative effect of age and smoking on taste sensitivity in males and females, J. Gerontol. **20**:334, 1965.

43. Klinger, J.L., Frieden, F.H., and Sullivan, R.A., eds.: Mealtime manual for the aged and handicapped, New York, 1970, New York University Medical Center, Institute of Rehabilitation Medicine.

44. Kohrs, M.B., and others: Title VII-Nutrition Program for the Elderly, J. Am. Diet. Assoc. **75**:537, 1979.

45. Krondl, M., and others: Food use and perceived food meanings of the elderly, J. Am. Diet. Assoc. **80**:523, 1982.

46. Learner, R.M., and Kivett, V.R.: Discriminators of perceived dietary adequacy among the rural elderly, J. Am. Diet. Assoc. **78**:330, 1981.

47. LeBovit, C., and Baker, D.A.: Food consumption and dietary levels of older households in Rochester, New York, Home Economics Research Rep. No. 25, Washington, D.C., 1965, U.S. Department of Agriculture.

48. Leichter, J., Angel, J.F., and Lee, M.: Nutritional status of a select group of free-living elderly people in Vancouver, Can. Med. Assoc. J. **118**:40, 1978.

49. Leslie, J.: Nutrition and diet, the elderly, Nurs. Mirror p. 31, Aug. 25, 1977.

50. Lonergan, M.E.: Nutritional survey of the elderly, Nutrition **25**:30, 1971.

51. Lonergan, M.E., and others: A dietary survey of older people in Edinburgh, Br. J. Nutr. **34**:517, 1975.

52. Lyons, J.S., and Trulson, M.F.: Food practices of older people living at home, J. Gerontol. **11**:66, 1956.

53. MacLennan, W.J., Martin, P., and Mason, B.J.: Energy intake, disability, disease and skinfold thickness in a long-stay hospital, Gerontol. Clin. **17**:173, 1975.

54. Manning, A.M., and Means, J.G.: A self-feeding program for geriatric patients in a skilled nursing facility, J. Am. Diet. Assoc. **66**:275, 1975.

55. Mason, J.B., and Bearden, W.O.: Profiling the shopping behavior of elderly consumers, Gerontologist **18**:454, 1978.

56. Miller, M.B.: Unresolved feeding and nutrition problems of the chronically ill aged, Gerontologist **11**:329, 1971.

57. Mumma, R.D., and Quinton, K.: Effect of masticatory efficiency on the occurrence of gastric distress, J. Dent. Res. **49**:69, 1970.

58. Neill, D.J., and Phillips, H.I.B.: The masticatory performance, dental state, and dietary intake of a group of elderly army pensioners, Br. Dent. J. **128**:581, 1970.

59. Nizel, A.E.: Role of nutrition in the oral health of the aging patient, Dent. Clin. North Am. **20**:569, 1976.

60. Ohlson, M.A., and others: Dietary practices of 100 women from 40 to 75 years of age, J. Am. Diet. Assoc. **24**:286, 1948.

61. Pao, E.: Food patterns of the elderly, Fam. Ec. Rev., U.S. Department of Agriculture, p. 16, December 1971.

62. Pelcovits, J.: Nutrition for older Americans, J. Am. Diet. Assoc. **58**:17, 1971.

63. Physicians desk reference, ed. 34, Oradell, N.J., 1980, Medical Economics Company.

64. Piper, G.M., and Smith, E.M.: Geriatric nutrition, Nurs. Outlook **12**:51, 1964.

65. Rawson, I.G., and others: Nutrition of rural elderly in southwestern Pennsylvania, Gerontologist **18**:24, 1978.

66. Rountree, J.L., and Tinklin, G.L.: Food beliefs and practices of selected senior citizens, Gerontologist **15**:537, 1975.

67. Schafer, R.B., and Keith, P.M.: Influences on food decisions across the family life cycle, J. Am. Diet. Assoc. **78**:144, 1981.

68. Schafer, R.B., and Keith, P.M.: Social-psychological factors in the dietary quality of married and single elderly, J. Am. Diet. Assoc. **81**:30, 1982.

69. Schiffman, S.: Food recognition by the elderly, J. Gerontol. **32**:586, 1977.

70. Schiffman, S.S., Hornack, K., and Reilly, D.: Increased taste thresholds of amino acids with age, Am. J. Clin. Nutr. **32**:1622, 1979.

71. Schiffman, S.S., and Pasternak, M.: Decreased discrimi-nation of food odors in the elderly, J. Gerontol. **34**:73, 1979.

72. Schlenker, E.D.: Nutritional status of older women, Ph.D. thesis, Lansing, 1976, Michigan State University.

73. Sexauer, B.: Food problems of the low income elderly and disabled, Nat. Food Rev. **6**(2):19, 1980.

74. Sexauer, B.H., and Mann, J.S.: Food expenditure patterns of single-person households, Agricultural Economics Report No. 428, Washington, D.C., 1979, U.S. Department of Agriculture.

75. Sheraton, M.: Memories of hot cereal mornings, Modern Maturity **23**(1):21, Feb.-March 1980.

76. Sherman, E.M., and Brittan, M.R.: Contemporary food gatherers: A study of food shopping habits of an elderly urban population, Gerontologist **13**:358, 1973.

77. Sherwood, S.: Sociology of food and eating: Implications for action for the elderly, Am. J. Clin. Nutr. **26**:1108, 1973.

78. Stafford, T.H.: The convenience store industry, Nat. Food Rev. **5**(3):19, 1979.

79. Swanson, P., and others: Food intakes of 2189 women in five North Central states, North Central Regional Publ. No. 83, Ames, 1959, Iowa Agricultural and Home Economics Experiment Station, Iowa State College.

80. Templeton, C.L.: Nutritional counseling needs in a geriatric population, Geriatrics **33**:59, 1978.

81. Timmreck, T.C.: Nutrition problems: A survey of the rural elderly, Geriatrics **32**:137, 1977.

82. Tiven, M.B.: Older Americans: Special handling required, Washington, D.C., 1971, National Council on the Aging.

83. Troll, L.E.: Eating and aging, J. Am. Diet. Assoc. **59**:456, 1971.

84. United States Department of Agriculture: Food and nutrient intakes of individuals in 1 day, low-income households, November 1977–March 1978. Nationwide Food Consumption Survey 1977-1978, Preliminary Report No. 11, Washington, D.C., 1982, U.S. Government Printing Office.

85. United States Department of Agriculture: Food and nutrient intakes of individuals in 1 day, low-income households, November 1979–March 1980. Nationwide Food Consumption Survey 1977-1978, Preliminary Report No. 13, Washington, D.C., 1982, U.S. Government Printing Office.

86. United States Department of Agriculture: The thrifty food plan, Fam. Ec. Rev., p. 7, Fall, 1981.

87. United States Department of Health, Education and Welfare: Health, 1978, DHEW Publication No. (PHS) 78-1232, Hyattsville, Md., 1978, U.S. Government Printing Office.

88. United States Department of Health, Education and Welfare: Basic data on dental examination findings of persons

1-74 years. United States, 1971-1974, DHEW Publication No. (PHS) 79-1662, Hyattsville, Md., 1979, U.S. Government Printing Office.

89. United States Department of Health, Education and Welfare: Dietary intake source data. United States, 1971-74, DHEW Publication No. (PHS) 79-1221, Hyattsville, Md., 1979, U.S. Government Printing Office.

90. United States Senate Special Committee on Aging: Single room occupancy: A need for national concern, Washington, D.C., 1978, U.S. Government Printing Office.

91. Vincent, M., and Gibson, R.S.: Dietary intake of a group of chronic geriatric psychiatric patients, Gerontology **28:**245, 1982.

92. Weinberg, J.: Psychologic implications of the nutritional needs of the elderly, J. Am. Diet. Assoc. **60:**293, 1972.

93. Wilson, C.W., and Nolan, C.: The diets of elderly people in Dublin, Ir. J. Med. Sci. **3:**345, 1970.

SELECTED RESOURCES

Institute of Rehabilitation Medicine, New York University Medical Center and Campbell Soup Company: Mealtime management for people with disabilities and the aging, ed. 2, New York, 1978, Campbell Soup Co.

Klinger, J.L.: Self-help manual for arthritis patients, New York, 1980, Arthritis Foundation.

Sargent, J.V.: An easier way: Handbook for the elderly and handicapped, Ames, 1981, Iowa State University Press.

Chapter 12

Nutritional Contribution of Food Delivery Programs

Providing food for older people is an activity described in early folklore. In the well-known fairy tale, Little Red Riding Hood was visiting her grandmother and bringing a gift of food. When the extended family was the general rule older people lived with relatives who provided assistance as needed. If parents chose not to live with their adult children they were still nearby, either in the same town or on another section of the family farm. In recent years increased mobility has led to the establishment of the nuclear family. One consequence of this change is that some older people no longer have family members nearby to help with food-related problems. As a result other support systems have been developed by community organizations and government agencies to help meet this need. A health professional working with older clients should become familiar with (1) the food-related services available within the community, (2) the relative nutrient contribution of the food provided, and (3) the system for client referral.

FOOD DELIVERY PROGRAMS AND LONG TERM CARE

Need for Food Delivery

Confinement to Home. Food delivery programs serve clients with different needs, capabilities, and resources. Meals on Wheels has traditionally served homebound individuals, particularly those who also have difficulty moving about and preparing meals.[16] Meals served in a congregate set-ting provide an alternative for older people able to leave their homes.[19,67] The advantage of congregate meals is the opportunity for socialization adding to general well-being. Congregate meal programs may include a transportation component to provide for those who lack transportation and are unable to walk the distance required.[57]

Physical Disability. For the confined individual who is unable to prepare meals home-delivered meals can be a solution. For those who are able to move about easily within their homes but for one reason or another cannot leave their homes (e.g., spouse who cannot be left alone) delivery of groceries is a possibility.[26] In some communities homemaker services providing food shopping are available through a Home Health Agency or Visiting Nurses Association.[5]

Period of Time Using Service. Food delivery programs can provide assistance on a short term or long term basis. Home-delivered meals may be required on a temporary basis during recuperation from illness or permit the patient to be discharged from the hospital at an earlier date to complete convalescence at home.[11,16] Delivery of food to the home can provide long term maintenance (for a period of years) for an individual with some degree of disability who can safely remain at home.[16,41,69]

Congregate meal programs provide on-going nutrition and social services to older individuals in the community and thus support independent living.[42,67] People become eligible to participate in federally funded congregate meal programs (Title

III-C) at age 60 and can attend for the remainder of their lives. (The Title III-C program will be discussed in detail in a following section of this chapter.)

Concept of Long Term Care

Continuum of Support Services. Long term care refers to the medical and support services required to maintain the functionally impaired older individual at an optimum level of well-being.[58,62] An individual may require one service or a range of services. For the older person who can no longer handle bundles of groceries, delivery of groceries or help with grocery shopping may be the only service required. If the individual is unable to prepare meals, homemaker services or home-delivered meals may solve the problem. When help is needed with activities of daily living such as eating, dressing, or bathing, institutional care is most likely required.[53] This implies a need for a continuum of health services ranging from preventive measures such as regular physical examinations and congregate meals for the relatively healthy older person to the skilled nursing facility required for the individual with numerous medical problems who is confined to bed.[5]

Types of Support Services. Support services may be formal or informal.[58] Formal support services are provided by hospitals, home health agencies, or other community organizations, and payment either by the individual receiving the service or through personal or government insurance is required. Payment is not required for services provided under Title III-C of the Older Americans Act, which are available to all persons age 60 and over, although voluntary donations are encouraged.

Informal support services are provided by family members, friends, or neighbors usually at no cost. About 60% to 80% of disabled older persons are cared for by family members within the community.[58] Family care may continue for an extended period, until an acute illness or other crisis intensifies the burden making home care no longer possible. An older individual with impaired mobility may be cared for by a spouse or adult child who handles meal preparation and household chores. Debilitating illness requiring confinement to bed may result in institutionalization and loss of independence. Unfortunately, support services are not always available to aid a family attempting to care for an older person. Providing meals on weekends and delivering supplemental groceries might be easily handled by adult children if home-delivered meals or homemaker services are available Monday through Friday.

The importance and level of care provided for older parents by their children are frequently underestimated. According to a national survey, 46% of institutionalized individuals are childless.[53] Among those with children, institutionalization occurred when need for medical or nursing services made care at home impossible. The goal of community based food delivery programs is to support independent living as long as (1) this is consistent with the wishes of the client and (2) the mental and physical health of the client safely permits independent living with appropriate services.[36] For the individual wishing to remain at home lack of nutritional support can be a major obstacle.[64]

Formal support services provide help with housekeeping, shopping, or meal preparation; home delivery of meals; home health and medical services; or transportation.[7,51,71] Homemaker services can include preparation of meals to be reheated by the client, shopping, or personal services, such as help with bathing or dressing. Frequently, homemaker services are provided by a home health agency allowing coordination of medical and social services.

In some cases only limited help is necessary to support independent living. An evaluation of a homemaker service program in an urban location revealed that in 92% of the 165 cases examined services were required 4 hours per week or less.[5]

Among those individuals food preparation and meal planning were critical problems. When feasible, existing meal delivery programs were used or meals were prepared by the visiting homemaker and reheated by the client as needed. The need for service was greatest among low income persons 70 years of age and older, with no close relatives. It is obvious, however, that such individuals will have difficulty obtaining services unless community or federal financial support is available.

Home Versus Institutional Care. The relative benefits and cost effectiveness of home versus institutional care is a matter of controversy.[7,58,62-63] In recent years increasing emphasis has been placed on preservation of personal life-style.[51] The comfort of familiar surroundings strongly influences life satisfaction in the older individual.[10] Many older people are uneasy about moving to an unfamiliar location effect,'' or increased rate of morbidity and A further argument used for home care is the ''relocation effect'', or increased rate of morbidity and mortality observed in older people after admission to a nursing home.[7] It must be recognized, however, that many older people have serious medical problems when admitted to a nursing home, and this effect is not observed when patients are counseled prior to the move.

The fact remains, however, that a physically impaired individual with serious activity limitations can be more adequately cared for in an institutional setting where all meals are provided on a regular basis. A group living situation can also improve the quality of life for a lonely, isolated older person. Each situation must be evaluated according to the needs, resources, and capabilities of the particular client.

One consideration in the provision of long term care is cost effectiveness. Comparing the cost of institutionalization (nursing home, group home, or other extended care facility) with support services for home care, however, is not appropriate unless the relative quality of the services can be evaluated.[56] A second factor is the need for medical services that could make home care either inappropriate or impossible.

Studies attempting to examine the cost benefit of home versus institutional care have been inconclusive.[58,62] Community based services appear to serve a different clientele, people with less severe disabilities and fewer medical problems than those in nursing homes. Nevertheless, it is suggested that 10% to 40% of those now in extended care facilities could have remained in the community if support services had been available.[58] These individuals do not require help with activities of daily living (e.g., dressing, bathing, eating) or constant medical attention.

Unfortunately, homemaker services or home-delivered meals do not exist in many localities and costs are generally not reimbursed under existing insurance.[62] When such services do exist and are financially accessible people may not know about them. A survey of aged in the Chicago area revealed that the majority of those living in public housing were aware of a local home-delivered meals program, but only half of older suburban homeowners had heard of the program.[6] Even when older people know of available programs they may lack the resources to participate. Federal insurance reimbursement policies support institutionalization rather than community support services.[56] As the birth rate continues to decline (see Chapter 1) and adult children are not available to assume long term care, food delivery programs and support services in general will become increasingly important for meeting the needs of older people.

CONGREGATE MEAL PROGRAMS (TITLE III-C)

Pertinent Legislation

The Older Americans Act of 1965 as Amended[55,63] is the major piece of legislation providing programs for people age 60 and over. When establishing the nutrition program in 1972, Congress pointed to the special needs of this age group.

Many elderly persons do not eat adequately because 1) they cannot afford to do so; 2) they lack the skills to select and prepare nourishing and well-balanced meals; 3) they have limited mobility which may impair their capacity to shop and cook for themselves; and 4) they have feelings of rejection and loneliness which obliterate the incentive necessary to prepare and eat a meal alone. These and other physiological, psychological, social, and economic changes that occur with aging result in a pattern of living which causes malnutrition and further physical and mental deterioration.

The nutrition program, designed to provide meals at little or no cost in a social setting, was originally established under Title VII of the Older Americans Act and targeted to reach low income and minority aged.[55,68] In 1978 the nutrition program was reorganized under Title III-C, and is usually referred to as the Title III-C nutrition program. Social services are funded under Title III-B.[63] The 1978 amendments provided for (1) the integration of nutrition and social services including transportation services, which had previously functioned independently, and (2) the establishment of a home-delivered meals component with separate funding.[19] The general intent was to strengthen the nutrition program in terms of both visibility and funding and meet the need for home-delivered meals. Previous guidelines restricted the number of home-delivered meals, emphasizing meals served in a social setting. The nutritional impact of this program is obvious as in fiscal year 1982 over 140 million congregate meals were served reaching 2.8 million different persons.[61] Over 500,000 persons received a total of 50.5 million home-delivered meals. The overall nutritional contribution of this program to older Americans cannot be estimated.

General Organization

Development of Meal Sites. Under present legislation[19,55] states are required to establish area agencies on aging, which have responsibility for planning, organizing, and implementing nutrition and social services in a given geographic area. A nutrition project serving a designated area will administer the operation of a variable number of individual meal sites depending on the size of the area and population density.[57] Federal funds are appropriated using a formula based on the number of persons age 60 and over residing in the state. A small percentage of total operating funds (15%) must be contributed from state or local sources.[19] Participants are encouraged to make a donation toward the cost of the meal, although no one can be denied a meal for failure to contribute.[55]

Meal sites have been established in community or recreation centers, municipal buildings, public housing, senior citizens centers, and churches. Important criteria in selecting a location are accessibility and familiarity to the older people in the community. Programs located in facilities such as senior centers where there are on-going activities are more likely to be well attended.[21,39-40,49,57] An appropriate location is one having a major concentration of low income and minority older individuals within walking distance or able to take public transportation. Although over 85% of all meal sites provide transportation using Title III-B social service funds, the need for service is greater than what can be made available.[57] Transportation needs may increase program costs by 20% to 30%.[40]

Food Service Options. Under federal guidelines a hot (or cold when appropriate) meal is served 5 days each week at noon. In rural or sparsely populated areas meals may be served only 1 to 4 days per week.[61] Generally meal sites do not operate on weekends, presenting a serious problem for the participant whose personal food resources are extremely limited.

Nutrition projects may choose to prepare their own food or purchase food from an outside caterer.[34,59] This will depend on (1) facilities available at the individual meal sites, (2) proximity of meal sites to one another, and (3) availability of potential caterers. When there are several meal sites in a particular locality meals may be prepared in a central kitchen and distributed to nearby sites. Another option is purchase of meals from a centrally located caterer, such as a restaurant or hospital, school, or college food service. In one community a high school food service program served as the catering unit for the meal site.[22] One obvious problem was the need to find another caterer during the summer months. In any given area the savings accrued through volume buying or large scale food production must be evaluated in terms of the cost of transporting the prepared food to the serving locations.[34]

A recent study evaluated the meal cost (including food cost, labor, transportation, and administration costs) of 119 nutrition projects.[59] About half purchased food from caterers and the others prepared their own food either on-site or in a central kitchen. About 80% of the caterers were food service companies and the others, schools and nonprofit organizations. Meal cost was not related to the number of persons served, urban or rural location, or food preparation system.

Those authors concluded that selecting one system over another will not necessarily reduce costs. Projects with lower costs had (1) reduced labor and administrative costs by using personnel more efficiently, (2) sought better buys in food and supplies, and (3) shared facilities with other programs to decrease overhead.[59] Larger nutrition projects with a greater number of meal sites had reduced costs compared to projects with fewer sites, as a result of lower administrative costs per site. Balsam and Carlin[3,8] pointed out that regional cooperation among several nutrition projects resulted in a lower contract price for catered meals. Management practices to reduce or stabilize costs should be emphasized in both project research and staff training.

Transportation of Food. When food is prepared at a central location and transported either to meal sites (congregate meals) or to individual homes (home-delivered meals) loss of nutrients, deterioration in appearance and flavor, and microbial growth are potential dangers. Holding and transportation time includes (1) the time food is held at serving temperature at the preparation site before or after packaging, (2) the transportation time to serving location, and (3) the time food is held at the meal site before being served.[34] McCool and Posner[34] recommend that food be held less than 2 hours after final heating. Total holding time (including transportation time) is influenced by the size of the geographical area of the nutrition project or the length of the delivery route for home-delivered meals. Heavy traffic, poor roads in rural areas, and adverse weather conditions will significantly increase holding time. Transportation time can be reduced by increasing the number of delivery vehicles, thereby shortening the delivery routes. If existing constraints result in holding times beyond the 2 hour limit, hot meals should be discontinued and replaced with chilled, frozen, or shelf-stable items.[34]

Extended holding time results in loss of quality and general acceptability of the meal. Losses of ascorbic acid and the B complex vitamins accelerate when food is held at serving temperature for long periods.[34] A British evaluation of six home-delivered meals programs serving 4200 meals daily reported that cooked vegetables were held about 24 minutes before being placed in insulated delivery containers and were held in the containers for another 23 minutes before delivery of the first meal.[52] Total delivery time (between delivery of first and last meal) was about 90 minutes. Losses of vitamin C averaged 31% to 54% during the holding period before delivery and up to another 19% during delivery. Because of the loss of ascorbic acid from hot vegetables, a citrus juice or fruit may be a better menu choice as losses from those items are minimal. Potential nutrient losses as a result of holding time should be considered when developing menus for food delivery programs.

Packaging of Food. Packaging materials for transport of hot and cold food items must maintain food at safe and acceptable temperatures, prevent contamination, be reasonable in cost, and be easily handled by both staff and older recipients. Desirable characteristics of meal delivery packaging are listed below.

Food container
  Nonabsorbent
  Firm (will not bend easily)
  Easy to stack when filled with food
  Deep enough so that liquids do not spill
  Maintains temperature of food (or reheatable if for hot food)
  Easily sealed
  Disposable
  No sharp edges
  No transfer of odor or flavor to food
  Easily opened by older client
Carrying case
  Stain and grease resistant
  Lightweight and easy to handle
  Maintains temperature of food
  Easily opened and closed during delivery so that heat or cold is retained
  Appropriate size and shape for delivery vehicle
  Prevents food containers from tilting[34,38]

Food served at meal sites is usually transported in bulk containers and portioned on-site. Bulk containers that can be preheated and thermally controlled are currently available. Home-delivered meals are individually packaged keeping hot and cold items separate.[34] Hot packs that hold one meal are extremely expensive and must be collected and sterilized for reuse. As a result disposable styrofoam and aluminum containers are most commonly used. The need for long term investment and appropriate technology is particularly pertinent in relation to temperature control; hot and cold items are delivered in weather conditions ranging from 100° F in summer to −30° F in winter. To prevent microbial growth cold items must be maintained at a temperature below 45° F, and hot items at a temperature above 140° F.[34]

An English study suggests that even electrically heated carrying cases may not maintain hot foods at elevated temperatures when holding time is extended beyond 2 hours.[52] In that instance the temperature of the last hot meals delivered was 106° F. On the other hand, hot items may not have been heated to 150° F before being placed in the container. Cooperation between program leaders and industry in developing packaging and delivery strategies is urgently needed.

Table 12-1. Title III-C meal pattern

Food Type	Recommended Portion Size*
Meat or meat alternate	3 ounces of cooked edible portion
Vegetables and fruits	Two ½ cup servings
Enriched white or whole grain bread or alternate	One serving (one slice bread or equivalent)
Butter or margarine	1 teaspoon
Dessert	½ cup
Milk	½ pint (one cup)

*A vitamin C–rich fruit or vegetable is to be served each day; a vitamin A–rich fruit or vegetable is to be served at least three times per week.

From United States Department of Health, Education and Welfare: Guide to effective project operations: The Nutrition Program for the Elderly, Corvallis, 1973, Oregon State University.

Nutritional Aspects

Nutrient Requirements. Federal guidelines require that meals provide one third of the RDAs for this age group.[55] The three methods used for planning menus to meet this criterion are the Title III-C meal pattern,[54] the nutrient standard method (adapted from the National School Lunch Program),[20] and calculation using the RDAs.

Title III-C Meal Pattern. This plan (Table 12-1), indicating both the types and the amounts of food to be included in each meal, is most commonly used by Title III-C personnel.[34] Possible substitutions within the meal pattern allow for items basic to various ethnic and cultural tastes (Table 12-2).[49] Including a wide variety of foods not only increases the potential for providing the desired levels of all nutrients, but also for pleasing participants with differing food preferences. Obviously, the favorite meal of Spanish-American aged will differ markedly from those accustomed to New England fare.

The nutrient quality of meals can be enhanced by the selection of nutrient-dense items. Fruits and vegetables can add vitamins A and C, folic acid, potassium, and fiber to the diet. It is recommended that a vitamin C–rich food be served daily and a vitamin A–rich food be served three times weekly.[54] Fruits and vegetables are frequently omitted from the self-selected diets of older people[25,40] and the high cost of fresh produce limits its use by low income aged. Menus not including a vegetable high in vitamins A or C could include a citrus fruit or pumpkin dish for dessert.

Although bread products prepared from enriched white flour are acceptable, whole grain items will increase intakes of both fiber and trace minerals, such as chromium. This may be particularly important for those older people consuming highly processed foods at home. Whole grain breads and pasta may be introduced gradually to improve acceptance among those not accustomed to these items.

Rising food costs limit the frequency of servings of meat, fish, or poultry; therefore other sources

Table 12-2. Possible substitutions in the Title III-C meal pattern

I. Meat or meat alternate (3 ounces)—substitutions for 1 ounce cooked meat:
   1 ounce cooked fish or poultry
   1 egg
   1 ounce cheddar cheese
   ½ cup cooked dried beans, peas, or lentils
   2 tablespoons peanut butter
   ¼ cup cottage cheese
   Examples of combinations that meet the standard of 3 ounces of meat or equivalent:
   Cheeseburger made with 2 ounces of cooked beef plus a 1-ounce slice of cheese
   Italian lasagna (2 ounces meat, 2 tablespoons cottage cheese, and ½ egg per serving)
   Cheese enchilada (1 ounce cheese and 1 cup refried beans)
II. Fruits and vegetables (two ½ cup servings)—substitutions for ½ cup vegetable or fruit:
   ½ cup vegetable juice
   ½ cup fruit juice
III. Bread (one serving)—substitutions for one slice of bread or one roll:
   ½ cup cooked spaghetti, macaroni, or noodles (enriched)
   ½ cup cooked rice (enriched or whole grain)
   5 saltine crackers (enriched) or 2 graham crackers
   1 cornmeal muffin
   1 tortilla
IV. Dessert (½ cup)—suggestions for one serving of dessert:
   ½ cup fruit (fresh, canned, frozen)
   ½ cup pudding
   ½ cup ice cream, sherbet, or ice milk
   1 serving cake, pie, or cobbler
   2 cookies
V. Milk (1 cup)—substitutions for 1 cup of whole, skim, or buttermilk:
   1½ ounces natural cheese
   ½ cup cottage cheese and ⅓ cup milk
   ½ cup ice cream and ⅓ cup milk
   ⅓ cup dried milk (used in cooking)

From references 49 and 54.

of iron need to be emphasized. Legumes or lentils supplying iron and protein are one alternative. If cheese or another dairy product is the meat alternate or primary protein source, iron must be provided elsewhere within the meal. A whole grain item and dessert containing eggs or iron-rich fruits would contribute toward meeting the iron requirement.

Older people consume less than the recommended level of calcium (see Chapter 7); therefore participants should be strongly encouraged to drink the milk provided. Milk drinking may increase if whole, nonfat, and buttermilk are available; buttermilk was preferred by blacks and Spanish-Americans attending a Title III-C program in Texas (see Chapter 4). The calcium content of the meal can be enhanced by using milk and dairy products in cooking.[52] Nonfat dried milk or grated cheese can fortify soups or sauces increasing the calcium, protein, and riboflavin content. (Cheese is sometimes available to Title III-C programs as a government commodity.)

Dessert should be a significant source of nutrients as well as a pleasant climax to the meal. Fruit desserts such as a baked apple or apple crisp contribute important nutrients, particularly if made with whole grains. Pudding, custard, or ice cream provides calcium, as well as high quality protein for those who do not drink milk. In a home-delivered meals program, meals containing milk-based desserts fortified with dried skim milk had twice the calcium content of those with desserts of canned fruit or baked products prepared from a mix.[52] Moist, flavorful baked products prepared with whole grains, oatmeal, raisins, applesauce, pumpkin, or banana add iron, B complex vitamins, and trace minerals. Recipes containing sugar, fat, and little else should be avoided.

Nutrient Standard Method. The nutrient standard method (NSM) evaluates the menu content of calories, percentage of fat (not to exceed 40% of calories), and nine other nutrients (protein, vitamins A and C, thiamin, riboflavin, niacin, iron, calcium, and phosphorus).[20] In this system standardized recipes are expressed according to the number of units of each nutrient contained. Ten units of a nutrient equals one third of the RDA or the level to be included per meal. Standardized forms simplify the computation of units from all items to be served. Evaluation within the National School Lunch Program suggested this method is more likely to provide desired levels of nutrients than a method based on food types. Poor food choices, although providing servings within the designated groups, result in a meal low in nutrient density. The NSM is most limiting for thiamin and iron.

The NSM has application for monitoring the nutrient content of meals prepared by caterers who provide the recipes used for mixed dishes. Substitution of one vegetable for another (e.g., beets for broccoli) can significantly influence the vitamin content of the meal; therefore menus as well as the food actually delivered must be monitored regularly. Testing of the NSM with 10 nutrition project managers revealed that menu monitoring is more difficult than menu planning.[20] Managers with more formal education mastered the skill most quickly, although those with no education beyond high school learned to use and apply the method accurately. Participating managers had an average of 1.6 years of education beyond high school and 4.6 years of experience in food service. A limitation of the Title III-C program is the lack of staff with professional training in nutrition, foods, or dietetics.

Special Diets. Limited funding and lack of professionally trained personnel make modified diets impractical in most locations. It is possible, however, to provide some flexibility within the meal pattern to accommodate those with a general food restriction. Prescribed diets for older people usually involve limiting calories, sodium, or fat. For diabetics or others limiting calorie intake, the Title III-C pattern is likely to be acceptable if portion size is controlled, skim milk is available, and fruit is offered as an alternative to a high calorie dessert. No salt should be added in meal preparation; those wishing to add salt may do so at the table.

Serving procedures can influence adaptability to a variety of diets. Meats should be portioned and served before addition of gravy, broth, or sauce for the benefit of those avoiding sodium or fat. Salad dressing can be added at the table rather than in the kitchen. Margarine or butter should be added to vegetables in only limited amounts.

Appropriateness of the meal for those on modified diets is influenced by the menu items selected, as well as the method of preparation. Limiting fat, sugar, and salt and increasing fiber and complex carbohydrates should be goals in menu planning.[15] Convenience items including soups, gravy mixes, and prepared sauces add sodium and fat to the meal. Frozen vegetables should be selected when possible in preference to canned. Unfortunately, cost or the availability of a government commodity food often has to take precedence as funding has not kept pace with the number of people to be served.

In a study of 91 meal sites, 42% made some effort to provide for special diets; for about a third this involved only limited changes such as salt-free or sugar-free meals.[57] Twenty-five percent tried to meet individual requests for any type of diet. Low cholesterol, bland, and vegetarian diets were provided by 12% to 14% of those responding. Whether this option was provided by caterers or on-site preparation units was not indicated. Among Title III-C participants in Vermont, 36% had a dietary restriction although only 13% had problems selecting food within the meals served.[46] Unless meals are being catered by a food service system with qualified dietitians, such as a hospital, specific diets should not be attempted. General modifications limiting salt or fat are of potential benefit to all participants.

Evaluation of the Title III-C Program

Reaching Target Population. Original legislation establishing the nutrition program emphasized the needs of low income, minority, isolated, and phys-

ically handicapped aged.[55,57] According to a national survey of nearly 2800 Title III-C participants, the program has been successful in reaching both the poor and ethnic minorities.[57] Although minority groups comprise only 10% of the over-60 population, they represented 23% of Title III-C participants. About two thirds of these participants were poor, with incomes below $4000 per year. Participation was related to location of the meal site; enrollment increased with the relative proportion of these groups within the immediate area served. Poor and minority aged are also more likely to attend on a daily basis. Whether this reflects a greater need for services or the social atmosphere at the meal site is not known.

Participation by mobility-impaired and non-English-speaking people is low (2% to 3% of participants). Recruitment efforts have been relatively unsuccessful in attracting those with physical disabilities. This could relate to the physical characteristics or location of the meal site or to the degree of help offered to the handicapped (e.g., service at the table if meal is handled buffet-style).

Emotional and Social Contribution. Evaluation of the social component of the Title III-C program considers benefits to individual participants as well as success in reaching isolated aged. Available studies suggest that participants place equal importance on the nutritional benefits and social support provided.[24,42,57] Subjective evaluations point to the improved general well-being of many attenders as reflected in their appearance and mental outlook.[39-40] They begin to make friends and participate in group activities. Remarks such as ''I am a different person since I found this program'' are common.[40]

A recent survey suggests that about 25% of older persons feel they have no one to ask for help in time of sickness or need.[57] Friends at the meal site can become such a support group. Involvement of participants as volunteers promotes self-esteem and a sense of being needed. Many on-site employees of Title III-C are senior citizens.

The nutrition program may be particularly important to older people living alone as 58% of long term participants (attended at least 18 months) as compared to 43% of nonparticipating neighbors similar in socioeconomic status live alone.[57] However, individuals attending Title III-C are also more likely to belong to clubs and organizations and attend church regularly. It may be more difficult for shy individuals with limited social contact to join a group if they do not know anyone. On the other hand, some apparently isolated people may not want or need increased social activity.

Based on observation the majority of Title III-C participants (96%) engage in conversation before or during the meal.[57] Social interaction after the meal is often not possible because of transportation schedules or the need to reorganize the room for another purpose or vacate the facility if it is available only during meal hours. Small tables seating four or five rather than long tables promote conversation and social exchange.[21]

About three fourths of all meal sites sponsor recreation or social activities in addition to the noon meal.[57] Over half have at least one activity per week. Participation in social events other than the meal is more frequent among women, among those under 75 years of age, and at small (serving 10 to 50 persons) rather than large (serving 51 to 300 persons) sites. Those above age 75 have more physical problems such as impaired hearing or eyesight and may be more dependent on the site or others for transportation. Long term participants were more likely to be aware of social activities than recent entrants.

Nutritional Contribution. Although Title III-C meals are required to provide 33% of the RDA, the majority of meals provide more than this amount for many nutrients.[29,59] In an analysis of meals from 119 sites,[59] over three fourths of the meals contained 50% of the RDA (for men) for protein, calcium, phosphorus, vitamin A, and riboflavin; 40% of the RDA for iron and vitamin C; and about 33% of the RDA for energy, thiamin, and niacin. Half

of the meals provided at least 67% of the day's requirement for protein and vitamin A. Zinc was the nutrient most frequently below 33% of the RDA. Calories, vitamin A, thiamin, and niacin were more likely to be low for men than women, because their requirement is higher. Those authors suggest increasing serving sizes for men to adjust intake.[59]

Title III-C participants consume better diets on days that include a site meal and consume better diets than nonparticipating neighbors of similar age and socioeconomic background (see Table 12-3).[57] Calcium and vitamin A were most influenced by participation. This suggests that older people consume less milk and other dairy products and dark green and deep yellow fruits and vegetables at home. Individuals with better diets tended to be younger, were more socially active, and had higher incomes.

Factors related to the meal site also influenced dietary adequacy.[57] Those with better diets attended

Table 12-3. Percentage of Title III-C participants and nonparticipants with adequate daily intakes of selected nutrients*

	Participants		Nonpartic-ipating Neighbors
	Includes Site Meal	Does Not Include Site Meal	
Calories	73	68	63
Vitamin A	69	56	53
Vitamin C	81	73	70
Calcium	67	49	47
Iron	86	77	76
Thiamin	79	74	71

*At least two thirds of the RDA.

Modified from United States Department of Health and Human Services: Longitudinal evaluation of the National Nutrition Program for the Elderly: Report on first wave findings, DHEW Publication No. (OHDS) 80-20249, Washington, D.C., 1979, U.S. Government Printing Office.

meal sites considered by participants to serve adequate amounts of food, although 92% of all attenders reported "always" receiving adequate food. The association of health-related meal site activities and higher diet scores might indicate a positive effect of nutrition education. Finally, people making a financial contribution toward their meal consume better diets overall than those not making a donation. Individuals not contributing are most likely lower in income and consuming poorer meals at home. This emphasizes the importance of outreach directed toward the target population.

Kohrs and coworkers[29,31] evaluated the impact of Title III-C on the nutritional status of 466 rural aged in central Missouri. In that location menus provided considerably more than the minimum for all nutrients evaluated. For women the meals contained at least 80% of the RDAs for protein, vitamins A and C, and riboflavin and at least half the RDAs for energy, calcium, iron, and niacin. For men the Title III-C meal met at least 67% of the RDAs for protein and vitamins A and C and at least 40% of the RDAs for energy, calcium, iron, and the B vitamins. It cannot be assumed, however, that all food served is always consumed, including the cup of milk.

The proportion of nutrients contained in the menus was reflected in the dietary intakes of participants (Fig. 12-1). For most nutrients, women consumed nearly half of their daily intake at the meal site. Men received about half of their daily intakes of protein, calcium, iron, vitamin A, and vitamin C from the Title III-C meal. This confirms the value of the meal in helping participants obtain an adequate diet and the need to select menu items that are nutrient dense.

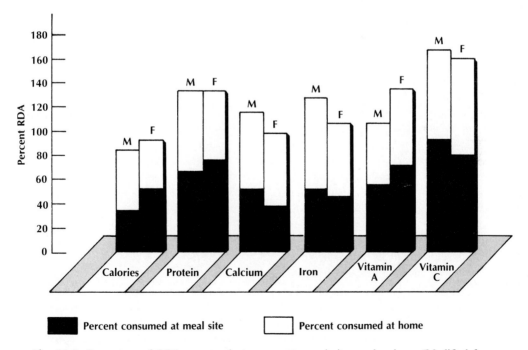

Fig. 12-1. Percentage of RDA consumed at congregate meal site or elsewhere. (Modified from Kohrs, M.B., O'Hanlon, P., and Eklund, D.: Title VII Nutrition Program for the Elderly. I. Contribution to one day's dietary intake, J. Am. Diet. Assoc. **72:**487, 1978.)

Socioeconomic factors influence the Title III-C contribution to the nutrient intake of participants. Women who lived alone consumed a higher proportion of their nutrients at the meal site.[29,30] Individuals with less education or previously employed as unskilled workers consumed a greater share of their nutrients at Title III-C than those with more schooling and a technical or professional occupation. Since education and occupation are closely related to income, this supports the conclusion that the program helps the economically disadvantaged. Those benefiting most were women over 75 years of age.

Nutritional benefit relates to frequency of attendance. The Missouri subjects were evaluated according to those who had discontinued participation, those who attended less than two times per week, and those who attended two to five times per week.[31] Intakes of foods rich in vitamins A and C were higher for attenders even if participation was less than twice per week. Forty-three percent of nonparticipants had less than acceptable levels of serum vitamin A as compared to only 4% of those who attended 2 to 5 days each week. Hemoglobin levels were not influenced by participation.

Those obtaining even limited numbers of meals at Title III-C need provide fewer meals for themselves with the resources they have available. Boston aged reported saving money on food by attending a site meal.[42] Meals consumed at home may improve in nutrient quality if some meals can be obtained elsewhere.

Frequency of Attendance. The nutritional impact of Title III-C is diminished by infrequent attendance. In a national survey of 2800 participants, 46% attended four to five times per week and 40% one to three times per week.[57] Frequent attenders were more likely to eat alone at home, have low incomes, and be over 75 years of age. Individuals who considered themselves to be in good health attended regularly. Those who enjoy food preparation may attend only occasionally as a diversion or to visit with friends. Nutrition projects should focus on the following aspects of their operation, which are known to influence attendance by the target population.

1. Accessibility of meal site
   Transportation problems hinder attendance; therefore meal sites should be established in locations easily accessible to the aged population.[39-40,57] This will continue to increase in importance, as transportation funds are inadequate to provide for all people needing assistance.

2. Method of handling contribution
   Federal law stipulates that no one can be denied a meal because of inability to contribute. When participants are given an envelope in which to place an anonymous donation, the person who cannot contribute or can contribute only a small amount avoids embarrassment. When a suggested fee is collected, the individual most in need of the program may choose not to participate rather than admit he cannot afford to pay.[57]

3. Frequent social activities
   Opportunity for social interaction attracts and maintains participation.[57] Having someone to talk with can be as important as the meal itself.[39-40]

4. Quality of meal service
   Participant satisfaction with food quality and portion size promotes regular and continued attendance. In the recent Title III-C survey, 92% expressed satisfaction with the meals and 86% attended at least once per week.[57] An efficient reservation system to ensure that people are not turned away without a meal should be developed in each location.

5. Effective outreach and referral
   Although individual meal sites engage in outreach activities, a coordinated community plan should be the goal. Physicians, visiting nurses, hospital social service workers, and other professionals who work with aged

clients on a daily basis need to be aware of both congregate and home-delivered meals services existing within the community.[18] Special efforts should be directed toward those units serving the mobility-impaired as this group has not been effectively reached by Title III-C.[57]

Need for Professional Staff. Present federal regulations do not specify professional qualifications for nutrition project managers, although individual states may develop professional criteria for these positions. A project manager may be responsible for the overall supervision of 2 or as many as 86 meal sites.[57] Poor management can result in meals of inferior quality or limit the number of individuals who can be served with the resources available. Furthermore, meals prepared by the nutrition project or obtained from a caterer must meet standards for nutrient content as well as food safety.

The nutritional quality of the meals served reflects the attention directed toward selection of a variety of foods to maximize the nutrients provided. This process demands that meal planners recognize not only the nutrient content of particular foods but also the overall nutrient requirements of older individuals as related to both physiologic and socioeconomic factors. This responsibility requires a professional background in nutrition, dietetics, and food service. Implementation of regulations at state and federal levels defining the educational background required of staff is essential if optimum nutrient content and food service practices are to be achieved.[28]

HOME DELIVERY OF MEALS

Early History

In the past when serious illness or chronic disease resulted in physical disability it was the role of the good neighbor to bring food to the home.[11] This role is to some extent being assumed by volunteer groups as well as state and federally supported agencies, as the need for home care continues to grow.

The formal concept of home-delivered meals, later given the popular designation of Meals on Wheels, began early in this century. In 1905 the invalid kitchens of London began sending hot meals to housebound patients.[27,36] In Great Britain home-delivered meals are still available through the government-supported social service system. The first Meals on Wheels program in the United States began in Philadelphia in 1954. The program operated through the Lighthouse, a settlement house serving an area of approximately 5 square miles, and served 50 homebound clients each day.[27,36] Since that time the number of programs in the United States has expanded rapidly. In 1971 there were about 350; the number is now estimated to be about 600.[35]

General Organization

Meal delivery programs have been organized by community nonprofit organizations and health and social service agencies such as hospitals, churches, nursing homes, and visiting nurses associations. Within community-sponsored programs meals are usually delivered by volunteers who pay their own transportation costs. People who deliver meals for the Title III-C program are usually reimbursed for both time and mileage.

Meal delivery programs usually operate Monday through Friday.[36] A hot meal is delivered at noon and is sometimes accompanied by a cold meal to be eaten later. Some programs include additional cold lunches on Friday or before a holiday to provide for days when meals are not delivered. Delivery of cold lunches requires that the recipient have a refrigerator to safely store the additional food. No program provides meals on all days or for all meals of the day.

Financial Resources

Meal delivery programs are classified on the basis of their funding sources and community affiliations.[35] The first kind of program consists of voluntary providers who receive no federal funds under Title III-C, relying completely on private contributions, community funding such as United Way, and fees from recipients. These programs are often associated with a nonprofit community organization and are not subject to any federal regulations regarding program participants or the nutritional content of meals served. Such programs depend heavily on volunteer help.

A second type of program combines both voluntary contributions and federal funding. Although community groups provide both financial support and volunteer help, federal funds are also received through the local Title III-C program. Acceptance of federal funds requires adherence to federal regulations regarding clients served and meal frequency and quality. In the third case meals are delivered by a Title III-C congregate program supported by federal funds.

There has been a reluctance on the part of many voluntary programs to accept federal funding.[35] Pride in their own achievements and autonomy over their operation are significant factors in their decision. Completely voluntary programs are more likely to be located in rural or suburban communities. Providers accepting federal funds are usually motivated by financial pressures and client needs. According to a recent survey of over 30 meal delivery programs, 78% accepting federal funds serve at least 100 clients as compared to 12% not accepting federal funds.[35] Federal funds often allow the expansion of meal delivery service to low income and minority aged who cannot afford to pay.

Cooperation between community meal delivery programs and the local Title III-C agency is essential to maximize resources and avoid duplication of effort. Title III-C agencies are expected to contract with existing community programs rather than establish a duplicate program.[19,44] Mutual support rather than competition between the two groups allows more clients to be served with the resources available.

Clients Served

Eligibility Requirements. Older people can request meal delivery directly or be referred by a family member, physician, visiting nurse, outreach worker, or social worker. Criteria for service need to be established to assure that the needs of the individual can be met by home-delivered meals.[36] For programs receiving federal funding, there are two requirements.[44]

1. The recipient must be age 60 or over, although spouses below age 60 can also be served.
2. The recipient must be unable to leave his home because of disability or other extenuating circumstances. Eligibility must be documented by Title III-C or health personnel and recertified every 6 months.[44]

When meal delivery is not appropriate the client should be assisted in exploring other options. If the individual is able to leave his home, transportation to a Title III-C meal site provides an opportunity for social activity. A two person household may be in need of home-delivered meals if both individuals are limited in mobility or if one person is so burdened caring for an invalid partner that he has little time or incentive to prepare adequate meals. Home-delivered meals should not perpetuate a dangerous or inadequate living situation,[36] as in serious illness requiring nursing care or medical supervision that cannot be provided appropriately on an outpatient basis.

Mental or emotional problems may preclude remaining at home. I recall visiting an older woman, age 73 and living alone, who had received both a telephone call and a letter regarding a community nutrition project. When I arrived, the client recalled nothing about the previous communications yet encouraged me "to come in and see my house." At the time she was heating water with curtains blowing dangerously close to the gas flame. All prospective clients should be visited and evaluated before service is initiated. Meal delivery is equally inappropriate for the individual who wishes to be relieved of all personal responsibility for meal preparation without good reason.[44]

A meal delivery program should serve all income groups.[36] A person in comfortable financial circumstances who lacks human resources may have as great a need for meal delivery as a low income individual. For those who have the ability to pay, the fee should about equal the cost of the meal. Federal regulations prohibit a required payment from recipients funded by Title III-C.[55] Those clients may give a donation as is the policy at congregate meal sites. Within voluntary programs not receiving government funds, contributions from individuals, civic organizations, churches, or the local United Fund can provide "food scholarships" for those who cannot afford the established fee. Individuals likely to require home-delivered meals as a result of deteriorating physical health and no family often have inadequate incomes as well.[5]

Profile of Recipients. Although home-delivered meals programs have been in existence for many years, descriptive information about recipients is extremely limited. A survey of 16 programs conducted some years ago suggested that the typical recipient was a woman above age 70; 70% of recipients lived alone although the majority had access to kitchen facilities; over half had received meals for at least 6 months.[41]

A recent survey of nearly 600 recipients of Title III-C home-delivered meals had similar findings.[60] Nearly half of the recipients were age 80 and over, although this age group comprises only 20% of the over-65 population. Two thirds lived alone and an equal number were women. Recipients in urban areas were more likely to be older and living alone. Although all income levels were represented, most recipients were considered to be low income. About half had been receiving meals for at least 1 year and 30% for 6 months or less. The need for more appropriate evaluation of prospective recipients is suggested by the fact that a significant number were not homebound and therefore could be better served by an alternative program such as congregate meals.

Meal Delivery Procedures. The success of a program depends to a great extent on the reliability and personal qualities of the volunteers delivering the meals; therefore their selection and training is an important responsibility.[70] Because volunteers will be entering the homes of older people who are vulnerable both physically and emotionally, all should be carefully screened. Those who deliver meals must be well informed about the program and operating procedures and be trained to handle any irregular situation.[70] If a recipient does not answer the door, the volunteer should be aware of the person or agency to contact as this could indicate an emergency. The need for referral is particularly acute if the older client lives alone. Delivery staff should also be alert to any physical or mental change in the recipient, which should be relayed to the appropriate individual.

Volunteers usually work in pairs, one driving and the other taking the meal to the door. Though it would be ideal to visit for a short time, this is not possible when many meals are to be delivered. An important aspect of recipients' attitudes toward the program appears to be the friendliness and attitude of the volunteer service.[36]

Nutritional Aspects

Nutritional Guidelines. Guidelines developed by the National Council on the Aging recommend that each meal provide at least one third of the RDA.[36] Adherence to this recommendation, however, is strictly voluntary on the part of programs receiving no federal funds. With careful food selection a program providing a hot meal plus a cold supper can provide two thirds of the RDAs or a significant proportion of the nutrient needs for the day. The meal pattern developed for the Title III-C program[54] can serve as a guide (see Table 12-1). As noted earlier, selecting menu items to maximize nutrient content should be a priority.

An issue in the nutritional management of home-delivered meals programs is providing modified diets. When meals are produced by the food service department of a hospital or extended care facility, sodium restricted, diabetic, or modified fat diets may be possible.[11,23] When food is provided by a food service company or independent kitchen without a dietitian on staff, stringent diet modifications are not available or appropriate. A large proportion of persons receiving home-delivered meals have some chronic illness or are in a stage of recuperation. With this in mind, gas-forming foods and items high in fat or sodium or difficult to digest should be avoided. Physicians need to be carefully informed when therapeutic diets are not available so they can make recommendations accordingly.

Food Preferences of Recipients. Information regarding the degree of satisfaction with food delivered is sparse. A food preference questionnaire administered by one program indicated that meat, potatoes, milk, and desserts were enjoyed the most and fish the least.[69] Other factors, in addition to the menu, influence whether or not the food is consumed or enjoyed. Among 107 recipients not all food was consumed because it was difficult to chew, poorly prepared, or portions were too large.[48]

Food temperature is important for both the safety and palatability of delivered meals. If the meal is to be enjoyed, hot foods should be "hot" and cold foods "cold." However, recipients do not always eat the meal as soon as it is delivered. A survey of 168 meal recipients revealed that less than half ate the entire meal at noon.[4] Others ate either the entire meal or a portion of it at a later time. This emphasizes the importance of available refrigeration for those receiving home-delivered meals and the need for nutrition education regarding meal storage. When refrigeration is not available, it must be made clear that perishable items not consumed immediately must be discarded.

Contribution to Daily Nutrient Intake. The adequacy of the diet of home-delivered meal recipients is dependent not only on the nutrient quality of the meal delivered but also on the food resources available on nondelivery days and for nondelivered meals.[48] At present there is no documentation of food intake of recipients on weekends. Although it is assumed that family members or neighbors provide assistance, this is certainly not true for all. Individuals who lack other resources may save less perishable items such as bread or fruit from the delivered meals for weekend days.

Although no studies are available from the United States, the nutritional impact of home-delivered meals was evaluated in 268 British recipients.[12-14,48] Both energy and vitamin intakes were improved by meal delivery.[12,14] The home-delivered meal supplied 70% of the vitamin A and 82% of the ascorbic acid consumed on that day.[12] Energy intake increased by about 120 kcal on delivery days. Mean energy intakes including both delivery and nondelivery days were 1694 kcal for women and 2174 kcal for men.[14] Meals as delivered contained only about 1100 mg potassium and the diets of recipients were generally low in this nutrient. (Mean daily intake of potassium equaled 2200 mg and did not differ on delivery versus nondelivery days.)

Overall nutrient contribution depends on the number of days meals are delivered. A delivery schedule of less than 4 days each week did not significantly improve the diet of recipients.[48] Twenty percent of those interviewed had severely reduced nutrient intakes (specific values were not reported) on days when meals were not delivered and help from neighbors was not available. In rural areas where meals are delivered by the Title III program, delivery can be less than 5 days per week and neighbors may be at some distance. Isolated homebound individuals appear to be especially vulnerable to poor nutrient intake on nondelivery days.

INNOVATIVE APPROACHES TO FOOD DELIVERY

Rising gasoline prices, problems in procuring volunteer drivers as more women are becoming employed, and the increasing numbers of clients to be served have led to evaluation of more cost-efficient methods of food delivery.[34] Daily delivery of a hot meal has been defended on the basis that it provides social contact as well as a supply of food, although the actual time spent with a client is often not more than a minute. The general well-being of a person living alone could be monitored by a daily telephone call from a responsible volunteer.[34]

Delivery of Frozen Meals

A successful alternative to daily delivery of hot meals has been weekly delivery of five frozen meals.[37] Thirty-one homebound aged who had been receiving a hot meal 5 days per week were asked to evaluate over a 5-week period the taste, texture, appearance, convenience, and healthfulness of the frozen meals. The hot meals and fresh items delivered previously were also rated using the same criteria. The majority of recipients considered the frozen meals to be equal if not superior to the conventional hot meals and over 80% either preferred or would accept frozen meals. Recipients appreciated the choice of what to eat on a particular day and the ability to set their own time for meals. Client satisfaction when converting from one system to another may relate to time spent in introducing the program and giving complete information and instructions for storing and reheating foods. Frozen meals were less well received in another group of older people who resented the effort involved in reheating the food.[33] Delivery of five frozen meals once per week reduced costs by 16% as compared to delivery of a hot meal 5 days per week.[37] With increased efficiency in delivery of frozen meals, costs might be reduced by as much as 50%.

Supplementing one or two home-delivered meals each week with several frozen meals presents another alternative. When a hot meal is not delivered, a frozen meal can be heated. Milk, fruit, and canned or freeze-dried items could accompany the frozen meals.[34] This approach is dependent on the availability of suitable equipment in the home. Recipients must have a freezer for storing meals until time for use, as well as an oven for reheating. Nutrition programs might purchase and lend toaster ovens to recipients of frozen meals who lack a working oven.[34] Exploration of frozen meal delivery should be continued, particularly in rural areas where daily meal delivery is prohibited by cost.

Delivery of Groceries

For homebound people able to move about within their homes, groceries can supplement either frozen or hot meals. In a recent evaluation groceries supplemented two home-delivered hot meals each week.[26] The groceries were selected to provide five meals, each containing one third of the required nutrients for the day. Recipes and preparation suggestions were included with the groceries, planned on an 8-week cycle. Because the 20 recipients (age 76 to 91) were capable of meal preparation, fresh and less processed items were delivered with emphasis on fruits and vegetables, dairy products, and high protein foods. Over the 6-month evaluation period deficient serum levels of vitamins A and C increased to normal and those participants low in vitamin B_6 showed some improvement. Weekly delivery of perishable items allowed these people to manage with only one shopping trip per month to obtain staple items.

High Technology Foods

Canned, dehydrated, and freeze-dried foods developed for use in the space program are also applicable to home delivery. These foods can be stored at room temperature for a year or more. Results from a pilot study with nearly 200 older volunteers suggest a high level of acceptance of these items.[43,65] Twenty-one different single meals were developed; each met one third of the RDA. Each included a main dish, two side dishes, dessert, and beverage. The menu cycle provided one meal per day over a 3-week period. A 1-week supply of seven meals, when packaged, weighed less than 10 pounds and was suitable for mailing, allowing delivery by the Postal Service.

Packaging and preparation requirements for these meals were appropriate for those with physical limitations such as impaired vision or stiffness in the hands. Cans could be opened by a pull-tab device or a can opener. Packages had perforated edges for ease in opening and instructions were provided in both written and graphic form. Required kitchen equipment included only utensils to measure, stir, and serve food, and the capacity to boil water and heat or cool items.

Recipients were positive about the program in general and the quality of the food. Meals were considered to be convenient, palatable, and easy to prepare. Sixty percent of the recipients considered the delivered meals equal or superior in quality to the hot meals they could prepare for themselves. Few expressed any difficulty with opening the food packages or food preparation. Three-fourths expressed a desire to continue receiving meals and indicated a willingness to pay for the foods if available and reasonable in cost. Although shelf-stable foods could replace either a congregate or home-delivered meals program, they are also appropriate as a supplementary food source for weekends or other nondelivery days.[34] Analysis of the relative cost effectiveness and cost benefit of alternative food delivery systems should be a priority in planning for long term care.

MEAL DELIVERY IN INSTITUTIONS

Types of Institutions

Several types[32,45] of long term care facilities accommodate older people who are no longer able to remain at home as a result of physical disability, serious illness, or need for supervision.

The skilled nursing facility (SNF) provides 24-hour professional nursing care under the supervision of a physician. The majority of patients are confined to bed or wheelchair and require skilled nursing procedures and carefully supervised medication. Those who are ambulatory also need specialized medical attention.

The intermediate care facility (ICF) is not required to have professional nurses present at all times as patients do not need constant skilled nursing care. Other types of staff can provide any help required with personal needs. Patients are more likely to be ambulatory and able to handle their medications without direct supervision.

A domiciliary (DCF) provides only room, board, and supervision with no medical services. This type of facility does not qualify for Medicaid reimbursement.

Patients are assigned a level of care on the basis of confinement to bed, mental state (confusion or disorientation), incontinence, and need for medical and nursing care.[45] About 40% of all institutionalized people need help with bathing and dressing and an equal number are totally dependent on others for these activities.[53] Nine percent need some help at meal time and 13% must be fed.[53]

Facilities eligible for reimbursement under Medicare or Medicaid (SNF and ICF) are required to have available additional services including physical therapy, social services, and social activities. Data suggest, however, that not all patients in need of particular services actually receive them.[32] About one third of those requiring physical therapy were being treated. Although about half of certified nursing homes surveyed reported employing social workers or activity coordinators, the qualifications and level of training required for these positions is not specified in federal regulations. Cards, bingo games, parties, religious activities, and television were activities offered in most facilities, although participation ranged from 19% for arts and crafts to 62% for television.

Nutrient Content of Meals Served

An important consideration in the evaluation of institutional meals is nutrient density. In a recent survey of 14 nursing homes requirements for calcium, iron, thiamin, riboflavin, and niacin were not met unless individuals consumed over 2000 kcal.[47] At median energy intakes (1620 kcal for men; 1361 kcal for women) only protein and vitamins A, C, and B_{12} met the RDAs for both sexes. Menus planned on the basis of an energy intake of 2000 kcal still contained less than recommended levels of magnesium, zinc, pyridoxine, and folic acid. Over half of the 108 women studied consumed less than 55% of the RDAs for those four nutrients.

Of further concern is the range of caloric intakes observed. Men consumed from 983 to 3007 kcal and women from 513 to 2613. In another report mean energy intakes were 1720 and 1330 kcal for men and women, respectively.[50] Sempos and coworkers[47] concluded that nursing home menus should be planned to meet the RDAs at low levels of energy intake and suggested that 1400 kcal be used as a base. Conversely, patients who are ambulatory and active should not be limited to 1400 kcal.

Allington and coworkers[1-2] developed a model food plan based on 16 food groups that defines the number of pounds of each food category that must be used per month per 100 patients if the RDA is to be met for all nutrients including trace minerals, pyridoxine, and folic acid. In order to remain within 100% of the energy requirement, cake and pastry desserts (about 14% of total calories in calculated nursing home menus) were reduced or omitted. Food items to be increased included meat, fish, and poultry; dried peas, beans, and nuts; green leafy vegetables; bananas; and dry cereals including wheat germ and bran flakes. As pointed out by those authors, such changes are also likely to influence costs.[2]

Nursing home residents in Kansas (n = 99) reported consuming less meat, eggs, and fruits and vegetables than they consumed 2 years earlier.[9] It was not indicated when these individuals entered the nursing home so it cannot be determined whether this reflects a change in food availability. Changes in food patterns could also result from decreasing mobility and chronic disease. People with greater changes in their food patterns were older (age 80 or above) and had poorer nutritional scores. In any case reduced use of these food items compromises intakes of trace minerals and vitamins such as zinc and folic acid. In light of the high use of prescription drugs by nursing home residents, vitamin and mineral status appears to be extremely precarious.

Patient Acceptance of Meals Served

A recent national survey reported that 83% of nursing home residents liked the meals served whereas 14% disliked the food presented.[53] Patients may refuse food because of boredom, from lack of appetite as a result of prescription drugs or inactivity, or because the meal schedule differs from their accustomed meal pattern. Ford and Neville[17] observed food acceptance among 26 pairs of patients residing in homes offering either three or five meals daily. The home offering three meals and two snacks served food between 8:15 A.M. and 8:00 P.M. In the facility providing 5 meals a continental breakfast was served at 6:30 A.M. and the final light meal at 8:00 P.M. Refusal of the early breakfast or late supper frequently related to sleeping patterns.

On a five meal pattern 77% refused at least one meal or part of a meal during the week; on the three meal pattern 77% refused part of at least one meal. In general nutrient intake was similar in both groups whether patients refused a portion of a large meal or all of a small meal. An important consideration when following a three meal pattern is the extended time between the evening snack and breakfast (about 12 hours). Moreover, with three main meals scheduled so close together (8:15 A.M.; 12:00 P.M.; 4:45 P.M.) individuals may not be hungry when the next meal arrives. Items such as sandwiches, milk, fruit, and juice should be available as evening snacks, particularly for frail aged who can consume only a small amount of food at a time.

SUMMARY

Various food delivery systems exist to provide nutritional support for older people who are unable to meet their food needs without help. For the confined individual who is physically and mentally able to remain at home, formal and informal support systems can provide long term care. Informal support services by family members or neighbors could include grocery shopping or bringing meals on weekends when other services are not available. Formal support services consist of home-delivered meals or homemaker services providing food shopping or meal preparation.

For individuals able to leave their homes, the congregate meal program organized under Title III-C of the Older Americans Act provides a hot meal at noon planned to contain at least one third of the RDA. An integral part of the Title III-C program is the social component and most meal sites sponsor social activities in addition to the served meal. Title III-C participants tend to consume about half of their daily nutrients at the meal site and have better diets than neighbors of similar age and socioeconomic background who do not participate. Title III-C meals are more likely to meet the target nutrient levels for women than men.

Home-delivered meals programs can be community-sponsored or operate under Title III-C funds. In general a hot meal is delivered 5 days per week at noon and may be accompanied by a cold meal to be consumed later. A current problem is attracting volunteer drivers as more women are entering the work force. Food safety becomes critical if holding and transportation time extend beyond 2 hours and ideal food temperatures are not maintained. A problem associated with both home-delivered and congregate meals is that food is not provided on all days or for all meals of the day; therefore additional sources of food are required.

Although nursing home menus are developed to contain adequate levels of nutrients, patients may not eat all food served. Meals should be planned to provide all necessary nutrients within 1400 kcal. Model systems for nutritional evaluation based on food inventories provide a reasonable means of monitoring the nutritional quality of meals served to assure high nutrient density. In all food delivery systems trace minerals, pyridoxine, and folic acid are the nutrients most likely to fall below standards.

REVIEW QUESTIONS

1. What are the programs and services funded under Title III of the Older Americans Act? Describe the target populations to whom these services are directed.
2. What are the nutritional requirements for Title III-C meals? In general do most meals meet these standards? What nutrients are most likely to be lacking (a) in Title III-C sponsored meals and (b) in nursing home meals?
3. What is the impact of Title III-C meals on the overall dietary intake of participants?
4. What are problems related to both food safety and nutrient retention that must be considered in home delivery of hot meals? Describe alternative methods of food delivery to homebound aged.
5. Develop recommendations to ensure optimum nutrient quality and client acceptance of meals served in (a) Title III-C programs and (b) nursing homes.

REFERENCES

1. Allington, J.K., and others: A short method to ensure nutritional adequacy of food served in nursing homes. 1. Identification of need, J. Am. Diet. Assoc. **76:**458, 1980.
2. Allington, J.K., and others: A short method to ensure nutritional adequacy of food served in nursing homes. 2. Development of a model food plan, J. Am. Diet. Assoc. **76:**465, 1980.
3. Balsam, A., and Carlin, J.M.: Consortium contracting, Community Nutritionist **2:**9, 1983.
4. Barker, R.A., and Martin, J.: Feeding the elderly, 1. The Auckland meals on wheels service, J. N.Z. Diet. Assoc. **26:**10, 1972.
5. Berg, W.E., Atlas, L., and Zeiger, J.: Integrated homemaking services for the aged in urban neighborhoods, Gerontologist **14:**388, 1974.

6. Bild, B.R., and Havighurst, R.J.: Senior citizens in great cities: The case of Chicago, Gerontologist **16**:76, 1976.

7. Brody, E.M.: Long-term care for the elderly: Optimums, options and opportunities, J. Am. Geriatr. Soc. **19**:482, 1971.

8. Carlin, J.M.: Nutrition service needs of the elderly: A look into the future, Annual Meeting of the American Public Health Association, Montreal, Nov. 16, 1982.

9. Clarke, M., and Wakefield, L.M.: Food choices of institutionalized vs. independent-living elderly, J. Am. Diet. Assoc. **66**:600, 1975.

10. Conner, K.A., Powers, E.A., and Bultena, G.L.: Social interaction and life satisfaction: An empirical assessment of late-life patterns, J. Gerontol. **34**:116, 1979.

11. Cox, D., and Neumann, F.K.: Hospital sponsors door to door dietary, Mod. Hosp. **108**:178, 1967.

12. Davies, L., Hastrop, K., and Bender, A.E.: Methodology of a survey on meals on wheels, Mod. Geriatr. **3**:385, 1973.

13. Davies, L., Hastrop, K., and Bender, A.E.: Potassium intake of the elderly, Mod. Geriatr. **3**:482, 1973.

14. Davies, L., Hastrop, K., and Bender, A.E.: The energy benefit of meals on wheels, Mod. Geriatr. **4**:220, 1974.

15. Food and Nutrition Board: Recommended dietary allowances, ed. 9, Washington, D.C., 1980, National Academy of Sciences.

16. Ford, C.S., Kaplan, J., and Gremling, D.: Home delivered meals help aged and ill live independently, Hospitals **42**:80, 1968.

17. Ford, M.G., and Neville, J.N.: Nutritive intake of nursing home patients served three or five meals a day, J. Am. Diet. Assoc. **61**:292, 1972.

18. Greene, J.: Nutritional care considerations of older Americans, J. Natl. Med. Assoc. **71**:791, 1979.

19. Greene, J.M.: Coordination of Older Americans Act programs, J. Am. Diet. Assoc. **78**:617, 1981.

20. Harper, J.M., and others: Menu planning in the Nutrition Program for the Elderly. Modified nutrient standard menu method, J. Am. Diet. Assoc. **68**:529, 1976.

21. Holmes, D.: Nutrition and health-screening services for the elderly: Report of a demonstration project, J. Am. Diet. Assoc. **60**:301, 1972.

22. Huiatt, A., and Hockin, B.L.: Nutrition programs for senior citizens, J. Home Econ. **63**:683, 1971.

23. Jernigan, A.K.: Home-delivered meals as a hospital service, Hospitals **43**:90, 1969.

24. Joering, E.: Nutrient composition of a meals program for senior citizens, J. Am. Diet. Assoc. **59**:129, 1971.

25. Jordan, M., and others: Dietary habits of persons living alone, Geriatrics **9**:230, 1954.

26. Keeney, D.B., and others: Nutrition evaluation of a grocery delivery program for rural homebound elderly, Fed. Proc. **42**:829, 1983.

27. Keller, M.D., and Smith, C.E.: Meals on wheels: 1960, Geriatrics **16**:237, 1961.

28. Kohrs, M.B.: The nutrition program for older Americans. Evaluation and recommendations, J. Am. Diet. Assoc. **75**:543, 1979.

29. Kohrs, M.B., O'Hanlon, P., and Eklund, D.: Title VII Nutrition Program for the Elderly, 1. Contribution to one day's dietary intake, J. Am. Diet. Assoc. **72**:487, 1978.

30. Kohrs, M.B., and others: Title VII Nutrition Program for the Elderly, 2. Relationship of socioeconomic factors to one day's nutrient intake, J. Am. Diet. Assoc. **75**:537, 1979.

31. Kohrs, M.B., and others: Association of participation in a nutritional program for the elderly with nutritional status, Am. J. Clin. Nutr. **33**:2643, 1980.

32. Lawton, M.P.: Environment and aging, Monterey, Calif., 1980, Brooks/Cole Publishing Co.

33. Lyons, E.T.: Seniors say no to frozen meals, Aging, Nos. 329-330, p. 40, July-Aug., 1982.

34. McCool, A.C., and Posner, B.M.: Nutrition services for older Americans: Foodservice systems and technologies. Program management strategies. Chicago, 1982, American Dietetic Association.

35. Monier, C.P., Makowiecki, M.M., and Yessian, M.R.: Follow-up on the home delivered meals program service delivery assessment, Washington, D.C., 1982, U.S. Dept. of Health and Human Services.

36. National Council on the Aging: Home-delivered meals for the ill, handicapped, and elderly, Am. J. Public Health **55**(suppl.):1, 1965.

37. Osteraas, G., and others: Developing new options in home-delivered meals: The SMOC demonstration elderly nutrition project, J. Am. Diet. Assoc. **82**:524, 1983.

38. Page, L.: Nutrition programs for the elderly: A guide to menu planning, buying and the care of food for community programs, Agricultural Research Publication No. 62-22, Washington, D.C., 1972, U.S. Government Printing Office.

39. Pelcovits, J.: Nutrition for older Americans, J. Am. Diet. Assoc. **58**:17, 1971.

40. Pelcovits, J.: Nutrition to meet the human needs of older Americans, J. Am. Diet. Assoc. **60**:297, 1972.

41. Piper, G.M., Frank, B., and Thormer, R.M.: Survey of home-delivered meals, Public Health Rep. **80**:432, 1965.

42. Posner, B.M.: Nutrition and the elderly, Lexington, Mass., 1979, D.C. Heath & Co.

43. Rhodes, L.: NASA food technology: A method for meeting the nutritional needs of the elderly, Gerontologist **17**:333, 1977.

44. Rosenzweig, L.: Coordination of private and public home delivered meals programs, Annual Meeting of the National Association of Meals Programs, Syracuse, N.Y., April 29, 1982.

45. Rossman, I.: Environments of geriatric care. In Rossman, I., ed.: Clinical geriatrics, ed. 2, Philadelphia, 1979, J.B. Lippincott Co.

46. Schlenker, E.D.: Nutrition and aging, Research Report No. 364, Lansing, 1978, Michigan State University Agricultural Experiment Station.

47. Sempos, C.T., and others: A dietary survey of 14 Wisconsin nursing homes, J. Am. Diet. Assoc. **81**:35, 1982.

48. Stanton, B.R.: Feeding the elderly: Meals on wheels in London, J. N.Z. Diet. Assoc. **26**:11, 1972.

49. Staton, M., and others: Handbook for site operations: The Nutrition Program for the Elderly, Corvallis, 1975, Oregon State University.

50. Stiedemann, M., Jansen, C., and Harrill, I.: Nutritional status of elderly men and women, J. Am. Diet. Assoc. **73**:132, 1978.

51. Trager, B.: Home care: Providing the right to stay home, Hospitals **49**:93, 1975.

52. Turner, M., and Glew, G.: Home delivered meals for the elderly, Food Technol. **36**:46, 1982.

53. United States Bureau of Census: 1976 Survey of institutionalized persons: A study of persons receiving long term care, Curr. Pop. Rep., Series P-23, No. 69, Washington, D.C., 1978, U.S. Government Printing Office.

54. United States Department of Health, Education and Welfare: Guide to effective project operations. The Nutrition Program for the Elderly, Corvallis, 1973, Oregon State University.

55. United States Department of Health, Education and Welfare: Older Americans Act of 1965, as amended, DHEW Publication No. (OHD) 76-20170, Washington, D.C., 1976, U.S. Government Printing Office.

56. United States Department of Health, Education and Welfare: Health. United States, 1978, DHEW Publication No. (PHS) 78-1232, Hyattsville, Md., 1978, U.S. Dept. of Health, Education and Welfare.

57. United States Department of Health and Human Services: Longitudinal evaluation of the national Nutrition Program for the Elderly. Report on first-wave findings, DHEW Publication No. (OHDS) 80-20249, Washington, D.C., 1979, U.S. Government Printing Office.

58. United States Department of Health and Human Services: Long term care: Background and future directions, HCFA 81-20047, Washington, D.C., 1981, U.S. Government Printing Office.

59. United States Department of Health and Human Services: Analysis of food service delivery systems used in providing nutrition services to the elderly. Executive summary, Washington, D.C., 1982, U.S. Government Printing Office.

60. United States Department of Health and Human Services: The home delivered meals program: A service delivery assessment, Washington, D.C., 1981, U.S. Government Printing Office.

61. United States Department of Health and Human Services: National summary of program performance fiscal year 1982, Washington, D.C., 1983, U.S. Dept. of Health and Human Services.

62. United States General Accounting Office: Entering a nursing home, costly implications for Medicaid and the elderly, Report to the Congress of the United States, PAD-80-12, Washington, D.C., 1979, U.S. Government Printing Office.

63. United States House of Representatives Committee on Education and Labor: Compilation of the Older Americans Act of 1965 and related provisions of law as amended through December 29, 1981, Washington, D.C., 1982, U.S. Government Printing Office.

64. United States Senate Committee on Human Resources: Home delivered meals for the elderly, Washington, D.C., 1977, U.S. Government Printing Office.

65. United States Senate Select Committee on Nutrition and Human Needs: National meals on wheels program, Washington, D.C., 1977, U.S. Government Printing Office.

66. United States Senate Special Committee on Aging: Developments in aging: 1976, Part I, Washington, D.C., 1977, U.S. Government Printing Office.

67. Watkin, D.M.: The Nutrition Program for Older Americans: A successful application of current knowledge in nutrition and gerontology, World Rev. Nutr. Diet. **26**:26, 1977.

68. Wells, C.E.: Nutrition programs under the Older Americans Act, Am. J. Clin. Nutr. **26**:1127, 1973.

69. Williams, I.F., and Smith, C.E.: Home delivered meals for the aged and handicapped, J. Am. Diet. Assoc. **35**:146, 1959.

70. Wolgamot, I.: Mobile meals, Washington, D.C., no date given, National Council on the Aging.

71. Youry, M., ed.: Hospitals and home care for the elderly, Washington, D.C., 1978, National Council on the Aging.

SELECTED RESOURCES

Carlin, J.M.: A food service guide to nutrition programs for the elderly, Publication No. 7058, Durham, N.H., 1975, New England Gerontology Center.

McCool, A.C., and Posner, B.M.: Nutrition services for older Americans: Foodservice systems and strategies, Program management strategies, Chicago, 1982, American Dietetic Association.

Page, L.: Nutrition programs for the elderly. A guide to menu planning, buying and the care of food for community programs, Agricultural Research Publication No. 62-22, Washington, D.C., 1972, U.S. Department of Agriculture.

United States Department of Health, Education and Welfare: A guide to nutrition and food service for nursing homes and homes for the aged, DHEW Publication No. (HSM) 71-6701, Washington, D.C., 1971, U.S. Government Printing Office.

Chapter 13

Development of Nutrition Education Programs

Dietary intake is influenced by nutrition knowledge and ability to select a nutritionally adequate diet from the food choices available. Although efforts have been made to reach older people with nutrition education,[2] these programs have not always been successful. One aspect of the problem is the relevance of the material being presented. One older man with complete dentures told of the nutritionist who spent an hour telling him about the importance of milk and calcium in maintaining strong teeth.[19] Nutrition education should build on the nutrition knowledge clients may already have and provide appropriate information useful in the daily food situation.

NUTRITION KNOWLEDGE OF OLDER PEOPLE

People acquire a basic pattern of food selection and knowledge of food through a lifetime of experience. For those older individuals with few years of formal schooling, nutrition knowledge has generally been acquired through informal sources such as newspapers or magazines and friends or acquaintances.[16,25] In some instances food beliefs are based on traditional concepts about food (e.g., milk is primarily for children) that may not be accurate.[20] Factual knowledge regarding nutrient requirements and appropriate food sources is limited among most adults.

Food Knowledge and Related Behavior

In 1975 the Food and Drug Administration evaluated the nutrition knowledge and food beliefs of 1664 adult food shoppers.[13] Nutrition knowledge related to both age and years of schooling. Low scores were most common among those with less than a high school education, those above age 50, and men. Sixty-five percent of the older persons with low knowledge scores belonged to a lower socioeconomic group.

Most participants were not familiar with good food sources of vitamins and minerals. Individual foods if correctly identified for nutrient content were not always associated with the appropriate physiologic function. Milk was considered important for building red blood cells, whereas beef and enriched bread were thought to be related to strong bones and teeth. Most shoppers knew foods that could be substituted in place of bread; however, milk and pork and beans were not recognized as protein sources that could be substituted for meat.

The majority of older people appear to have only limited knowledge of good food sources of the nutrients required for good health. The inability to substitute one nutrient source for another is particularly serious for the person who is low income or following a modified diet. If meat, fish, or poultry cannot be included in the diet on a daily basis because of cost, lack of information regarding other sources of protein such as milk or legumes will compromise nutrient intake. If dairy products become the major protein source, other foods must supply the iron usually obtained from meat. Individuals avoiding acid or gas-forming fruits or vegetables need to recognize alternative sources of vitamins or fiber. Alternative sources of nutrients should be an integral part of a nutrition education program.

Nutrition knowledge is essential for planning an adequate diet; however, nutrition knowledge may not be reflected in actual practice. Although older people know what foods should be included in the diet, cost or physical disability may interfere in food selection or preparation[43] (see Chapter 11).

Rountree and Tinklin[45] tested the nutrition knowledge of 104 independent-living aged (Table 13-1) and compared their answers with actual practices described in a dietary interview focusing on food purchasing, preparation, and frequency of intake. Although 95% knew that a balanced diet

Table 13-1. Responses of older people (n = 104) to nutrition knowledge questions

Statement	Percent Correct
Meat is a good source of protein.	80%
Protein is needed to build and replace cells.	65%
Gelatin is one of the best sources of protein.	50%
Adults need to drink milk.	83%
Carbohydrate foods provide energy.	52%
Breads and cereals are rich in carbohydrate.	54%
Whole grain breads and cereals are higher in nutritive value than enriched white flour products.	60%
Vitamin A is needed for night vision.	45%
Dark green leafy vegetables are a good source of vitamin A.	48%
Citrus foods are good sources of vitamin C.	75%

Data from Rountree, J.L., and Tinklin, G.L.: Food beliefs and practices of selected senior citizens, Gerontologist **15**:537, 1975.

should contain foods from all four food groups, not all groups were actually included in the daily pattern. In some cases food selection did reflect food beliefs. Most participants included beef or other meat in their diet several times per week, supporting their belief in the importance of protein. The positive response to the statement that gelatin is a good source of protein points to the need for information regarding protein sources. Although 83% agreed that adults need milk, only 67% actually consumed milk or other dairy products on a daily basis.

Beliefs and practices were least consistent for grain products and fruits and vegetables. About 30% consumed white bread or rolls daily, and only 9% consumed whole grain products, despite the belief that whole grains provide more nutrients. Avoidance of carbohydrate foods may reflect an effort to decrease calorie intake or the general feeling that carbohydrate is a nutrient of lesser importance. Although 75% and 45% recognized the need for vitamins C and A, respectively, fruits and vegetables were consumed in low amounts. Frozen orange juice was used by 72%, although over half believed that fresh juice was higher in nutritive value. Similarly, 77% used canned vegetables, although canned items were considered to contain lower levels of nutrients than fresh.

Variables other than nutrition knowledge influence food choices. Cost, convenience of preparation, and storage facilities affect the type of food purchased regardless of food beliefs. For the older person dependent on one store for food shopping, the availability or quality of particular items will influence the choices made. Nutrition educators must recognize the importance of these factors when developing program content.

Ability to Evaluate the Diet

Many older individuals overestimate their nutrition knowledge.[3,16] This could make them less likely to take advantage of nutrition education opportunities or less receptive to information presented.

Among 64 urban aged, 16% considered themselves as well informed in nutrition as a professional dietitian, although none had a perfect score on a nutrition knowledge test.[16] Lack of knowledge influences the ability to evaluate one's own diet. In that study participants were asked to rate their diets as excellent (containing at least 100% of the RDA for all nutrients); good (containing 66% to 99% of the RDA for all nutrients); fair (containing less than 66% of the RDA for one to two nutrients); or poor (containing less than 66% of the RDA for three or more nutrients).[16] Although 65% considered their diets to be excellent or good, less than one-third actually met these criteria. Seventy percent of the diets were fair or poor, although few individuals perceived their diets to be less than adequate.

Meal planning guides commonly used in nutrition education may contribute to the problem. Older individuals who refer to meal planning guides of some type tend to rate their diets as higher in nutrient content than people who are not using any nutrition materials.[3] The fact that these diets do not contain the level of nutrients assumed raises questions concerning the accuracy and appropriateness of nutrition guides now in use. The nutrient content of actual foods within a certain food group or the adequacy of a particular portion size may be exaggerated. The selection process based on a limited number of food groups is, for some nutrients, oversimplified (see Chapter 10). Meal planning guides now in use require continued evaluation.

Nutrition Attitudes and Food Beliefs

Food misinformation is a problem among older people.[9,16,22,35,45] The aged are especially vulnerable to advertising claiming cures for well-known chronic complaints that cannot be healed by available medicines. Health maintenance is of real concern to the older individual, and it may seem less threatening and costly to try patent medicines or vitamin supplements than to visit a physician.[4,51] Such a decision will postpone the treatment necessary for the health problem. A further danger of food misinformation is a detrimental effect on nutrient intake, resulting from avoidance of particular foods or categories of food thought to be harmful to health. Money required to purchase "health foods" or costly vitamin or mineral supplements might be used more wisely to purchase wholesome food.

An evaluation of nutrition beliefs in the general population[22] (n = 340) suggested that questionable beliefs are more common among older people (above age 60) with limited education.[22] Individuals having less nutrition education consumed high levels of vitamin and mineral preparations, considered particular foods to have special significance for health, and had exaggerated concerns about the general wholesomeness of foods. Serious health problems existing within the family often contributed to the anxiety. Items emphasized in the diets of those individuals are listed below.

Vitamin and mineral supplements
Wheat germ
Molasses
Honey
Brewers' yeast

Although food items such as molasses or brewers' yeast may add particular vitamins or minerals to the diet, the danger lies in exaggerated emphasis on these items with exclusion of other foods containing important nutrients. Nutritional supplements are high in cost leaving less money for the purchase of other food items.

It is important for the nutrition educator to understand why some older people purchase nutritional supplements.[16] In one older group such items were associated with general well-being and expected to give a person more energy, improve health, prevent colds, or prevent arthritis. More than a third of older supplement users, however, indicated these items were included in the diet "just to be safe."[16] Those emphasizing food items of questionable value or with unrealistic views about particular foods tended to have lower nutrition knowledge scores.

Despite the potential for misuse or abuse of particular foods or supplements by older people with questionable food beliefs, they often select items higher in nutrient density and consume a more adequate diet (excluding the contribution of vitamin and mineral supplements) than people with little or no interest in dietary choices.[9] In an older urban population those who believed that nutrition was important were better informed about nutrition and tended to have better diets.[16] The approach to nutrition education should be to build on those aspects of the dietary pattern that are related to sound nutrition principles. A totally negative attitude will accomplish nothing and very likely lead the client to reject all further attempts at nutrition counseling.

Maintaining health and vitality and preventing disease appear to be the bases of food selection for many older individuals.[16] Nutrition educators should consider health as a positive motivating factor for the older client. Concern for health and weight status was associated with better quality diets among older married couples.[46-47] Interest in health can provide the basis for food behavior promoting better health.

Sources of Nutrition Information

In general older people rely on less formal sources of nutrition information including television, physicians, magazines, cookbooks, and newspapers.[6,16,22] Information relating to new food products is often obtained from television and newspapers.[6,34] Food labels are used less frequently by older people.[16] Health professionals are an important source for this age group; individuals seeking nutrition information from their physicians had fewer misconceptions concerning weight loss regimens or the value of foods or supplements in treating disease. Among those urban aged (n = 64), individuals using diet books were more likely to see a need for vitamin and mineral supplements.[16] Although use of magazine articles and cookbooks as sources of nutrition information was positively related to nutrition knowledge, those individuals also considered nutrition to be important, which may have influenced their seeking out information in the first place.[16]

Older people differ according to sex and living situation in their response to formal or informal sources of nutrition information.[47] Among older married men (n = 82) the quality of the diet was positively related to information received from both casual sources, such as the mass media, and selective sources, such as food classes or extension bulletins. For single women only food classes and government information, or more reliable sources of nutrition information, were associated with a better diet.

These findings suggest that older individuals do seek out and respond to positive sources of nutrition education including government releases, university materials, and food classes. It is not known whether the food classes attended were offered by an educational institution or a health professional or home economist serving the lay public. This method of teaching does appear, however, to attract some older individuals. Others make use of printed educational materials when appropriate to their needs.

THE LEARNING PROCESS IN OLDER PEOPLE

Learning in the older adult is influenced by both physiologic and environmental factors. At one time professional educators considered the potential learning ability of older individuals to be very poor.[1,23,32] This erroneous opinion was based on studies comparing the performance of old and young learners in formal testing situations in which older people were at a disadvantage because of limited time and decreased familiarity with standard tests.[1,23] Older people do have potential for learning in a favorable environment. The nutrition educator must be aware of both the teaching methods and climate which enhance learning in the older adult.

Physiologic Aspects of Learning

Reaction Time and Control Processes. As one grows older, the body responds more slowly to both physiologic and verbal stimuli. Messages pass less rapidly through the brain and nervous system. Control processes that aid in the retrieval of stored information are less efficient. Older learners are disadvantaged when given only a limited amount of time to respond because they perceive, think, and react more slowly.[23] Because the older adult is more concerned about the correctness of his answer than is the young adult, he takes more time to respond. In the older individual speed of response and correctness of response are not related. Although the rate of learning may be slowed, the accuracy of performance may be unchanged in older versus younger learners. Although individual differences are significant, the learning ability of some individuals age 70 does not differ from that of individuals age 30.

Sensory Perception. Learning by older adults is enhanced by both visual and auditory stimuli; therefore sensory changes can significantly affect the degree of learning that takes place.[32] Establishing the proper conditions in the teaching situation can compensate for changes in sensory perception and maximize learning potential.

Visual Problems. Changes occurring in the eye as a result of normal aging influence several visual processes. The older person is less able to see objects clearly without blurring, distinguish between colors, focus rapidly from one object to another, or adapt easily from bright light to dim light.[31] Lofton and coworkers[31] have developed practical suggestions for helping the learner with poor vision.

- Keep visual aids simple. Include only one or two ideas because many words or pictures can be confusing. Attach real objects when possible, as they can be seen more easily. Use large block letters combining upper and lower case letters; letters all the same size are difficult to read. Prepare one visual aid for every 6 to 10 persons to minimize distance from viewers. Print should be large enough to be read at a distance of 10 feet.[18] Emphasize warm colors such as orange, red, and yellow, which are easier to see than cool colors or tints.
- Avoid ditto materials if duplication quality is poor. Black lettering on nonglossy white paper is best for handouts.
- Arrange for good lighting; older people require more light for reading than younger people. Place chairs away from sources of glare such as windows, bright lights, or flickering lights.
- Avoid using blackboards, which can be difficult to read because of glare. A broad-tipped felt marker on an easel pad is more easily read.
- Use actual food items as visual aids whenever possible. An older person can relate more easily to a ½-cup portion if he can see it.

Hearing Problems. Loss of hearing can be age related or result from prolonged exposure to loud concentrated sounds as in a factory with a high noise level. Despite hearing loss most people can hear a spoken voice reasonably well.[31] At the same time, the individual becomes very sensitive to background noise and is less able to separate sounds. When selecting a location for a nutrition education program, one should avoid an area with distracting noises. The following recommendations may facilitate communication with people who have some hearing impairment.[31]

- Stand still facing the group. This helps those who may be lip reading.
- Speak slowly and clearly.
- Speak in short sentences.
- Use words familiar to the group and easily recognized. New words should be defined and printed on an easel pad.
- Try to project your voice but do not shout. A microphone may be necessary with a large group.
- Repeat comments or questions that may not have been heard.

Physical Aspects of the Learning Situation. Learning can be enhanced by a favorable physical environment. Having chairs arranged in a U-shape or circle promotes eye contact with participants. A constant temperature with adequate ventilation is essential for comfort. Sessions should be limited to 15 or 20 minutes or less. It is better to end a session before interest fades or participants become bored. Material not covered can be included another time. Keeping each session short encourages continuing attendance.[31,55]

Psychologic Aspects of Learning

Attitudes Influencing Learning. The older individual brings to a learning situation a set of attitudes developed over a lifetime. If conditioned by the prevailing popular opinion that older people cannot or will not accept new ideas, the individual may be discouraged from even attempting a situation that could possibly result in failure. Moreover, childhood school experiences may not have been positive.[17] In the past teaching environments with strictly authoritarian standards were considered most effective. If previous educational activities were unpleasant, the older person may avoid joining a class. Therefore the first step in encouraging an older adult to participate is to emphasize the informality of the session.[23,48,57]

Need for Relevance. Learning reflects an effort on the part of an individual to meet needs as he perceives them.[23] Although children are resigned to learning facts that they may or may not consider important to their personal situation, the older learner hopes to make immediate use of the material presented.[23,48] The aged woman on a limited income will have little interest in the nutritional value of high cost foods that are beyond her budget. Older individuals see, hear, and perceive information on a selective basis. Unless one is fully involved in the process, the information will not be acted on.[48] The ability of the listener to act on the suggestions being presented should be an important criterion when selecting material for a nutrition education lesson.

Environmental Aspects of Learning

Older people often approach the learning situation with considerable anxiety. Therefore a favorable emotional climate is paramount in encouraging participation. Factors contributing to the environment include the location of the class, the qualities of the teacher, and the degree of participation expected or required of attenders.[15,17,48,57]

Location of Class. Opportunities for learning can be formal or informal and can take place in a variety of locations. Educational institutions within the community such as public school systems, community colleges, or other universities or colleges often make courses available to older people with tuition waived or reduced. Less formal educational activities are sponsored by senior citizens groups, congregate meal sites, or residential housing facilities. A survey of 86 independent-living aged from both rural and urban locations revealed that 85% preferred continuing education activities held in less formal facilities such as senior centers or senior housing.[17] The educational level of this group was above average, as 37 were former teachers. Therefore lack of formal education did not influence preference of informal activities. For 25%, lack of transportation interfered with participation in educational programs.

Emotional Climate. Older adults bring to a learning situation perceptions of themselves, their abilities, and limitations. It is important therefore to create positive experiences.[57] This is best accomplished in a relaxed, noncompetitive atmosphere in which material is presented at the pace appropriate for the learner rather than the teacher. Participants should be encouraged to express themselves and be made to feel that their opinions are important. The shy adult who does not volunteer to answer should not be forced to respond.[48] If active participation becomes mandatory, those most in need of information may not remain a part of the group. A supportive environment directed toward individual needs and capabilities is most likely to attract the older learner.

IMPLEMENTATION OF NUTRITION EDUCATION

Recognizing Client Needs

The first step in developing a successful nutrition education program is to become acquainted with the client group. In some communities it may be necessary for a nutrition educator to be bilingual in order to communicate with the program participants. In that situation visual aids or handouts must be available in the language of the people served.[41]

Learning experiences for aged coming from differing economic, ethnic, and racial backgrounds require innovative methods. Nutrition education programs organized along traditional lines have, for the most part, been unsuccessful with older people.[19,54] Nutrition lectures are not attended and talks given during congregate meals are usually ignored as participants chat among themselves.[19,21] For a program to be successful it must focus on the real life situation of participants, keeping in mind income, housing arrangements, and physical condition.[41-42]

The goal of nutrition education is to improve or enhance nutritional status, health, and well-being.[48] For the individual at risk this may require a change in food habits to improve nutrient intake. If the present diet is adequate, nutrition education can encourage the most effective use of resources to maintain that intake.

Among 680 older persons attending a health clinic, over one third expressed a need for nutrition information.[53] Areas of interest (in descending order of importance) were planning a balanced diet, tips on food buying, food preparation and storage procedures, new food products, and information on food stamps. About 75% of those participants requesting information on planning a balanced diet were consuming diets inadequate in at least one nutrient. An informal survey of the client group to establish areas of interest will help in developing a program that meets client needs.

Developing Curriculum for Nutrition Education

Selecting Behavioral Objectives. Behavioral objectives for nutrition education can be cognitive or affective.[8] Cognitive objectives relate to thinking skills and acquisition of knowledge. A cognitive objective for older adults could be learning to use nutrition labels to recognize foods high in sodium content. Affective objectives relate to values and attitudes toward food. Although individuals recognize foods high in sodium content, they may continue to select these items for their daily diet. Cognitive learning is not always translated into practice. Eppright and coworkers[10] in their classic work on nutrition education pointed out that changing the way people think may be less important than changing the way they feel.

The complex relationship between previous experience and new information within the decision making process is schematically presented in Fig. 13-1. Olson and Sims[38] suggest that new information is processed in relation to one's previous knowledge, beliefs, attitudes, and intentions. Information received may be modified or eliminated at any stage as a result of psychologic (internal) or environmental (external) factors. Therefore exposure to a nutrition message may not necessarily have an influence on decision making or actual selection of a food.

New information is processed and assigned a meaning based on previous knowledge. Learning the sodium content of particular foods will have little meaning if the health related aspects of sodium have not been explained. Building on previous nutrition knowledge and attitudes will enhance both learning and the decision making process.

Developing the Learning Sequence. If the learner is to be prepared to use the facts presented in making day to day food decisions, theories and generalizations must be applied to practical situations in appropriate sequence. Educators have defined four sequential levels of learning.

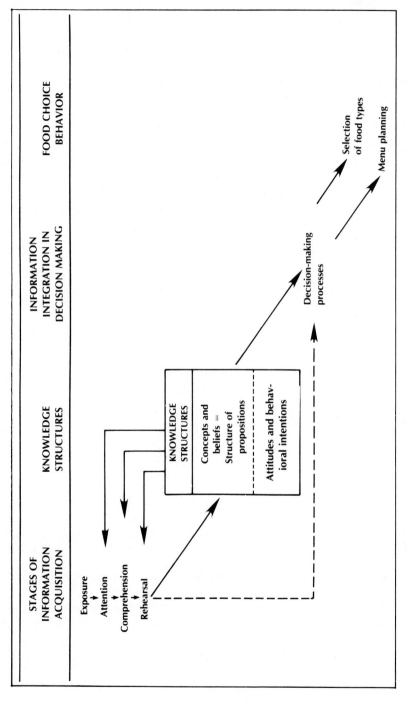

Fig. 13-1. Model for processing nutrition information. (Reprinted from the *Journal of Nutrition Education*, Olson, J.C., and Sims, L.S.: Assessing nutrition knowledge from an information processing perspective, J. Nutr. Ed. **12:**157, 1980, © Society for Nutrition Education.)

Knowledge: Acquiring facts, theories, and general information, which serve as a foundation for future learning.

Comprehension: Understanding and integrating facts with previous knowledge, beliefs, and attitudes.

Application: Using facts and ideas in practical life situations.

Problem solving: Analyzing and evaluating a situation and selecting an appropriate course of action.[5,8]

This sequence should be considered when developing modules for nutrition education. Teaching methods should include activities in which the learner can practice the skills to be acquired. Lessons with suggestions for appropriate visual aids can be found in references 31 and 55.

Selecting Teaching Methods

Group Discussion. Group discussion, based on process rather than the didactic approach,[19] has been successful with older persons.[19,21,24,41-42] Although the discussion leader should prepare information relating to a general topic, the actual ideas discussed should be guided by the interests of those attending.[19] Such a group could function as a recreational activity.

Learning Activities. Adults learn more easily if several senses are stimulated simultaneously.[32] Therefore combining several learning techniques is more effective than using only one. A film followed by discussion or a presentation describing the nutritional importance of dairy foods followed by tasting of milk-based recipes is a combination that can lead to changes in behavior. The activity-oriented experiences described in Table 13-2 can be adapted for use at a congregate meal site, a senior center, or a long term care facility, or with individuals at home.[24,27,31,41-42]

Handouts contribute to a teaching situation by reinforcing learning after the participants have returned to their homes. Handouts poorly prepared or not easily understood are usually discarded without being read. Recipes, nutrient food sources, and a low cost shopping list to be used at a later time are extremely helpful handouts.[31]

Table 13-2. Learning activities for nutrition education

Type of Activity	Example
Demonstration	Prepare a low calorie or low cost recipe or new food for tasting with recipe handout for people to try at home.
Skits; role playing	Volunteers from the client group or visitors from a nearby school or community group present problems of several people who have been trying to lose weight.
Problem solving	Using newspapers with weekly food specials, select groceries for the week considering both nutritional adequacy and cost; have participants keep diet diaries and evaluate for nutritional adequacy.
Field trip	Visit a grocery store that provides shopping assistance or a local food co-op (this may be a special treat for an individual who lacks personal transportation).
Panel	Have several "experts" (group participants or visitors) briefly discuss a topic, then continue discussion with the entire group. Topic might be a food-buying problem or use of food stamps.
Group activity	Develop and duplicate a "cooking for one or two" recipe book; plant a vegetable garden or plant vegetables in containers for those unable to go outdoors; prepare a consumer exhibit for the senior center. (Provides a way for participants to get to know each other.)

Developing a Standard of Performance. The behavioral objective should include a standard of performance to demonstrate that the learner has mastered the task.[8] Unfortunately, emphasis is often placed on the correct recitation of nutrition facts or the percentage of questions answered correctly in a posttest. Developing a positive attitude toward nutrition or selecting an appropriate food for lunch is even more important. Outcomes involving a change in behavior, however, are more difficult to evaluate than a change in nutrition knowledge. (Types of evaluation will be discussed in a later section.)

Selecting Nutrition Education Materials

A nutrition educator may not have either the time or resources to prepare original materials. Instead existing materials must be adapted for use with the client group. Because few materials have been developed specifically for older people, health professionals are often forced to rely on films or handouts planned with younger people in mind. Another problem relates to the validity of the information presented. Attractive, well designed materials are often available free from companies or trade associations selling particular food products. In some cases the food and nutrition information is biased to promote the organization's products to best advantage. Other commercially produced materials contain factually sound consumer information. Materials obtained from any source should be examined carefully as to content and presentation.[37] Criteria to be considered when selecting or developing materials are presented below.

Do the materials present a favorable image of older persons? The attitude of many is that most aged individuals are sick, incapacitated, and unable to care for themselves. These inaccurate stereotypes are sometimes carried over into published materials. Sketches of older people may present a gaunt, tired image. Such materials detract from the learning environment.

Are the materials appropriate for older persons?

Both content and visual display enter into the evaluation of nutrition materials. Cartoons or stick figures, acceptable for a school age group, can be insulting to the older audience. Nutritional needs and problems also differ between old and young. I recall visiting a nutrition education workshop at a congregate meal site that used posters designed to encourage children to "make your own milkshake" adding ice cream, syrup, juices, and fruits. Although promoting use of milk and dairy products among older people is vitally important, those with limited energy needs cannot afford to consume a high calorie milkshake as a snack. Some materials may be appropriate with clarification of when and how particular food choices can be included in the diet.

Is information presented with a positive approach? The aged are more receptive to learning principles that are positive in nature.[48] Negative or unpleasant associations are shut out and tend to be forgotten. Food choices should be presented as options within the individual's control, not as a set of edicts. For many older individuals the realities of disease and disability are frightening enough without the association of these threats with the food one eats. Presenting nutritional advice from the standpoint of "keeping well," or "feeling better," or "having energy to go for a walk or play with your grandchild" will be considerably more effective than focusing on the physical consequences of poor eating habits. Poor attendance at nutrition education sessions can result from too much emphasis on "telling me not to eat foods that I like."[37]

Is the information presented accurate? Extravagant claims regarding the nutrient contribution of any one particular food or food group can be misleading. Generalizations that present only part of the picture lead to inaccurate conclusions. For example, the comment that "high calorie foods should be eliminated from a weight reduction diet" does not address the issue of serving size. Furthermore, meat items relatively high in calories do provide essential nutrients including protein, iron, and zinc. The concept presented should be reinforced with examples and any exceptions to the rule should be clearly defined.

Is the information practical? Nutritional advice is of no value unless it can be put into practice. Therefore aspects of cost, time, cooking skills, and available cooking facilities must be considered when selecting both lesson content and materials.[37] Recipes containing mushrooms, black olives, or other expensive condiments may be appropriate if such items can be omitted if necessary. When working with individuals who rely on convenience items because of physical disability or poor cooking skills, lessons suggesting more nutritious choices among convenience items or foods that might effectively complement a convenience main dish will be more helpful than merely pointing out the nutrient limitations of some convenience foods. Providing information to solve immediate problems should be the priority in any nutrition education program.

Are the materials attractive and well designed? A common mistake in preparing nutrition education materials is including too many details and too many pictures. As a result, posters or handouts look crowded and confused. Wording should be kept as brief as possible and illustrations simple.[18]

EVALUATION OF NUTRITION EDUCATION PROGRAMS

Types of Evaluation

Evaluation procedures should be developed when the nutrition education program is initiated. Frequently, evaluation is not considered until after the program has been completed and opportunities to obtain feedback from participants have been lost.

Several forms of evaluation are applicable to nutrition education programs.[28,52] *Continuous* evaluation provides on-going information indicating whether changes are needed and, if so, what kinds of changes should be introduced. *Periodic* evaluation is carried out at specific stages and monitors progress and effectiveness. *Follow-up* evaluation is conducted some time after completion of a project and determines the extent to which desired outcomes are being implemented or continued. Because both time and personnel are usually limited, simple indicators or easily collected data are preferred.[28] Continued attendance or increased attendance, suggesting that participants are inviting others, is one indication that a nutrition education series is meeting needs of the client group.

Methods of Evaluation

Nutrition Knowledge. The most common evaluation procedure in nutrition education is testing nutrition knowledge.[48] Although children may be accustomed to being tested, older people may resent the traditional pretest, posttest approach. A pretest can serve as a teaching tool if class members keep their tests as a basis for the discussion to follow. In that case it should be made clear at the beginning that tests will not be collected and only the individual will be aware of the number of right and wrong answers. If knowledge tests are used, they should be pretested with individuals of similar age and background so that misunderstandings can be avoided.[48]

Nutrition Attitudes. One alternative to knowledge tests is evaluating attitudes toward the information presented.[48] Grotkowski and Sims[16] found that attitudes regarding the relative importance of nutrition were strongly correlated with nutrition knowledge in older subjects. Curry[7] successfully used an indirect approach in evaluating training workshops for older participants. Questions might include:

What information presented today was most helpful to you?

What information presented today was least helpful to you?

Will the information presented today be of use to you (in doing your food shopping, watching your weight, etc.)? If not, why not?

On what topics would you like to have more information?

Such a format would be acceptable to participants and still provide valuable feedback for future programs.

Food Selection Patterns. The most desirable criteria for evaluating the effectiveness of a nutrition education program are demonstrated changes in clients' food behavior. Methods used to determine food intake include food frequency tabulations, 24-hour recall records, or written records (see Chapter 10). In many situations formal evaluation is not feasible in terms of the time and professional expertise required.

Observation of food selection or consumption at a congregate meal site or long term care facility is an appropriate informal evaluation of nutrition practices. The number of persons accepting and consuming the cup of milk served, before and after a nutrition education series, provides a measure of success in bringing about positive change. A plate waste study of the vegetables served will give some indication of acceptance.

Encouraging participants to share their ideas as part of a problem-solving lesson may be another way of evaluating nutrition practices in a nonthreatening manner. At a session following a lesson on nutrition labeling, the leader might ask if anyone encountered any problems with the labels they observed the last time they went food shopping.[39] If food shopping is a group activity sponsored by the congregate meal site, the leader may informally observe the food selection process and choices made. Food purchasing patterns and use of vitamin or mineral supplements have been suggested as practices that could serve as indicators of the effectiveness of nutrition education.

Nutritional Status. If nutrition education is one component of a broad nutrition intervention program, an evaluation of nutritional status based on dietary and biochemical measurements may be possible. The problems associated with these procedures have been described previously (see Chapter 10). Because of the many uncontrollable factors influencing both the dietary intake and biochemical status of the aged, it is often difficult to draw conclusions regarding the success of a nutrition intervention program.

In a recent program[14] evaluating the effect of iron supplementation and dietary counseling on Boston aged, hemoglobin values improved in both groups receiving counseling regardless of the level of iron in the foods provided. Those authors concluded that the personal attention received by control subjects contributed to improved food selection and the apparent nutritional benefit.[14] The personal concern of the nutrition educator as perceived by the client may be as important as the actual information shared.

INNOVATIVE APPROACHES TO NUTRITION EDUCATION

Integrating Nutrition Education and Meal Programs

Effective nutrition education for people of all ages integrates nutrition knowledge and food behavior. Therefore an ideal setting is a meal program where food is prepared or served.[21,26,30,41-42] Home-delivered meals are a way to extend nutrition education to homebound aged.

Using the Served Meal. Nutrition education should begin with the presentation of good food. Parham[40] suggests that the food experiences of the aged are not always pleasant. Cost, convenience, or eating alone may lead to a monotonous diet consisting of relatively few foods (see Chapter 11). Being presented with a variety of nutritious foods in a social setting can be a positive educational experience. New foods can be introduced and common foods high in nutritional value reinforced within the meal pattern.

In one program menus were revised to include more dairy foods such as cheese and pudding, when participants were found to have low intakes of calcium, riboflavin, and vitamin A.[44] Those individuals seldom drank the milk served with the congregate meals and consumed few dairy foods at home. It was the intent that meal patterns including more dairy foods would be carried over into meals and snacks prepared at home, although there was no follow-up evaluation.

Other items to be stressed in program menu planning are dark green and deep yellow vegetables. New ways of preparing vegetables introduced in the program meal may be adopted for home use. Serving vegetables with a milk-based sauce could add needed calcium to the diet. Liver and other iron-rich foods could be presented on a more frequent basis. The meal as served should provide positive reinforcement of the major food groups and good food sources of particular nutrients.[41-42]

Involving Participants in Menu Planning. Having a small group work with the nutritionist in planning the menus has been a successful approach.[19] The planners were expected to be reasonably knowledgeable about the foods selected and to interpret their findings to others. When a cycle menu covering several weeks or months is implemented for a city or region, actual participation in menu planning may not be feasible; however, participants should be given an opportunity for input and all suggestions accepted in a positive manner.

One older participant when asked about his suggestions for improvement of the congregate meal menus recommended that pie be served every day for dessert. It could be pointed out that a high calorie dessert is appropriate on an occasional but not daily basis for those with limited calorie needs. If meals as served do not represent high nutritional standards, participants should be encouraged to make recommendations for improvement.

Nutrition Education in the Home

Many older individuals who need information are homebound as a result of rural location, lack of transportation, or physical disability. Others may be too shy or embarrassed to participate in a group situation. Methods tested for reaching older people at home have included one-to-one visitation and the mass media.

Nutrition Aide Program. Paraprofessionals trained in food preparation, food shopping, and meal planning have been used successfully with families of various ages to bring about changes in food behavior.[27,29,56,58] For the isolated aged the nutrition aide can be a source of emotional support serving as both teacher and friend.[29,56]

This one-on-one method was successfully used in rural Mississippi; older people with some understanding of food and nutrition were recruited to work with their peers.[58] Each was assigned a specific neighborhood with the responsibility of becoming acquainted with the aged living there. On home visits the nutrition aide shared nutrition information and looked for signs that pointed to nutrition problems, such as a poor supply of food on the shelf or physical indications of malnutrition. Once each week aides met with professional staff to discuss the problems observed and receive advice and referral.

Through this program older clients not only learned more about nutrition and community food-related resources but also improved their general outlook on life. This method of teaching can be extremely effective; however, the cost limits the number of clients reached. A telephone call or letter might supplement an occasional visit. In light of the increasing number of older households needing food-related assistance, these alternatives should be tested with this age group.

Peer counseling, at a congregate meal site or in the client's home, has been implemented in some communities under the Retired Senior Volunteer Program (RSVP). Retired volunteers with professional training in nutrition and foods are ideally suited for helping peers deal with prescribed diets, weight control, or general food problems. Counselors who have only a general background in nutrition, need to recognize their limitations and the types of problems that should be referred to a health professional.

Use of Television. Manoff[33] has pointed to the mass media as an untapped resource for disseminating nutrition information. Television watching is a favorite pastime of many retired people, especially those who are confined to their homes.[6] An effective use of television may be the short sequence, 1 minute or less, inserted as a public service announcement. Such a message requires no viewer interest or motivation, reaching its objective through repetition over days and weeks.

Public Service Announcements. Nutrition public service announcements (PSAs) have been evaluated as a method of nutrition education for reaching older people. In an Iowa study four 30- to 60-second announcements, emphasizing food sources of protein, calcium, and vitamin A and the nutritional value of enriched bread, were broadcast 112 times within a 2-month period.[11,12] The majority of the 65 older persons interviewed before and after the PSA broadcasts, however, had no recall of the televised messages. Moreover, there was no apparent relationship between recall of the PSAs, nutrition knowledge of the nutrients described in the PSAs, or changes in reported intakes of specific foods.

In commercial advertising a 20% recall of a message shown once during prime time is considered good; therefore the recall of the vitamin A and protein PSAs (8% each) and the enrichment PSA (14%) suggests that this method deserves further consideration. Since all persons interviewed were attenders of a congregate meal program they could represent a more socially active group of aged who spend less time watching television. It was not known how many people actually saw the announcements.

PSAs may be most useful for simple messages, such as announcing congregate meal programs or giving information about food stamps. A health message may be too general or abstract to hold attention.[11] PSAs could be effectively reinforced with printed materials.[12]

Television Series. A television cooking series directed toward older adults in a metropolitan area attracted many viewers as indicated by the number of requests received for booklets advertised on the air.[59] Each show demonstrated two low cost, nutritious recipes requiring only limited preparation time and incorporated information on meal planning, food buying, and nutrition. Recipes were designed for one to two persons and required no elaborate equipment. Items from other food groups that would complement the recipes demonstrated and make a complete meal were suggested. Although nutritionists may wish to deemphasize "cooking," per se, the fact remains that people not interested in nutrition may be attracted to such a program. Important food and nutrition information can be developed in an entertaining food-related format. Older people living in senior housing or visiting a senior center might watch a nutrition-related television program as a group and follow it with discussion or questions. This requires, however, a discussion leader with some background in nutrition and foods.[36,59]

Recommendations for Effective Use of Television

Length of Program. Television programs evaluated for effectiveness have varied in length from 5 minutes to 1 hour.[36,49,59] A program of 10 minutes or less did not permit adequate discussion of the topic and viewers felt that the time was too short. An hour, on the other hand, was too long for continued interest. A 30-minute program seems to be a good compromise.

Publicity. The viewing audience can be increased significantly by prior publicity.[59] Newspaper advertisements regarding time and channel, an announcement in newsletters distributed to older people, or posters displayed at senior housing or senior centers aid in attracting viewers.[12,36,59]

Audience Participation. Providing an opportunity for older people watching the program to participate fosters learning. Conducting a recipe contest or encouraging viewers to submit questions that could be answered on the air strengthens involvement with the program.[59] If materials are available, a telephone number in addition to a mailing address is helpful.[12] Concurrent classes conducted by an adult education group reinforce learning from both activities.

Program Development. Each show should have a simple and direct message. Information is less likely to be understood if the show moves rapidly from one idea to another. Fitzgibbons and co-workers[12] recommend pretesting the program to determine whether the message is perceived as intended. When both good and poor sources of vitamin A were mentioned on one program, viewers assumed that all foods mentioned were good sources.[49]

Feature Older Individuals. Information becomes more attractive and relevant if older people are presenting it.[12] A series of highly successful food demonstration programs featured an older man who, although not a professional, related well to his target audience.[59] The benefit derived from a ''teacher'' with whom the audience can identify may outweigh any errors in presentation resulting from limited experience.[12]

Most local commercial television stations are required to provide time for nonprofit programming. Public television stations are also a source of air time for educational purposes. Pooling of resources by various community groups such as state or local agencies on aging, state or local departments of health, or the cooperative extension service can make possible development of informative programming.

Team Approach to Nutrition Education

A multidisciplinary approach to health education including a physician, nutritionist, health educator, and home economist was successful in motivating older people to alter their food behavior.[50] One-day workshops held in senior centers in several locations presented information on the relationships between diet and chronic disease, calorie balance, and nutrient requirements with practical aspects of food selection.

Participants were urged to set personal goals for improvement of dietary practices. Most wished to either lose weight or resist weight gain. Seventy percent of those responding to a postcard questionnaire mailed 2 weeks following the conference indicated they had implemented changes in their diet based on the conference and several had begun to lose weight.

Those workshops, scheduled for 7 hours with 1 hour for lunch, were very tiring for some participants (ages ranged from 40 to 92). Another approach might be to schedule two sessions, each 2 to 3 hours in length. If classes were several weeks apart, participants would have time to make dietary changes and share progress and problems at the second session.

SUMMARY

Older people are poorly informed as to required nutrients, their functions in the body, and good food sources. Furthermore, those who do recognize the need for particular nutrients may because of cost or convenience not include those foods in their diets. Older people rely on less formal sources of nutrition information such as newspapers, television, or cookbooks.

Although older individuals are as able to learn as younger individuals, they think and respond more slowly. Visual materials should be in large print with good contrast to compensate for decreased sensory perception. Leaders should speak slowly and distinctly, facing the audience, to facilitate participation by those with hearing problems. A nonthreatening, positive approach is most likely to attract participants.

Nutrition education objectives should be relevant and address client needs. Active learning and problem-solving activities provide reinforcement and comprehension of the facts presented. Evaluation can address changes in attitudes or food habits as well as recall of nutrition information.

Congregate meal programs offer opportunities to

integrate nutrition education with a served meal. For persons confined to their home nutrition aides can offer help with meal planning and, under the direction of a health professional, monitor general well-being. Use of television to reach older people with nutrition education appears to be successful and should be expanded.

REVIEW QUESTIONS

1. Based on available evidence, what areas of food and nutrition information should be emphasized in nutrition education programs for older people?
2. Describe visual and hearing changes occurring over adulthood. How can a nutrition educator compensate for these changes with appropriate visual materials, room arrangement, and speaking techniques?
3. Are older people able to learn as easily as younger people? Explain. Define psychologic, emotional, and environmental factors that can influence learning in the older adult.
4. Prepare a series of three 15-minute nutrition education lessons for use at a Title III congregate meal site. Include objectives, outline of subject matter, description of visual aids and/or handouts, evaluation techniques, and reference materials.
5. Develop a list of suggested nutrition and food related learning activities for use by a Title III program director, keeping in mind time and budgetary constraints.

REFERENCES

1. Arenberg, D., and Robertson-Tchabo, E.A.: Learning and aging. In Birren, J.E., and Schaie, K.W., eds.: Handbook of the psychology of aging, New York, 1977, Van Nostrand Reinhold Co. Inc.
2. Brazzarre, T.L.: Aging and nutrition education, Educ. Gerontol. 3:149, 1978.
3. Brown, E.L.: Factors affecting food choices and intake, Geriatrics 31:89, 1976.
4. Butler, R.N.: Why are older consumers so susceptible, Geriatrics 23:83, 1968.
5. Chamberlain, V.M., and Kelly, J.: Creative home economics instruction, New York, 1975, McGraw-Hill Book Co.
6. Clancy, K.L.: Preliminary observations on media use and food habits of the elderly, Gerontologist 15:529, 1975.
7. Curry, R.C.: Training guide for trainers: Nutrition program for the elderly, Corvallis, 1976, Oregon State University.
8. Cyrs, T.E.: You, behavioral objectives and nutrition education, Rosemont, Ill., 1977, National Dairy Council.
9. Davidson, C.S., and others: The nutrition of a group of apparently healthy aging persons, Am. J. Clin. Nutr. 10:181, 1962.
10. Eppright, E., Pattison, M., and Barbour, H.: Teaching nutrition, ed. 2, Ames, 1963, Iowa State University Press.
11. Fitzgibbons, J.J., and Garcia, P.A.: TV, PSAs, nutrition and the elderly, J. Nutr. Ed. 9:114, 1977.
12. Fitzgibbons, J.J., Garcia, P.A., and Connolly, C.P.: Nutrition education for the elderly: Using television PSAs, J. Home Econ. 71:43, 1979.
13. Fusillo, A.E., and Beloian, A.M.: Consumer nutrition knowledge and self reported food shopping behavior, Am. J. Public Health 67:846, 1977.
14. Gershoff, S.N., and others: Studies of the elderly in Boston: 1. The effects of iron fortification on moderately anemic people, Am. J. Clin. Nutr. 30:226, 1977.
15. Goodrow, B.A.: Limiting factors in reducing participation in older adult learning activities, Gerontologist 15:418, 1975.
16. Grotkowski, M.L., and Sims, L.S.: Nutrition knowledge, attitudes, and dietary practices of the elderly, J. Am. Diet. Assoc. 72:499, 1978.
17. Hiemstra, R.P.: Continuing education for the aged: A survey of needs and interests of older people, Adult Ed. 22:100, 1972.
18. Holmes, A.C.: Visual aids in nutrition education, Food and Agriculture Organization, Rome, 1968, United Nations.
19. Holmes, D.: Nutrition and health-screening services for the elderly, J. Am. Diet. Assoc. 60:301, 1972.
20. Howell, S.C., and Loeb, M.B.: Nutrition and aging: A monograph for practitioners, Gerontologist 9(suppl.):1, 1969.
21. Huiatt, A., and Hockin, B.L.: Nutrition programs for senior citizens, J. Home Econ. 63:683, 1971.
22. Jalso, S.B., Burns, M.M., and Rivers, J.M.: Nutritional beliefs and practices, J. Am. Diet. Assoc. 47:263, 1965.
23. Kidd, J.R.: How adults learn, Chicago, 1973, Follett Publishing Co.
24. Kim, S., Schriver, J.E., and Campbell, K.M.: Nutrition education for nursing home residents, J. Am. Diet. Assoc. 78:362, 1981.
25. Klippel, R.E., and Sweeney, T.W.: The use of information sources by the aged consumer, Gerontologist 14:163, 1974.
26. Kocher, L.M., and Peterson, G.S.: Nutrition education: One state's experience, J. Am. Diet. Assoc. 81:64, 1982.
27. Lasswell, A.B., and Curry, K.R.: Curriculum development for instructing the elderly in nutrition, J. Nutr. Ed. 11:14, 1979.
28. Latham, M.C.: Planning and evaluation of applied nutrition programmes, Food and Agriculture Organization, Rome, 1972, United Nations.
29. Leong, Y.: Nutrition education for the aged and chronically ill, J. Nutr. Ed. 1:18, 1970.

30. Light, L.: Cameras help the elderly to improve food patterns, J. Nutr. Ed. **8:**80, 1976.

31. Lofton, J., Staton, M., and Crisp, A.: Nutrition education resources: Program planning and activities, Corvallis, 1975, Oregon State University.

32. Manney, J.D.: Aging in American society, Institute of Gerontology, Ann Arbor, 1975, University of Michigan.

33. Manoff, R.K.: Potential uses of mass media in nutrition programs, J. Nutr. Ed. **5:**125, 1973.

34. Mason, J.B., and Bearden, W.O.: Profiling the shopping behavior of elderly consumers, Gerontologist **18:**454, 1978.

35. McBean, L.D., and Speckmann, E.W.: Food faddism: A challenge to nutritionists and dieticians, Am. J. Clin. Nutr. **27:**1071, 1974.

36. Medved, E.: Television in nutrition education, J. Home Econ. **58:**167, 1966.

37. Natow, A., and Heslin, J.: Nutrition education in the later years, J. Nutr. Elderly **1:**101, 1981.

38. Olson, J.C., and Sims, L.S.: Assessing nutrition knowledge from an information processing perspective, J. Nutr. Ed. **12:**157, 1980.

39. Pao, E.M., and Hill, M.M.: Diets of the elderly, nutrition labeling and nutrition education, J. Nutr. Ed. **6:**96, 1974.

40. Parham, E.S.: Nutrition education for the elderly, J. Home Econ. **72:**24, 1980.

41. Pelcovits, J.: Nutrition for older Americans, J. Am. Diet. Assoc. **60:**297, 1972.

42. Pelcovits, J.: Nutrition education in group meals programs for the aged, J. Nutr. Ed. **5:**118, 1973.

43. Rae, J., and Burke, A.L.: Counselling the elderly on nutrition in a community health care system, J. Am. Geriatr. Soc. **26:**130, 1978.

44. Rawson, I.G., and others: Nutrition of rural elderly in southwestern Pennsylvania, Gerontologist **18:**24, 1978.

45. Rountree, J.L., and Tinklin, G.L.: Food beliefs and practices of selected senior citizens, Gerontologist **15:**537, 1975.

46. Schafer, R.B., and Keith, P.M.: Influences on food decisions across the family life cycle, J. Am. Diet. Assoc. **78:**144, 1981.

47. Schafer, R.B., and Keith, P.M.: Social-psychological factors in the dietary quality of married and single elderly, J. Am. Diet. Assoc. **81:**30, 1982.

48. Shannon, B., and Smiciklas-Wright, H.: Nutrition education in relation to the needs of the elderly, J. Nutr. Ed. **11:**85, 1979.

49. Shannon, B., Thurman, G., and Schiff, W.: Foodsense: A pilot TV show on nutrition issues, J. Nutr. Ed. **11:**15, 1979.

50. Sorenson, A.W., and Ford, M.L.: Diet and health for senior citizens: Workshops by the health team, Gerontologist **21:**257, 1981.

51. Stare, F.J.: Three score and ten plus more, J. Am. Geriatr. Soc. **25:**529, 1977.

52. Talmage, H., Hughes, M., and Eash, M.J.: The role of evaluation research in nutrition education, J. Nutr. Ed. **10:**169, 1978.

53. Templeton, C.L.: Nutrition counseling needs in a geriatric population, Geriatrics **33:**59, 1978.

54. United States Department of Health and Human Services: Longitudinal evaluation of the National Nutrition Program for the Elderly. Report on first-wave findings, DHEW Publication No. (OHDS) 80-20249, Washington, D.C., 1979, U.S. Government Printing Office.

55. Virginia Council on Health and Medical Care: Nutrition education for the elderly, ed. 2, Richmond, 1978, Virginia Council on Health and Medical Care.

56. Wang, V.L.: Changing nutritional behavior by aides in two programs, J. Nutr. Ed. **9:**109, 1977.

57. Wass, H., and West, C.A.: A humanistic approach to education of older persons, Educ. Gerontol. **2:**407, 1977.

58. Williams, L.: Experiences in systematic training in a rural program for elderly Mississippians, Am. J. Clin. Nutr. **26:**1138, 1973.

59. Wolczuk, P.: The senior chef, J. Nutr. Ed. **5:**142, 1973.

SELECTED RESOURCES
For the Professional

California Dietetic Association: A dozen diets for better or for worse, Los Angeles, 1974, California Dietetic Association.

Carlin, J.: Nutrition education for the older American, Durham, N.H., 1975, New England Gerontology Center.

Cooperative Extension Service, Rutgers University: Nutrition for the elderly mini-lesson kit, New Brunswick, 1975, Cooperative Extension Service, Cook College, Rutgers University.

Crisp, A., and Cale, B.: Nutrition education resources: An annotated bibliography, Corvallis, 1975, Oregon State University.

Hoops, L.L.: List of nutrition education materials for the elderly, Moorhead, Minn., 1981, Moorhead State University.

ITT Continental Baking Co.: Nutrition education for older Americans, Rye, N.Y., 1982.

Keown, G.M., and Klippstein, R.N.: Concerns of the aging: Nutrition. Abstracts and reference material for professionals, Ithaca, N.Y., 1976, Cornell University.

Lofton, J., Staton, M., and Crisp, A.: Nutrition education resources: Program planning and activities, Corvallis, 1975, Oregon State University.

Society for Nutrition Education: Aging and nutrition, Nutrition Education Resource Series No. 5, Berkeley, 1980, Society for Nutrition Education.

United States Department of Agriculture: How to buy food: Lesson aids for teachers, Agriculture Handbook No. 443, Washington, D.C., 1975, U.S. Government Printing Office.

United States Department of Agriculture: Nutritive value of foods, Home and Garden Bulletin No. 72, Washington, D.C., 1981, U.S. Government Printing Office.

Virginia Council on Health and Medical Care: Nutrition education for the elderly, ed. 3, Richmond, 1983.

For the Layperson

American Association of Retired Persons, National Retired Teachers Association: Your retirement food guide, Long Beach, 1970.

American Diabetes Association, American Dietetic Association: Exchange lists for meal planning, Chicago, 1976.

American Dietetic Association: Food 2—getting down to basics: A dieter's guide, Chicago, 1982.

American Dietetic Association: Food 3—eating the moderate fat and cholesterol way, Chicago, 1982.

American Heart Association: The way to a man's heart, Dallas, 1972, American Heart Association Communications Division.

Bohan, M., and others: Food without fuss for senior adults, Tallahassee, 1975, Florida Department of Health and Rehabilitative Services.

Briley, M.: Your retirement health guide, Long Beach, 1977, American Association of Retired Persons, National Retired Teachers Association.

Cooperative Extension Service, Cornell University: Cooking for two, Ithaca, N.Y., (no date given).

Darling, M.: Potassium: Its function and sources, St. Paul, 1982, Cooperative Extension Service, University of Minnesota.

Florida Division of Aging: Nutrition for older adults, Tallahassee, 1975, Florida Department of Health and Rehabilitative Services.

Hamilton, L.: Choose to stay healthy, University Park, 1982, Cooperative Extension Service, Pennsylvania State University.

Hamilton, L.: Stretch your protein $$: Use more vegetable protein, University Park, 1982, Cooperative Extension Service, Pennsylvania State University.

Hoerr, S., and Troftgruben, J.: Choices in the marketplace, Urbana-Champaign, 1977, Cooperative Extension Service, University of Illinois.

Irwin, T.: Better health in later years, New York, 1981, Public Affairs Committee, Inc.

Johnson, N.: Beverages count too, Madison, 1981, Cooperative Extension Service, University of Wisconsin.

Katz, M.: Vitamins, food, and your health, New York, 1982, Public Affairs Committee, Inc.

Lavender, M.: Facts about fiber in food, Madison, 1979, Cooperative Extension Service, University of Wisconsin.

Margolius, S.: Health foods: Facts and fakes, New York, 1980, Public Affairs Committee, Inc.

Maryland High Blood Pressure Coordinating Council: Health is in salt is out, Maryland Department of Health and Mental Hygiene (no date given).

Mennes, M., and Rygasewicz, K.: Food for folks over 55: Overcoming special problems in the kitchen, Madison, 1979, Cooperative Extension Service, University of Wisconsin.

Mennes, M., and Rygasewicz, K.: Food for folks over 55: Storing foods safely, Madison, 1979, Cooperative Extension Service, University of Wisconsin.

Mennes, M., and Rygasewicz, K.: Food for folks over 55: Supermarket strategies, Madison, 1979, Cooperative Extension Service, University of Wisconsin.

Mennes, M., and Rygasewicz, K.: Cooking with less effort, Madison, 1981, Cooperative Extension Service, University of Wisconsin.

Mennes, M., and Rygasewicz, K.: Meal planning for one or two, Madison, 1981, Cooperative Extension Service, University of Wisconsin.

National Dairy Council: For mature eaters only: Guidelines for good nutrition, Rosemont, 1982, National Dairy Council.

National Institutes of Health: Everything doesn't cause cancer, NIH Publication No. 80-2039, Washington, D.C., 1980, U.S. Government Printing Office.

Page, L., and Raper, N.: Food and your weight, Home and Garden Bulletin No. 74, Washington, D.C., 1977, U.S. Government Printing Office.

Peterkin, B.: Your money's worth in food, Home and Garden Bulletin No. 183, Washington, D.C., 1973, U.S. Government Printing Office.

President's Council on Physical Fitness and Sports: The fitness challenge in the later years. An exercise program for older Americans, DHEW Publication No. (OHD-AOA) 73-20802, Washington, D.C., 1973, U.S. Government Printing Office.

Stark, C.: Till we meat again: A guide to complementary proteins, Madison, 1981, Cooperative Extension Service, University of Wisconsin.

Stark, C.: Vegetarian diets: The choice is yours, Madison, 1981, Cooperative Extension Service, University of Wisconsin.

Tybring, J., and Johnson, N.: Break the fat barrier: Keep a daily food diary, Madison, 1977, Cooperative Extension Service, University of Wisconsin.

United States Department of Agriculture: Vegetables in family meals, Home and Garden Bulletin No. 105, Washington, D.C., 1971, U.S. Government Printing Office.

United States Department of Agriculture: Food guide for older folks, Home and Garden Bulletin No. 17, Washington, D.C., 1973, U.S. Government Printing Office.

United States Department of Agriculture: Food safety in the kitchen, Washington, D.C., 1974, U.S. Government Printing Office.

United States Department of Agriculture: Nutrition: Food at work for you, Washington, D.C., 1975, U.S. Government Printing Office.

United States Department of Agriculture: Nutrition labeling: Tools for its use, Agriculture Information Bulletin No. 382, Washington, D.C., 1975, U.S. Government Printing Office.

United States Department of Agriculture: Cooking for two, Program Aid No. 1043, Washington, D.C., 1977, U.S. Government Printing Office.

United States Department of Agriculture: Building a better diet, Program Aid No. 1241, Washington, D.C., 1979, U.S. Government Printing Office.

United States Department of Agriculture: Family food budgeting—for good meals and good nutrition, Home and Garden Bulletin No. 94, Washington, D.C., 1979, U.S. Government Printing Office.

United States Department of Agriculture: Nutrition and your health. Dietary Guidelines for Americans, Home and Garden Bulletin No. 232, Washington, D.C., 1980, U.S. Government Printing Office.

United States Department of Agriculture: Ideas for better eating: Menus and recipes to make use of the dietary guidelines, Washington, D.C., 1981, U.S. Government Printing Office.

Vermont Department of Health: Avoid sodium—use your imagination, Burlington, 1980, Vermont Department of Health.

Voichick, J.: Protein, Madison, 1975, Cooperative Extension Service, University of Wisconsin.

Voichick, J., and Lavender, M.: Promises, promises: Today's food myths, Madison, 1978, Cooperative Extension Service, University of Wisconsin.

Voichick, J., and Kjentvet, M.: Managing a modified diet, Madison, 1978, Cooperative Extension Service, University of Wisconsin.

Voichick, J., and Rygasewicz, K.: Food for folks over 55: Food for health: Misconceptions and fallacies, Madison, 1979, Cooperative Extension Service, University of Wisconsin.

Voichick, J., and Rygasewicz, K.: Food for folks over 55: Special diets, Madison, 1979, Cooperative Extension Service, University of Wisconsin.

Voichick, J., and Rygasewicz, K.: Food for folks over 55: Vitamin and mineral supplements, Madison, 1979, Cooperative Extension Service, University of Wisconsin.

Voichick, J., and Rygasewicz, K.: Evaluating nutrition information sources, Madison, 1980, Cooperative Extension Service, University of Wisconsin.

Washington State Bureau of Aging: Now I can eat nutritious low cost convenient food in my room, Olympia, 1980, Washington State Department of Social and Health Services.

Appendix A

Agencies and Professional Organizations Serving the Aged

AGENCIES—UNITED STATES GOVERNMENT

Administration on Aging
  Office of Human Development Services
  U.S. Dept. of Health and Human Services, North Bldg.
  330 Independence Ave., S.W.
  Washington, DC 20201
National Institute on Aging
  National Institutes of Health, Bldg. 31
  9000 Rockville Pike
  Bethesda, MD 20014
Gerontology Research Center—National Institute on Aging
  Baltimore City Hospitals
  4940 Eastern Ave.
  Baltimore, MD 21224
Social Security Administration
  Office of Research and Statistics
  1875 Connecticut Ave., N.W., Room 1120
  Washington, DC 20009
Veterans Administration
  Vermont Ave. and H Street, N.W.
  Washington, DC 20420
Select Committee on Aging
  U.S. House of Representatives
  House Annex # 1, Room 712
  Washington, DC 20515
Special Committee on Aging
  United States Senate
  Dirkson Office Building, Room G-223
  Washington, DC 20510
ACTION
  806 Connecticut Ave., N.W.
  Washington, DC 20525
  (Administers programs serving the aged including RSVP and
    Foster Grandparents Program)
United States Department of Agriculture
  Office of Information
  14th Street and Independence Ave., S.W.
  Washington, DC 20250

PROFESSIONAL ORGANIZATIONS
General Aspects of Aging

National Council on the Aging
  600 Maryland Ave., S.W.
  West Wing 100, Suite 208
  Washington, DC 20024
Gerontological Society of America
  1835 K Street
  Suite 305
  Washington, DC 20006
American Aging Association
  c/o Dr. Denham Harman
  College of Medicine
  University of Nebraska
  Omaha, NE 68105
National Caucus and Center on Black Aged
  1424 K Street, N.W.
  Suite 500
  Washington, DC 20005
International Federation on Ageing
  1909 K Street, N.W.
  Washington, DC 20049
International Center for Social Gerontology
  453 13th Street, N.W.
  Suite 826
  Washington, DC 20004
National Interfaith Coalition on Aging
  P.O. Box 1924
  Athens, GA 30603
National Retired Teachers Association
  1909 K Street, N.W.
  Washington, DC 20049
National Senior Citizens Law Center
  1424 16th Street, N.W.
  Suite 301
  Washington, DC 20036

Association for Gerontology in Higher Education
600 Maryland Ave., S.W., West Wing
Suite 204
Washington, DC 20024

Physical Health

Committee on Aging, American Medical Association
535 N. Dearborn Street
Chicago, IL 60610
American Geriatrics Society
10 Columbus Circle
New York, NY 10019
American Cancer Society
777 3rd Ave.
New York, NY 10017
American Diabetes Association
2 Park Ave.
New York, NY 10016
American Heart Association
7320 Greenville Ave.
Dallas, TX 75231
American Parkinson Disease Association
116 John Street, Suite 417
New York, NY 10038
Arthritis Foundation
3400 Peachtree Road, N.E.
Atlanta, GA 30326
American Lung Association
1740 Broadway
New York, NY 10019
American Society for Geriatric Dentistry
1121 W. Michigan Street
Indianapolis, IN 46202
National Safety Council
444 North Michigan Ave.
Chicago, IL 60611

Health Care Facilities and Services

American Health Care Association
1200 15th Street, N.W.
Washington, DC 20005
American Hospital Association
840 North Lake Shore Drive
Chicago, IL 60611
National Association for Home Care
311 Massachusetts Ave., N.E.
Washington, DC 20002
National Homecaring Council
67 Irving Place
New York, NY 10003
American College of Nursing Home Administrators
4650 East-West Highway
Washington, DC 20014

American Association of Homes for the Aging
1050 17th Street, N.W.
Suite 770
Washington, DC 20036
National Association for Jewish Homes for the Aged
2525 Centerville Road
Dallas, TX 75228
Health Insurance Association of America
1850 K Street, N.W.
Washington, DC 20006

Physical Rehabilitation Services

Institute of Rehabilitation Medicine
New York University Medical Center
400 East 34th Street
New York, NY 10016
National Rehabilitation Association
633 S. Washington Street
Alexandria, VA 22314
American Occupational Therapy Association
1383 Piccard Drive
Suite 301
Rockville, MD 20850
American Foundation for the Blind
15 W. 16th Street
New York, NY 10011
National Society To Prevent Blindness
79 Madison Ave.
New York, NY 10016
American Association of Workers for the Blind
1511 K Street, N.W.
Suite 637
Washington, DC 20005
American Speech-Language-Hearing Association
10801 Rockville Pike
Rockville, MD 20852
National Hearing Aid Society
20361 Middlebelt
Livonia, MI 48152

Nutrition

American Dietetic Association
430 North Michigan Ave.
Chicago, IL 60611
American Institute of Nutrition
9650 Rockville Pike
Bethesda, MD 20814
American Society for Clinical Nutrition
9650 Rockville Pike
Bethesda, MD 20814
Society for Nutrition Education
1736 Franklin Street, 9th Floor
Oakland, CA 94612

The Nutrition Society (British)
  Chandos House
  2 Queen Anne Street
  London WIM 9LE, England
Nutrition Today Society
  703 Giddings Ave.
  Annapolis, MD 21404

Nutrition and Social Services

National Association of Meal Programs
  Box 6959
  604 W. North Ave.
  Pittsburgh, PA 15212
National Association of Area Agencies on Aging
  600 Maryland Ave., S.W.
  Suite 208
  Washington, DC 20024
Jewish Association for Services for the Aged
  40 W. 68th Street
  New York, NY 10023
National Institute of Senior Centers
  600 Maryland Ave., S.W.
  West Wing 100, Suite 208
  Washington, DC 20024

American National Red Cross
  17th and D Streets, N.W.
  Washington, DC 20006
Score and Ace (Retired Executives Service Corps)
  822 15th Street, N.W.
  Washington, DC 20416
Legal Services for the Elderly
  132 W. 43rd Street, 3rd Floor
  New York, NY 10036

ADVOCACY GROUPS—GENERAL MEMBERSHIP

American Association of Retired Persons
  1909 K Street, N.W.
  Washington, DC 20049
Gray Panthers
  3635 Chestnut Street
  Philadelphia, PA 19104
International Senior Citizens Association
  11753 Wilshire Boulevard
  Los Angeles, CA 90025
National Council of Senior Citizens
  925 15th Street, N.W.
  Washington, DC 20005

Appendix B

Tools for Evaluating Dietary Status

SAMPLE CONSENT FORM

I do hereby consent to participate in a study of nutritional status of senior citizens conducted by ____. I understand that as part of the study I will record my food intake for a 3-day period and measurements of my height, weight, triceps skinfold thickness, and arm circumference will be taken. A registered nurse from the Visiting Nurse Association will come to my home to obtain a venous blood sample (20 ml), on which biochemical tests will be performed. *I understand that I may withdraw from the study at any time.* All records will be held in confidence. I can request that my records be released to my personal physician. I will receive (amount of honorarium, if any) when the dietary records, physical measurements, and blood collection have been completed.

_____   _____
Date   Signature—Participant

_____   _____
Date   Signature—Investigator

DIET HISTORY FORM FOR OLDER ADULTS

Name _____ Address _____

What type of housing do you live in?

Public housing for senior citizens _____ Single family house _____ Rented apartment _____

Rented room–kitchen privileges _____ Rented room–no kitchen privileges _____

Is this a satisfactory arrangement for you? Yes _____ No _____

If not, why not? _____

Do you live alone? Yes _____ No _____

Do you prepare your own meals? Yes _____ No _____ Partially _____

If not, who does? _____

With whom do you usually eat your meals? Alone _____ Spouse _____ Other _____

What kind of facilities are available for cooking your food?

None _____ A stove and oven that work _____ A hotplate only _____ Small appliances only _____

Is this a satisfactory arrangement for you? Yes _____ No _____

If not, why not? _____

Do you have a refrigerator in working condition in your living unit?

Yes _____ No _____ Other _____

Do you have adequate storage space for food supplies?

Yes _____ No _____

Some people have problems with shopping. How do you usually get to the food store?

Walk to and back _____ Walk to, public transit back _____ Walk to, taxi back _____

Public transit both ways _____ Ride from friend/neighbor/relative _____ Use own car _____

Adapted from Christakis, G., ed.: Nutritional assessment in health programs, Washington, D.C., 1973, American Public Health Association and Dietary Interview Questionnaire, Vermont Agricultural Experiment Station, University of Vermont, Burlington, Vt.   *Continued.*

DIET HISTORY FORM FOR OLDER ADULTS—cont'd

Is this arrangement satisfactory for you? Yes _____ No _____

If not, why not? _____

Where do you do your major food shopping? Neighborhood grocery _____ Supermarket _____

Co-op _____ Convenience store (24-hour store) _____ Health food store _____

Is there any other store in which you would rather shop?

Yes _____ No _____

If yes, why? _____

What keeps you from shopping there? _____

Is your choice of food restricted because of problems with chewing?

Yes _____ No _____

If yes, what foods can't you eat? _____

How would you describe your appetite? Excellent _____ Good _____ Poor _____ Varies _____

Never get hungry _____

Has your weight changed in the last year? No change _____

Approximate number of pounds gained _____ Approximate number of pounds lost _____

Explanation for weight change, if known _____

Have you been on a special diet of some kind in the past 12 months?

None _____ Low residue (diverticulitis) _____ Low sodium _____ Low cholesterol _____

Diabetic _____ Bland _____ Low fat _____ Weight reduction _____ Other _____

Did a doctor put you on this diet? Yes _____ No _____

If not, how did you decide to follow this diet? _____

Some people have problems following their diet. Do you find your diet difficult to follow? Very difficult _____ Moderately difficult _____ No problem—easy to follow _____ Not following diet _____

DIET HISTORY FORM FOR OLDER ADULTS—cont'd

Do you participate in any of the following nutrition programs?

Title III congregate meal program _____

If yes, how frequently do you attend? _____

Home-delivered meals program _____

If yes, how frequently are meals delivered? _____

Food stamps _____ Commodity food distribution _____

If yes, what food do you receive? _____

If not participating now, would you like to participate in any of these nutrition programs?

Yes _____ Program(s) _____

Do you smoke? Yes _____ No _____

Do you take any vitamin, mineral, or protein supplements? Yes _____ No _____

If so, what do you take? _____

(Ask to see container if possible.)

Were these supplements recommended by a physician? Yes _____ No _____

How frequently do you take them? _____

Do you use any of the following over the counter drugs on a regular basis?

Aspirin _____ Antacids _____ Laxatives _____ "Water" pills _____ Pain pills _____

Sleeping pills _____ Anti-diarrhea preparations _____

If so, were these drugs recommended by your doctor? Yes _____ No _____

Do you take any prescription drugs regularly? Yes _____ No _____

If so, what drugs? (Ask to see container if possible.)

Drug _____

Drug _____

Continued.

DIET HISTORY FORM FOR OLDER ADULTS—cont'd

About how many glasses or cups of fluids do you drink each day?

Number _____

Do you eat at regular times each day? Yes _____ No _____

Describe a typical daily pattern of when you eat _____

_____

What types of food do you usually eat at those times? _____

_____

What specific kinds of the following foods do you eat most often?

Fruit _____ About how often _____ Never Eat _____

Fruit juices _____ About how often _____ Never Eat _____

Dark green or deep yellow vegetables _____ About how often _____ Never eat _____

Other vegetables _____ About how often _____ Never eat _____

Meat, fish, or poultry _____ About how often _____ Never eat _____

Milk _____ About how often _____ Never eat _____

Other dairy products _____ About how often _____ Never eat _____

Bread, rolls, muffins _____ About how often _____ Never eat _____

Cereal _____ About how often _____ Never eat _____

Legumes or nuts _____ About how often _____ Never eat _____

Is your physical activity restricted in any way? Yes _____ No _____

Nature of restriction _____

Does this interfere with food preparation? Yes _____ No _____

Does this interfere with food shopping? Yes _____ No _____

FOOD FREQUENCY QUESTIONNAIRE

Directions:
1. Please indicate how many times per week you eat each of the following foods.
2. What size portion do you have of each food when you eat it?

	No. of Times per Week	Usual Portion Size
Protein Foods:		
Chicken, turkey	_____	_____
Beef, hamburger	_____	_____
Pork, ham	_____	_____
Luncheon meats, frankfurters, sausage	_____	_____
Liver, braunschweiger	_____	_____
Eggs	_____	_____
Peanut butter or nuts	_____	_____
Fish	_____	_____
Dried peas or bean dishes	_____	_____
Dairy Foods:		
Milk: Type _____	_____	_____
Cottage cheese	_____	_____
Other cheese or cheese dishes	_____	_____
Custard, pudding, cream soup	_____	_____
Ice cream, ice milk	_____	_____

Adapted from Christakis, G., ed.: Nutritional assessment in health programs, Washington, D.C., 1973, American Public Health Association and Wisconsin Department of Health and Social Services: Nutrition screening and assessment manual, Madison, 1980.

Continued.

FOOD FREQUENCY QUESTIONNAIRE—cont'd

	No. of Times per Week	*Usual Portion Size*
Fruits and Vegetables:		
Beet greens, turnip greens, spinach	_____	_____
Carrots	_____	_____
Mixed vegetables	_____	_____
Cabbage, brussel sprouts	_____	_____
Broccoli	_____	_____
White potato (other than potato chips)	_____	_____
Sweet potato	_____	_____
Tomatoes, tomato juice	_____	_____
Prunes, raisins, dates	_____	_____
Peaches	_____	_____
Watermelon, cantaloupe	_____	_____
Oranges, orange juice	_____	_____
Grapefruit, grapefruit juice	_____	_____
Strawberries	_____	_____
Fruit drink (vitamin C–fortified)	_____	_____

FOOD FREQUENCY QUESTIONNAIRE—cont'd

	No. of Times per Week	Usual Portion Size
Breads and Cereals:		
Whole grain bread	_____	_____
Whole grain cereal	_____	_____
Enriched bread	_____	_____
Enriched cereal	_____	_____
Enriched macaroni, spaghetti, rice	_____	_____
Enriched or whole grain crackers	_____	_____
Cake, doughnuts, sweet rolls	_____	_____
Cookie	_____	_____
Pie, pastry	_____	_____
Other:		
Butter	_____	_____
Margarine	_____	_____
Potato chips, corn curls	_____	_____
Candy	_____	_____
Coffee, tea	_____	_____
Beer, wine	_____	_____

HINTS FOR INTERVIEWERS

Check carefully for the following information:

Additions to foods already recorded such as:

1. Fats: Butter, margarine, honey-butter, peanut butter, mayonnaise, lard, meat drippings, cheese spreads or others.
   Used on toast, bread, rolls, buns, cookies, crackers, sandwiches.
   Used on vegetables.
   Used on potatoes, rice, noodles.
   Used on other foods.
2. Sugars: Jam, jelly, honey, syrup, sweetening.
   Used on breads, sandwiches, vegetables, fruit, cereal, coffee, tea, other foods.
3. Other spreads: Catsup, mustard, relish.
4. Milk: Cream, half and half, skim milk.
   Used on cereal, coffee, tea, desserts, other foods.
5. Gravies: Used on bread, biscuits, meat, potatoes, rice, noodles, other foods.
6. Salad dressings: Used on vegetables, salads, sandwiches, other foods.
7. Chocolate or other flavoring to milk.

Food preparation

1. Preparation of eggs, (i.e., fried, scrambled, boiled, poached).
2. Preparation of meat, poultry, fish, (i.e., fried, boiled, stewed, roasted, baked, broiled).
3. Preparation of mixed dishes—major ingredients used (e.g., tuna fish and noodles, macaroni and cheese).
4. Special preparation of food—strained, chopped

Special additional detail about food items

1. Kinds of milk (whole, partially skim, skim, powdered, chocolate).
2. Kinds of carbonated beverages (regular, low-calorie).
3. Kinds of fruits (canned, frozen, fresh, dried, cooked with sugar added).
4. Kinds of fruit juices, fruit drinks or juice substitutes.

From Fomon, S.J.: Nutritional disorders of children. Prevention, screening and follow-up. DHEW Publication No. (HSA) 77-5104, Washington, D.C., 1977, U.S. Government Printing Office.

Glossary

ad libitum feeding Allowed to eat as much as desired.

Alzheimers-type senile dementia Progressive irreversible degenerative changes in the brain resulting in loss of neuromuscular coordination and mental function.

anemia Below normal levels of hemoglobin or red blood cells per unit of whole blood.

anorexia Loss of appetite.

antioxidant A substance that inhibits oxidation of unsaturated fatty acids and formation of free radicals.

biologic age The relative age of an individual based on physiologic measurements.

cardiac output Total amount of blood pumped by the heart per minute.

cathartic A drug that hastens and increases the emptying of the bowels.

cerebral hemorrhage Rupture of an artery in the brain; stroke.

cholecystectomy Surgery to remove the gallbladder.

chronologic age Age of an individual based on the number of years lived.

cohort Individuals falling within a specified age range.

congregate meals Group meals served in a social setting usually funded under Title III-C of the Older Americans Act.

constipation Infrequent and difficult passage of excessively dry stool.

dependency ratio The number of individuals age 65 and over divided by the number of individuals of working age (age 18 to 64).

dysgeusia Loss of or alteration in taste.

dyspepsia Upset stomach.

dysphagia Difficulty in swallowing.

edentulous Without teeth.

erythrocyte Mature red blood cell.

feed efficiency Weight gain divided by amount of food consumed.

flatulence Excessive gas in the stomach and intestine resulting in discomfort.

functional disability Disability that interferes with daily activities (e.g., bathing, dressing, shopping, preparing meals).

geriatrics The branch of medicine concerned with chronic disease and physical health in older people.

gerontology The study of aging including biologic, physiologic, psychologic, and sociologic aspects.

heartburn Burning sensation in the esophagus usually after eating.

home health agency A community, nonprofit organization providing nursing services, personal care services and/or homemaking services to homebound aged under the supervision of a physician.

hypochromic Low in hemoglobin concentration (in reference to red blood cells).

ideal weight Optimal weight for an individual of a given height, sex, and age.

kyphosis Abnormal curvature of the spine; humpback.

life expectancy The average remaining lifetime for a person of a given age.

long term care Medical, personal, or homemaking services provided in an institution or in the community to older people who are no longer able to care for their own needs; services are usually continued for the remainder of the life span.

mastication Chewing of food.

mean Average value.

mean corpuscular hemoglobin concentration Index to express the hemoglobin content of red blood cells (grams of hemoglobin per 100 ml red blood cells); used in diagnosis of anemia.

median The middle value in a distribution with half of the values falling above and half of the values falling below.

microcytic Small in size (in reference to red blood cells).

mortality ratio Total number of deaths divided by the total population.

parietal cells Cells lining the stomach that secrete HCl.

patient care plan A strategy developed by health care professionals for the maintenance or treatment of an individual patient.

poverty line The minimum income (as determined by the federal government) required to provide basic necessities of food, clothing, and shelter.

residual volume Air remaining in the lungs after the individual has exhaled.

secular Occurring as a function of time.

tachycardia Rapid heart beat.

taste threshold The lowest concentration of a substance that can be detected by the taste buds.

Title III The statute of the Older Americans Act authorizing congregate and home-delivered meals and social services for persons age 60 and above.

viscera Large internal organs located in the chest and abdomen.

vital capacity Volume of air moved in and out of the lungs with each breath.

Index